the Brain

A **SCIENTIFIC** *Book*
AMERICAN

the Brain

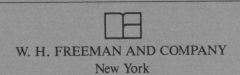

W. H. FREEMAN AND COMPANY
New York

The Cover

The picture on the cover is a computer-generated display of the normal human brain. The surface of the cerebral cortex is dark blue, that of the cerebellum purple and that of the brain stem light blue (or yellow where other structures are not superposed on it). Here the front of the brain is rotated slightly toward the viewer. The display was created by a group in the laboratory of Robert B. Livingston at the University of California at San Diego. It is based on images of the cut surface of a brain sliced in a giant microtome. Images of the surface made at regular intervals were traced into a computer memory and displayed as a three-dimensional object on an Evans and Sutherland picture system.
Sponsored by Roche Laboratories. The group included Roy E. Mills, William Atkinson, Guy Tribble III, David Rempel, John MacGregor, John Cornelius, Roger Sumner, and Philip Cohen.

Cover photograph courtesy of Robert B. Livingston

Library of Congress Cataloging in Publication Data

Main entry under title:

The Brain.

"A Scientific American book."
"The chapters . . . originally appeared as articles in the September 1979 issue of Scientific American."
Bibliography: p.
Includes index.
1. Brain—Addresses, essays, lectures.
I. Scientific American. [DNLM: Brain—Physiology—Collected works. W1300.3 B 814]
QP376. B695   612.82   79-21012
ISBN 0-7167-1150-8
ISBN 0-7167-1151-6 pbk.

The eleven chapters in this book originally appeared as articles in the September 1979 issue of *Scientific American*.

Printed in the United States of America
Printed on recycled paper

9 8 7

Contents

Foreword

This book does not explain how the brain works. That remains the most alluring and baffling of all questions on the frontier of understanding. The occasion for the publication of this book is provided by the convergence of work in many fields that has begun to show us how to frame questions about the brain that yield accumulative answers. Knowledge about the brain, gathered at an accelerating rate in recent years, shows this organ to be marvelously designed and capacitated beyond the wonders with which it was invested by innocent imagination.

The plan of the book corresponds to the informal organization of the enterprise of brain research that engages talent and energy on many lines of attack and at many places around the world. To begin with, it is necessary to understand the nerve cell and the chemical physics of the nerve impulse. Systems of no more than a few nerve cells in invertebrates present objects of study that are prospectively more comprehensible than the human brain and may serve as models of its subsystems. Neurosurgeons long ago began to map the localization of function on the cortex. The embryonic growth of the brain offers other clues to its anatomy and higher organization. Lately, the identification of more than 30 different transmitter molecules that jump the impulse across the synapse between one nerve cell and the next has beggared the reductionist model of the brain as a mere switchboard.

Function has been studied at the scale of the subsystem, perhaps with highest precision through study of the sensory mode of vision. Linguistics now provides approaches to the subsystems that most distinguish the human brain among those of other animals. To the leads offered by defect and damage to motor and sensory function, the study of emotional disorder has begun to add other kinds of insight.

The most elusive questions about brain function concern the capacities of memory and learning. Theoretically, the number of pieces of information that the brain can acquire or store exceeds the number of elementary particles in the universe. The actual number of stored facts and impressions is smaller but still stupendous. It is different for each of us, and it sums the singularity of our brief existence.

The chapters in this book were first published in the September 1979 issue of SCIENTIFIC AMERICAN, which was the thirtieth in the series of single-topic issues published annually by the magazine. The editors herewith express appreciation to their colleagues at W. H. Freeman and Company, the book-publishing affiliate of SCIENTIFIC AMERICAN, for the enterprise that has made the contents of this issue so speedily available in book form.

THE EDITORS*

September 1979

*BOARD OF EDITORS: Gerard Piel (Publisher), Dennis Flanagan (Editor), Francis Bello (Associate Editor), Philip Morrison (Book Editor), Judith Friedman, Brian P. Hayes, Paul W. Hoffman, Jonathan B. Piel, John Purcell, James T. Rogers, Armand Schwab, Jr., Jonathan B. Tucker, Joseph Wisnovsky.

I

The Brain

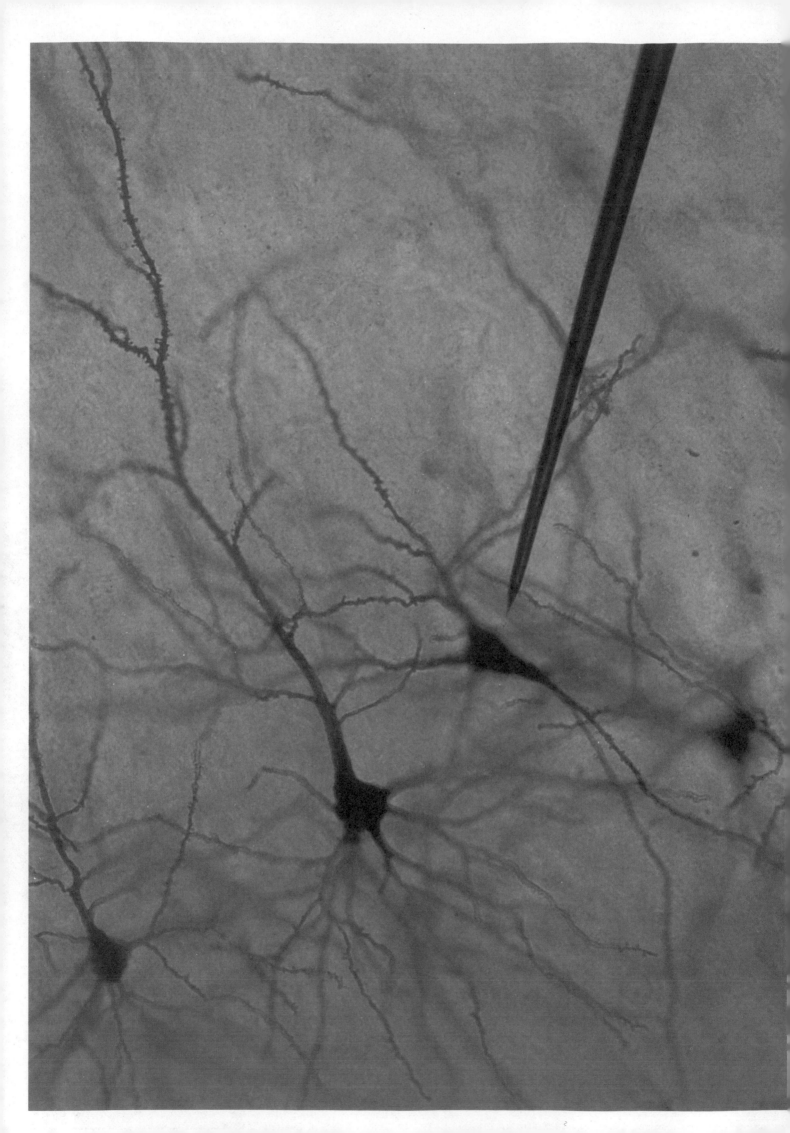

The Brain

BY DAVID H. HUBEL

Introducing a volume about neurobiology and its central problem: How does the human brain work? Although notable progress has been made, the question remains one of the profoundest confronting modern science

Can the brain understand the brain? Can it understand the mind? Is it a giant computer, or some other kind of giant machine, or something more? These are questions that are regularly asked, and it may help to get them out of the way. When someone maintains that brains cannot be expected to understand brains, the analogy is to the aphorism that a person cannot lift himself by his own bootstraps. The analogy is not compelling. Certainly even a brief glimpse of what has been accomplished toward understanding the brain will convince any reader of this *Scientific American* book that much progress has been made since the phrenologists. The pace of progress at the moment is rapid. For all practical purposes, then, neurobiologists are working on the hunch that they can understand the brain, and for the moment they are doing well.

I think the difficulties with questions such as these are semantic. They are loaded with words such as "understand" and "mind," useful words for many purposes but fuzzy at the edges and out of place when they are applied to questions such as these, which they render either meaningless or unanswerable.

The brain is a tissue. It is a complicated, intricately woven tissue, like nothing else we know of in the universe, but it is composed of cells, as any tissue is. They are, to be sure, highly specialized cells, but they function according to the laws that govern any other cells. Their electrical and chemical signals can be detected, recorded and interpreted, and

their chemicals can be identified; the connections that constitute the brain's woven feltwork can be mapped. In short, the brain can be studied, just as the kidney can.

The problem comes when we ask about understanding, because such a word carries with it the implication of a sudden revelation or dawning, the existence of a moment when we might be said to leave the darkness of the tunnel. It is not clear to me that there can be such a moment, or that we will know when it comes.

Brain research is a very old field of investigation—and before that of speculation. Its pace accelerated greatly at the end of the 19th century; since World War II new techniques have brought significant advances, and in the past decade or so neurobiology has become one of the most active branches in all science. The result has been a virtual explosion of recent discoveries and insights. Brain research is nonetheless only at its beginning. The incredible complexity of the brain is a cliché, but it is a fact.

The problem of understanding the brain is a little like that of understanding proteins. There must be millions of those ingeniously complicated molecular inventions in every organism, one protein quite different from the next. To work out the structural details of even one of them seems to take years, to say nothing of knowing exactly how it works. If understanding proteins means knowing how all of them work, the pros-

pects are perhaps not good. In an analogous way the brain consists of very large numbers of subdivisions (although not millions), each with a special architecture and circuit diagram; to describe one is certainly not to describe them all. Hence understanding will be slow (if only for practical reasons of time and manpower), steady (one hopes) and asymptotic, certainly with breakthroughs but with no likely point of terminus.

Mind is similarly a useful word but alas even fuzzier. Since its definition is elusive, to talk of understanding it (not just the word but the thing the word refers to) is to talk about an exercise in mental gymnastics that seems to fall outside of natural science. The mathematician G. H. Hardy is supposed to have said a mathematician is someone who not only does not know what he is talking about but also does not care. Those who discuss in depth subjects such as the physiology of the mind probably care, but I cannot see how they could ever know.

The number of nerve cells, or neurons, that make up man's three pounds or so of brain is on the order of 10^{11} (a hundred billion) give or take a factor of 10. The neurons are surrounded, supported and nourished by glial cells, whose number is also large. A typical neuron consists of a cell body, ranging from about five to 100 micrometers (thousandths of a millimeter) in diameter, from which emanate one major fiber, the axon, and a number of fibrous branches, the dendrites. The axon may give off branches near its beginning and it often branches extensively near its end. In general terms the dendrites and the cell body receive incoming signals; the cell body combines and integrates them (roughly speaking, it averages them) and emits outgoing signals, and it

THREE ESSENTIAL TOOLS of the neurobiologist are represented symbolically in the image on the opposite page. The three tools are the microscope, the selective staining of nerve tissue and the microelectrode. The image is a light micrograph of several Golgi-stained neurons in a section of brain tissue obtained from the visual cortex of a monkey; the long needle is the tip of a microelectrode poised as if to record the electrical impulses generated by one of the cells. The scene, which was photographed by Fritz Goro, is shown here enlarged some 500 diameters.

also serves for the general upkeep of the cell; the axon transports the outgoing signals to the axon terminals, which distribute the information to a new set of neurons.

The signaling system is a double one: electrical and chemical. The signal generated by a neuron and transported along its axon is an electrical impulse, but the signal is transmitted from cell to cell by molecules of transmitter substances that flow across a specialized contact, the synapse, between a supplier of information (an axon terminal or occasionally a dendrite) and a recipient of information (a dendrite, a cell body or occasionally an axon terminal). One neuron generally is fed by hundreds or thousands of other neurons and in turn feeds into hundreds or thousands of still other neurons.

This may be enough to make it possible to tackle the comparison between brains and computers. Most neurobiologists would agree, for the purposes of this discussion, that the brain can be regarded as a machine that is not endowed with properties lying beyond the reach of science. It is also true, however, that not all neurobiologists would agree with that proposition. On the other hand, everyone would surely agree that the computer is a machine and nothing more. And so, depending on one's taste and convictions, the brain and the computer are in one sense either fundamentally similar or radically different. Rational arguments will not, in my opinion, resolve the issue.

Assuming that the brain and the computer are both machines, how are the two to be compared? The exercise is interesting. Computers are invented by man and are therefore thoroughly understood, if human beings can be said to understand anything; what they do not know is what future computers will be like. The brain was created by evolution and is in many important ways not understood. Both machines process information and both work with signals that are roughly speaking electrical. Both have, in the largest versions, many elements. Here, however, there is an interesting difference. For cells to be manufactured biologically appears to be reasonably simple, and neurons are in fact produced in prodigious numbers. It seems to be not so easy to increase the elements of a computer, even though the numbers are expanding rapidly. If synapses rather than neurons are considered to be elements of the nervous system, however, I can hardly imagine computers catching up. No one would want to be held to a guess as to the number of synapses in a brain, but 10^{14} (100 trillion) would not be implausible.

A still more important difference is a qualitative one. The brain is not dependent on anything like a linear sequential program; this is at least so for all the parts about which something is known.

It is more like the circuit of a radio or a television set, or perhaps hundreds or thousands of such circuits in series and in parallel, richly cross-linked. The brain seems to rely on a strategy of relatively hard-wired circuit complexity with elements working at low speeds, measured in thousandths of a second; the computer depends on programs, has far fewer elements and works at rates at which millionths of a second are important. Among brain circuits there must be many devoted to keeping evolution going by means of competition and sex drives. So far the computer seems free of all that; it evolves by different means.

How is one to study an organ such as the brain? The major approach, of course, is to study its components and then try to learn how they function together. This is done primarily in animals rather than in man. The principles of neuronal function are remarkably similar in animals as far apart as the snail and man; most of what is known about the nerve impulse was learned in the squid. Even the major structures of the brain are so similar in, say, the cat and man that for most problems it seems to make little difference which brain one studies. Moreover, neurobiology is notable for the wide range of approaches and techniques that have been brought to bear on it, from physics and biochemistry to psychology and psychiatry. In no other branch of research is a broad approach so essential, and in recent years it has begun to be achieved.

The two great interlocking branches of neurobiology itself have traditionally been neuroanatomy and neurophysiology. Anatomy seeks to describe the various elements of the brain and how they are put together; physiology asks how the parts function and how they work together. Investigators in the two fields have tended to pursue separate courses and have even been housed in different departments in universities, but in fact they are interdependent. Most modern neuroanatomists are not content with a simple description of structure and spatial relations for their own sake but go on to ask what the structures and connections are for. Physiology, on the other hand, is impossible without anatomy.

At each stage of their development both neuroanatomy and neurophysiology have had to wait until the physical sciences could provide them with necessary tools and techniques. The neuron is too small to see with the unaided eye except as a mere speck and far too small for its signals to be recorded with ordinary wires. In order to advance beyond the most rudimentary stages anatomy required first the light microscope and then the electron microscope, and physiology required the microelectrode. Both fields of study have been dependent on the invention of increasingly selective methods of staining nerve tissue.

The fundamental achievements of the neuroanatomists of the early part of this century were the recognition that the neuron is the basic unit of nervous tissue and the discovery that neurons are interconnected with a high degree of order and specificity. The physiologists made a strong beginning by learning, in electrical and chemical terms, how the neuron transmits its messages. These two sets of accomplishments have by no means revealed how the brain works, but they provide an absolutely essential foundation. One way to see how far neurobiology has come (and, implicitly, how enormously far it has to go) is to consider some of the historical steps toward the present understanding of the brain and to briefly review the current status of research in some of the divisions of the field.

Why was it so hard to establish in the first place that the single neuron is the basic unit of nervous tissue? The main obstacles were the minute dimensions, the fantastic forms and the enormous variety of shapes of these cells and the fact that the branches of cells near one another are closely intermingled. The word "cell" conjures up a shape like that of a brick or a jelly bean, but a neuron

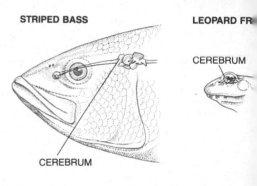

STRIPED BASS

CEREBRUM

LEOPARD FR

CEREBRUM

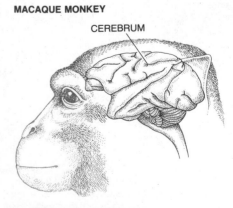

MACAQUE MONKEY

CEREBRUM

PROGRESSIVE INCREASE in the size of the cerebrum in vertebrates is evident in the

may look more like an elongated oak tree or a petunia—with a trunk or stem that is from 10 to 20 micrometers (thousandths of a millimeter) in diameter and from .1 millimeter to as much as a meter or so in length. To see individual neurons one needs not only a microscope but also a stain to contrast them with their surroundings. The neurons are normally packed together so intimately that in any one region the branching systems of hundreds of them intertwine in a dense thicket, with adjacent branches separated by films of fluid only about .02 micrometer thick, so that virtually all the space is occupied by cells and their various processes; when all the cells in a region are stained, one sees through an optical microscope only a dense and useless smear.

The most important single advance in neuroanatomy (after the microscope itself) was therefore a discovery by the Italian anatomist Camillo Golgi in about 1875. He came on a method by which, seemingly at random, only a very small proportion of the cells in a region are stained at one time, and those cells are stained in their entirety. Instead of a hopeless morass a good Golgi stain shows only a few neurons, each one complete with all its branches. By looking at many slices of Golgi-stained brain tissue the anatomist can build up an inventory of the various kinds of cells in that tissue. To this day no one knows how or why the Golgi method works, staining one cell in 100 completely and leaving the others quite unaffected.

Golgi's Spanish contemporary, Santiago Ramón y Cajal, devoted a lifetime of stupendous creativity to applying the new method to virtually every part of the nervous system. His gigantic *Histologie du système nerveux de l'homme et des vertébrés,* originally published in Spanish in 1904, is still recognized as the most important single work in neurobiology. In Cajal's day there was controversy over the extent of continuity between nerve cells. Were the cells completely separate entities or were they joined, axon to dendrite, in a continuous network? If there were protoplasmic continuity, signals generated by one cell could pass to an adjoining cell without interruption; if there were no continuity, there would have to be a special process for generating signals anew in each cell. Cajal's Golgi-stained preparations revealed large numbers of discrete, completely stained cells but never anything to suggest a network. His first great contribution, then, was to establish the notion of a nervous system made up of separate, well-defined cells communicating with one another at synapses.

Cajal made a second contribution, possibly even more important. He compiled massive evidence to show that the incredibly complex interconnections among neurons are not random, as has sometimes been supposed, but rather are the very antithesis of random: highly structured and specific. He described exhaustively the architecture of scores of different structures of the brain, in each case identifying and classifying the various cells and in some cases showing, as far as his methods would allow, how the cells are interconnected. From his time on it has been clear that to understand the brain the neurobiologist not only would have to learn how the various subdivisions are constructed but also would have to discover their purposes and learn in detail how they function as individual structures and as groups. Before that could be done it would be necessary to find out how a single neuron generates its signals and transmits them to the next cell. Cajal may never have

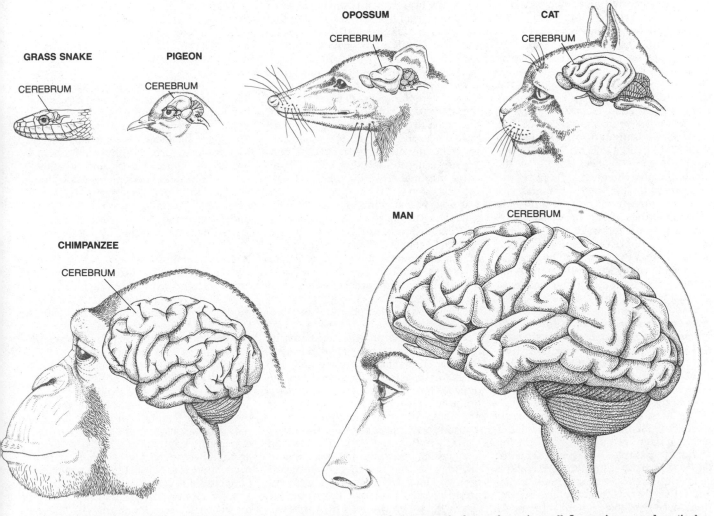

GRASS SNAKE
CEREBRUM

PIGEON
CEREBRUM

OPOSSUM
CEREBRUM

CAT
CEREBRUM

CHIMPANZEE
CEREBRUM

MAN
CEREBRUM

drawings on these two pages, which show a representative selection of vertebrate brains, all drawn to the same scale. In vertebrates lower than mammals the cerebrum is small. In carnivores, and particularly in primates, it increases dramatically in both size and complexity.

formulated the problems of understanding the nervous system explicitly in those terms, but one can hardly survey his work without taking that message from it.

For a long time neuroanatomists had to be content with increasingly detailed descriptions based on light microscopy, the Golgi stain and the Nissl stain (which picks out individual cell bodies but not their dendrites and axons). The first powerful tool for mapping the connections between different brain structures—between different parts of the cerebral cortex, for example, or between the cortex and the brain stem or the cerebellum—was a staining method invented in the Netherlands in the early 1950's by Walle J. H. Nauta, who is now at the Massachusetts Institute of Technology. The method capitalizes on the fact that when a neuron is destroyed (by mechanical or electrical means or by heat), the nerve fiber coming from it degenerates and, before disappearing altogether, can be stained differently from its normal neighbors. If a particular part of the brain is destroyed and the brain is stained by the Nauta method a few days later and then examined under the microscope, the presence of selectively stained fibers in some second and perhaps quite distant part means that the second region receives fibers from the destroyed part. The method has led to an enormous expansion in detail of the map of the brain.

In the past decade neuroanatomy has advanced at a higher rate, with more new and powerful techniques, than in the entire 50 years that preceded [see "The Organization of the Brain," by Walle J. H. Nauta and Michael Feirtag, page 40]. The advances are partly the result of better chemical tools and better understanding of how substances are taken up into neurons and are shipped in both directions along nerve fibers. A typical example is transport autoradiography. A radioactive chemical is injected into a brain structure; cell bodies take it up and transport it along their axons and it accumulates in the terminals. When a photographic emulsion is put in contact with a slice of brain tissue, microscopic examination of exposed silver grains in the emulsion reveals the destination of the axons. Other chemicals can be injected that are taken up instead by nerve terminals and transported back along the axons to the cell bodies, revealing the origin of the axons.

The latest in this series of advances is the deoxyglucose technique invented a few years ago by Louis Sokoloff of the National Institute of Mental Health. Glucose is the fuel for neurons, and the cells consume more glucose when they are active than when they are at rest. Radioactively labeled deoxyglucose is taken up by the cells as if it were glucose. It is broken down like glucose, but the product of the first step of metabolism cannot be further metabolized. Because it also cannot escape from the cell it accumulates there, and the extent of the radioactivity in particular cells shows how active they have been. For example, one can administer the chemical to a laboratory animal by vein and then stimulate the animal with a pattern of sound. Microscopic examination of the brain then reveals the various areas of the brain that are involved in hearing. Very recently a new technique called positron-emission transverse tomography has been developed that makes it possible to detect from outside the skull the presence of deoxyglucose or other substances labeled with positron-emitting radioactive isotopes. This promising technique makes it possible to map active brain structures in a living laboratory animal or in a human being.

Applying all the available techniques, to work out in a rough and undetailed fashion the connections in a single structure, say a part of the cerebral cortex or the cerebellum, may take one or two neuroanatomists five or 10 years. Accomplished neuroanatomists, a special breed of people, often compulsive and occasionally even semiparanoid, number only a few score in the entire world. Since the brain consists of hundreds of different structures, it is easy to see that an understanding of just the wiring of the brain is still many years away.

Moreover, to know the connections of a structure within the brain is a quite different thing from understanding the structure's physiology. To do that one needs to begin by learning how individual neurons work. How a single neuron generates electrical signals and conveys information to other cells has become reasonably well understood over the past three or four decades. The work was done by many individuals; Sir Henry Dale, Otto Loewi, A. L. Hodgkin, A. F. Huxley, Bernhard Katz, Sir John Eccles and Stephen W. Kuffler are some of the major contributors. One of the surprising findings was that neurons, in spite of their differences in size and shape, all use the same two kinds of electrical signals: graded potentials and action potentials.

The entire neuron—the cell body, its long axon and its branching dendrites—is polarized so that the inside is about 70 millivolts negative with respect to the outside. Two properties of the cell membrane are responsible for this "resting potential." First, the membrane actively transports ions, extruding positively charged sodium ions from the cell and bringing in positively charged potassium ions, so that the concentrations of the two kinds of ion are quite different inside the cell and outside it. Second, the ease with which the ions flow through the membrane is quite different for sodium and potassium.

It is changes in the resulting outside-to-inside resting potential that constitute the electrical signals of nerves. A change in the transmembrane voltage anywhere on the cell or its processes tends to spread quickly in all directions along the membrane, dying out as it spreads; a few millimeters away there is likely to be no detectable signal. This is the first kind of electrical signal, the graded potential. Its main function is to convey signals for very short distances.

The second type of signal, the action potential, conveys information for greater distances. If the membrane is depolarized (its potential decreased) to a critical level—from the resting level of 70 millivolts to about 50 millivolts—there is a sudden and dramatic change: the normal barriers to the flow of sodium and potassium ions are temporarily removed and there ensues a local flow of ions sufficient to reverse the membrane potential, which reaches about 50 millivolts positive inside and then is reversed again to restore the normal resting potential. All of this happens within about a millisecond (a thousandth of a second). Meanwhile the first reversal (to inside-positive) has produced a powerful graded signal that spreads and brings the adjacent region of the membrane to its critical level; that leads to a reversal in the next segment of membrane, which in turn leads to a reversal in the next segment. The result is a rapid spread of the transient reversal in polarity along the nerve fiber.

This propagating action potential, which travels the entire length of the fiber without attenuation, is the nerve impulse. All signaling in the nervous system over distances of a millimeter or more is in the form of impulses. Regardless of the type of fiber and whether it is involved in movement, vision or thought, the signals are virtually identical. What varies in a given nerve fiber under particular circumstances is simply the number of impulses per second.

When an impulse arrives at an axon terminal, the neuron next in line is influenced in such a way that its likelihood of in turn generating impulses is modified. A chemical transmitter substance is released from the presynaptic membrane of the terminal, diffuses across the narrow space separating the two cells and affects the postsynaptic membrane on the far side of the synapse in one of two ways. In an excitatory synapse the transmitter leads to a lowering of the postsynaptic-membrane potential, so that the postsynaptic cell tends to generate impulses at a higher rate. In an inhibitory synapse the effect of the transmitter is to stabilize the postsynaptic-membrane potential, making it harder for excitatory synapses to depolarize the postsynaptic cell and thereby either preventing new impulses from arising or reducing their rate.

Whether a given synapse is excitatory or inhibitory depends on what chemical transmitter the presynaptic cell makes and on the chemistry of the postsynaptic cell's membrane. Almost every neuron receives inputs from many terminals, usually many hundreds and sometimes thousands, some of which are excitatory and some inhibitory. At any instant some inputs will be active and some quiescent, and it is the sum of the excitatory and inhibitory effects that determines whether or not the cell will fire and, if it does fire, the rate at which it does so. In other words, the neuron is much more than a device for sending impulses from one place to another. Each neuron constantly evaluates all the signals reaching it from other cells and expresses the result in its own rate of signaling.

The propagation of the two types of signals along the neuron membrane and the chemical events at synaptic contacts are, then, understood at least in broad outline. What is still far from clear is the relation between a neuron's shape (oak v. petunia) and the way it summates and evaluates the inputs it receives. Two incoming signals, either of which may be excitatory or inhibitory, surely add up very differently depending on whether the synapses are adjacent (for example on the same dendritic branch) or one synapse is on one branch and the other on a remote one (perhaps a branch of a different limb) or one synapse involves a branch and the other the cell body. Shape, being very different in different classes of neurons, is bound to be important in neuronal function, but that is about all one can say with assurance.

A related set of questions concerns the implications of certain synapses (ordinary-looking synapses with presynaptic and postsynaptic components) that are junctions between two dendrites or between two axons rather than—as is usual—between an axon and either a dendrite or a cell body. To put it mildly, no one knows quite what to make of them. Finally, to complicate things even more, some synapses are profoundly different from the usual chemical type, depending on flow of current rather than diffusion of a transmitter. These were discovered in the 1950's by Edwin J. Furshpan and David D. Potter at University College London. Why nature resorts to chemical transmission for some synapses and electrical transmission for others is still a puzzle.

At a more fundamental level many of the important unanswered questions about nerve signals have to do with the fine structure and functioning of the neuron membrane, because it is still not known in molecular terms exactly how ions are transported across membranes or how the permeability to particular ions is influenced by changes in potential and by transmitter substances [see "The Neuron," by Charles F. Stevens, page 14]. A particularly exciting area

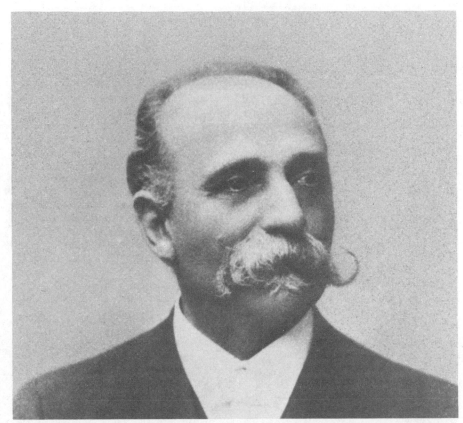

CAMILLO GOLGI (1844–1926) provided the key to the microscopic investigation of the nervous system by devising (in about 1875) a method of selectively staining nerve tissue so that only a very small fraction of the cells in a given sample are stained at one time, and those cells are stained in their entirety. This photograph was made sometime in the early 1880's, at which time Golgi served as professor of histology and general pathology at the University of Pavia.

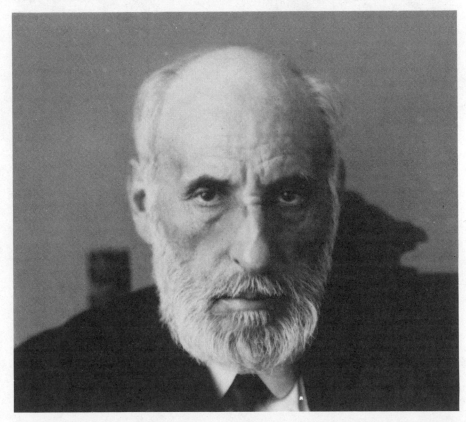

SANTIAGO RAMÓN Y CAJAL (1852–1934) applied Golgi's method to the lifelong scrutiny of virtually every part of the nervous system of many different animals. In recognition of their work on the structure of the nervous system Golgi and Cajal shared the Nobel prize in physiology and medicine in 1906. Cajal taught at several universities in Spain, spending most of his career at the University of Madrid. This photograph, a self-portrait, was made in the 1920's.

is the chemistry of synaptic transmission, with more than 20 transmitter substances already identified and the methods by which neurons make, release, take up and destroy the substances fairly well known [see "The Chemistry of the Brain," by Leslie L. Iversen, page 70].

The still incomplete but greatly improved understanding of synapse chemistry has had profound effects in psychiatry and pharmacology. Many disorders, ranging from Parkinson's disease to depression, appear to stem from disturbances of synaptic transmission, and many drugs act by increasing or decreasing transmission [see "Disorders of the Human Brain," by Seymour S. Kety, page 120].

In a decade or so the main activities of individual neurons should be known in great detail. At the present stage, with a reasonable start in understanding the structure and workings of individual cells, neurobiologists are in the position of a man who knows something about the physics of resistors, condensers and transistors and who looks inside a television set. He cannot begin to understand how the machine works as a whole until he learns how the elements are wired together and until he has at least some idea of the purpose of the machine, of its subassemblies and of their interactions. In brain research the first step beyond the individual neuron and its workings is to learn how the larger subunits of the brain are interconnected and how each unit is built up. The next step is to try to find out how the neurons interact and to learn the significance of the messages they carry.

One way to get a feel for the overall organization of the brain is to consider it in rough caricature [see illustration on opposite page]. On the input side there are groups of receptors: modified nerve cells specialized to transform into electrical signals the various forms of information that impinge on them from the outside world. Some receptors respond to light, others to chemicals (taste and smell) and still others to mechanical deformation (touch and hearing). The receptors make contact with a first set of neurons, which in turn contact others, and so on. At each step along the way axons branch to supply a number of the neurons next in line, each of which is supplied by a number of axons that converge on it. Each recipient cell integrates the excitatory or inhibitory impulses converging on it from lower-order cells. Sooner or later, after a number of steps, nerve axons terminate on gland or muscle cells: the outputs of the nervous system.

In brief, there is an input: man's only way of knowing about the outside world. There is an output: man's only way of responding to the outside world and influencing it. And between input and output there is everything else, which must include perception, emotions, memory, thought and whatever else makes man human.

The input-to-output flow described above, it need hardly be said, is oversimplified. Although the main flow of traffic is from left to right in the diagram, there are frequent lateral connections among cells at any one stage; often there are connections in the reverse direction, from output toward input, just as there is feedback in many electronic circuits. There is not just one pathway from input to output; there are many different arrays of receptors, specialized for the various senses and for particular forms of the energy affecting each sense, and there are countless different shunts, relays and detours. The number of synapses between receptors and muscles may be very many or only two or three. (When the number is small, the circuit is usually designated a reflex; the constriction of the pupil in response to light shining on the retina represents a reflex involving perhaps four or five synapses.) And it should be mentioned again that a synapse can be either excitatory or inhibitory; if both kinds of influence impinge on a cell at a particular moment, the result may be a complete cancellation of effects.

Physiologists now have some idea of the kinds of operation performed by the nervous system close to the input end and at the output. At the input end the system is apparently chiefly preoccupied with extracting from the outside world information that is biologically interesting. The receptors generally respond best at the onset or cessation of a stimulus such as pressure on the skin.

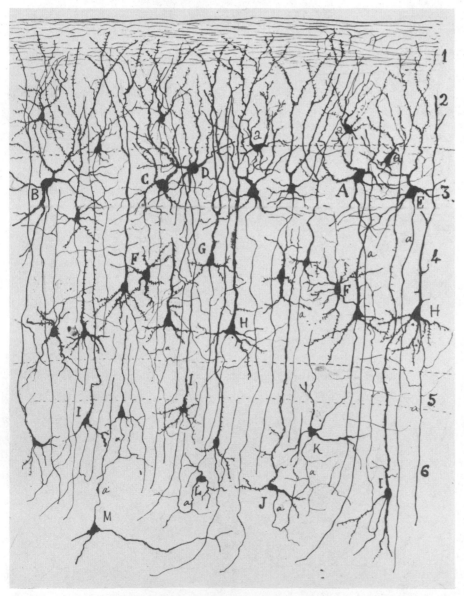

GOLGI-STAINED NERVE TISSUE from the visual cortex of a rat was sketched by Cajal in 1888. The numbers along the right-hand margin identify cellular layers; the capital letters label individual neurons. One of Cajal's most important contributions to neurobiology was to establish the neuron as a discrete, well-defined cell rather than as part of a continuous network.

We need above all to know about changes; no one wants or needs to be reminded 16 hours a day that his shoes are on.

In the visual system, to take one example, it is contrasts and movements that are important, and much of the circuitry of the first two or three steps is devoted to enhancing the effects of contrast and movement. At subsequent stages of the visual system the behavior of the cells becomes more complex, but it is always orderly, and fortunately it makes sense in terms of perception. By now information originating with the light-receptive cells of the retina has been followed into the brain to the sixth or seventh stage, to the part of the cerebral cortex concerned with vision [see "Brain Mechanisms of Vision," by David H. Hubel and Torsten N. Wiesel, page 84].

Although the visual system is now one of the best-understood parts of the brain, neurobiologists are still far from knowing how objects are perceived or recognized. Yet the amount that has been learned in the few years since microelectrodes became available does suggest that a part of the brain such as the cerebral cortex is, at least in principle, capable of eventually being understood in relatively simple terms.

At the output end of the nervous system the mechanism whereby a motor neuron delivers an impulse to a muscle fiber has been understood in its essentials for some time, and for 50 years or more the parts of the brain concerned with movement have been known. Just what these structures actually do when a human being moves or contemplates moving is still largely unknown, however. Progress has been slow mainly because investigating voluntary movement calls for working with an animal that is awake and that has been given elaborate training, whereas one can study sensory systems in anesthetized animals. One of the main efforts today is to trace the motor impulse back from the motor neuron to structures such as the motor cortex and the cerebellum to learn how the decision to execute a movement is influenced by various signals coming from the input end of the nervous system [see "Brain Mechanisms of Movement," by Edward V. Evarts, page 98].

What is important at the output end is not the contraction of an individual muscle but the coordinated contraction and relaxation of many muscles. In making a fist or grasping an object, for example, a person cannot merely flex the fingers by contracting flexor muscles in his forearm; he must also contract extensor muscles in the forearm to keep the finger-flexor muscles from flexing the wrist. This counteracting extension force at the wrist is exerted automatically and without thought (as one can verify by making a fist and feeling the exten-

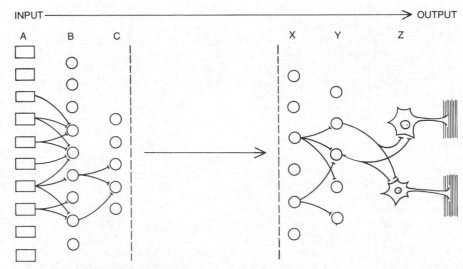

INPUT ——————————————————————————————→ OUTPUT

OVERALL ORGANIZATION of the brain is indicated in a rough caricature that suggests the flow of information from the input of sensory signals by receptor cells (A) to the eventual output by motor neurons (Z) terminating on muscle cells. The outputs of receptors and neurons usually branch to send diverging signals to the next stage. Most neurons receive converging inputs, both excitatory and inhibitory, from earlier stages. Something is known about the significance of the connections near the input end of the brain (B, C) and near the output end (X, Y). Far less is known about the workings of regions in between, which make up most of the brain.

sor muscles contract on the hairy side of the forearm).

Evidently a command from the brain to make a fist involves the firing of cells several stages removed from the output end of the nervous system, cells whose axons are distributed to the various motor neurons and inhibitory neurons that in turn supply all the muscles involved in executing the command. Other movements bring in different circuits that may well involve the same muscles but in different combinations.

It is not hard, then, to visualize a few of the kinds of functions that may be performed by the nervous system, particularly close to the sensory or the motor ends of the system. It is in the vast in-between region—in the frontal and parietal lobes, the limbic system, the cerebellum and so on and on—that knowledge of function is most lacking, although quite a bit is known about the anatomy. In some cases a kind of basic wiring-diagram physiology is known: which neurons excite or inhibit which, for example. In the case of the cerebellum not only is the wiring known in some detail but also it is now fairly clear which synapses are excitatory and which are inhibitory; for a few kinds of synapse the transmitters have been identified chemically with a moderate degree of confidence. Yet how the cerebellum works is known only in the vaguest terms. It surely has to do with the regulation of movements, muscle tone and balance, but how these functions are carried out by this magnificently patterned, orderly and fantastically complex piece of machinery is quite obscure.

The cerebellum is admittedly a diffi-

cult place to work; it lies at the watershed between sensory and motor processes, in the blankest part of the rough diagram above. The kinds of input it receives—the particular significance of impulses that come to the cerebellum from the cerebral cortex, the spine and so on—are imperfectly known; the neural structures to which it sends its output, which are in turn ultimately connected to the muscles, are also not well known. For similar reasons most other parts of the brain are still dimly understood. In spite of recent advances in technique, new and revolutionary methods are badly needed. To give just one example, there is now no known way of studying the signals of single cells in a human being without actually opening his skull on the operating table, and that is generally unacceptable from an ethical standpoint. Major advances have nonetheless been made in understanding some of the higher functions of the human brain [see "Specializations of the Human Brain," by Norman Geschwind, page 108], but in order to really understand something such as speech, which is peculiar to man, it will be necessary to find ways of recording from single neurons from outside the skull.

Knowledge of the wiring of neurons and their moment-to-moment workings represents only one ultimate goal in neurophysiology. Certain large aspects of brain function are beyond such a horizon. Memory and learning, for example, are surely cumulative processes involving change over a period of time, and very little is yet known about the mechanisms that underlie them.

Neurobiology seems to be particularly subject to fads that sometimes amount almost to a derailment of thought. A few years ago the notion was advanced that memories might be recorded in the form of large molecules, with the information encoded in a sequence of smaller molecules, as genetic information is encoded in DNA. Few people familiar with the highly patterned specificity of connections in the brain took the idea seriously, and yet much time was consumed in many laboratories teaching animals tasks, grinding up their brains and either finding differences in the brain chemistry of the trained animals or finding "statistically significant" improvement in the ability of other animals, into which extracts of the trained animals' brains were injected, to learn the same tasks. The fad has died out, but the fact is that neurobiology has not always advanced or even stood still; sometimes there is momentary backsliding.

In the final analysis an understanding of memory will probably involve two quite different components. One component is the changes that most likely take place in synapses as a result of the repeated use of neural circuits. For example, there could be an increase in the efficiency of one synapse at the expense of other synapses on the same cell. Particular combinations of stimuli, if repeated, might thus enhance one possible pathway among many in a neural structure.

Studies that might get at this aspect are rather difficult in higher animals; they are far easier in the small systems of neurons that constitute all, or large parts, of the nervous system of certain lower animals. Individual cells in these animals are often easy to poke with microelectrodes and, even more important, such cells often have unique identity; one can speak of cell No. 56 in a certain lobster ganglion and know that it will have virtually the same position and connections in other lobsters. (This is one profound difference between many invertebrate brains and man's. One can no more assign a number to a neuron of the human brain than one can to a hair of the head or a pore of the skin.) Elegant experiments are being done at the single-cell level on learning in these invertebrate systems [see "Small Systems of Neurons," by Eric R. Kandel, page 28]. It has even been shown, for example, that when an animal learns or forgets a response, identifiable changes take place in the transmission of signals across particular synapses. The learning here is obviously of a simple kind, but it appears to be true learning. (Again and again discoveries have been made in invertebrates that were later extended to higher forms. There is therefore little likelihood that investigators will be discouraged from working on such animals by the gibes of politicians about the implausible sound of such projects as, say, "Problem-solving in the Leech.")

The second component that will need to be grappled with in studying memory will be far more difficult. Things one remembers (in anything but the most rudimentary sense of that word) involve percepts or movements or experiences. To get at memory in any real sense it will be necessary to know what goes on when human beings perceive, act, think and experience, in order to know what of all that is recapitulated when they remember or learn. Of the two components the first—the synaptic—seems to me to be relatively easy, the second stupendously difficult.

To understand the brain of an adult animal is a hard enough task; to understand how a brain gets to be a brain is probably at least as difficult. How does the nervous system develop, both before birth and afterward? The central problem is to discover how the information encoded in molecules of DNA is translated into cell-to-cell connections within structures, the mutual spatial relations of those structures and the connections among them. The optic nerve, for example, contains about a million fibers, each originating in a tiny part of the retina. Each fiber in turn connects in an orderly way to the platelike lateral geniculate nucleus in the brain, so that in a sense the retina is mapped onto the geniculate. How, during development, do the fibers grow out of the retina, reach the plate and distribute themselves with absolute topographical precision? Similar specifically wired sets of cablelike connections between topographically mapped areas are common throughout the nervous system, and how this precise wiring is laid down remains one of the great unsolved problems [see "The Development of the Brain," by W. Maxwell Cowan, page 56].

Developmental studies are potentially important not only because they shed light on how the brain works but also because so many neurological diseases are, or seem likely to be, developmental in origin. These include most birth defects, Down's syndrome, certain kinds of muscular dystrophy, probably certain common epilepsies and a large number of rarer diseases.

How long it will be before one is able to say that the brain—or the mind—is in broad outline understood (those fuzzy words again) is anyone's guess. As late as 1950 anyone who predicted that in 10 years the main processes that underlie life would be understood would have been regarded as optimistic if not foolish, and yet that came to pass. I think it will take a lot longer than 10 years to understand the brain, simply because it is such a many-faceted thing: a box brimful of ingenious solutions to a huge number of problems. It is quite possible that human beings may never solve all the separate individual puzzles the brain presents. What one may hope is that, as each region of the brain is looked at in turn, it will become more and more established that the brain's functions are orderly and capable of being understood in terms of physics and chemistry, without appeal to unknowable, supernatural processes [see "Thinking about the Brain," by F. H. C. Crick, page 130].

There will be major individual milestones. For example, some single mechanism by which memory (the synaptic component) works may be revealed, or some one process that explains how nerve fibers find their proper destinations in development. This does not mean, however, that at some particular moment in the future a discovery or set of discoveries is likely to be made that completely explains the brain. Progress in brain research tends to be slow. Technical advances have produced a marked acceleration in the past few decades, and yet there have certainly not been any abrupt upheavals to compare with those brought about by Copernicus, Newton, Darwin, Einstein or Watson and Crick.

Each of those revolutions had the property of bringing some very fundamental aspect of man's study of nature into the realm of rational and experimental analysis, away from the supernatural. If Copernicus pointed out that the earth is not the center of the universe and Galileo saw stars and planets but not angels in the sky, if Darwin showed that man is related to all other living organisms, if Einstein introduced new notions of time and space and of mass and energy, if Watson and Crick showed that biological inheritance can be explained in physical and chemical terms, then in this sequence of eliminations of the supernatural the main thing science seems to be left with is the brain, and whether or not it is something more than a machine of vast and magnificent complexity.

It is a question that goes to the very center of man's being, so that fundamental changes in our view of the human brain cannot but have profound effects on our view of ourselves and the world. Certainly such advances will have significant effects on other fields of inquiry. The branches of philosophy concerned with the nature of mind and of perception will to some extent be superseded, and so, I think, will some parts of psychology that seek to obtain answers to similar questions by indirect means. The entire field of education will be affected if the mechanisms underlying learning and memory are discovered.

A revolution of truly Copernican or Darwinian proportions may never come in neurobiology, at least not in a single stroke. If there is one, it may be gradual, having its effect over many decades. Every stage will surely bring human beings closer to an understanding of themselves.

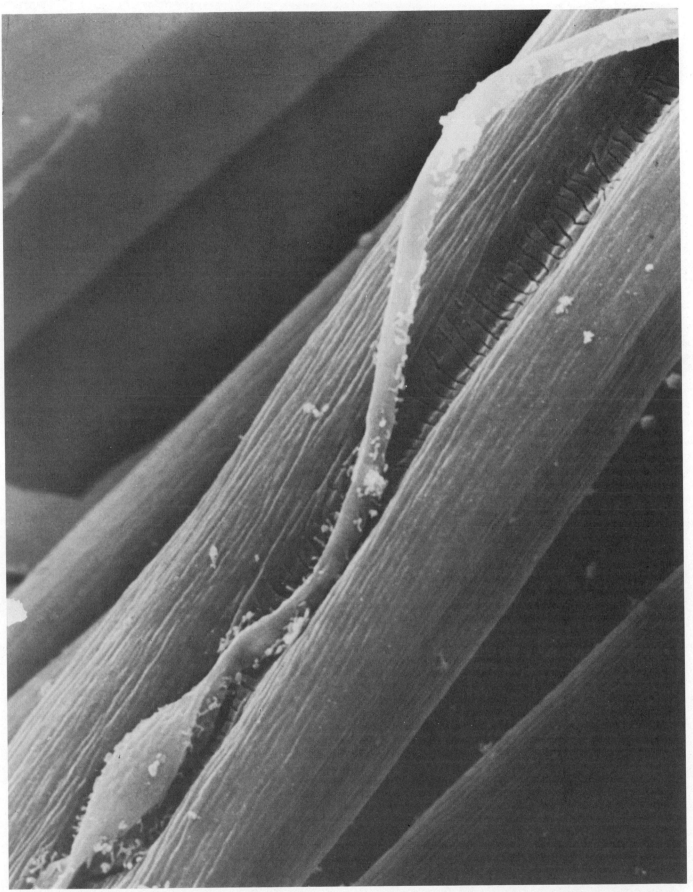

OUTPUT OF NERVOUS SYSTEM is the activation of a muscle fiber by the terminal branches of a motor-neuron axon. In this scanning electron micrograph made by Barbara F. Reese and Thomas S. Reese of the National Institute of Neurological and Communicative Disorders and Stroke one terminal branch lies in (and in places has been pulled away from) a junctional groove in a muscle fiber. The nerve fiber is largely enveloped by the sheath of a Schwann cell, the cell body of which is at the bottom left. The junctional groove is traversed by narrow folds in the postsynaptic muscle membrane. Each fold normally abuts an "active zone" in the nerve fiber, from which a chemical transmitter, acetylcholine, is released through "windows" in the Schwann-cell sheath when an impulse arrives at the synapse. Molecules of acetylcholine activate receptors on muscle membrane to initiate muscle contraction. Enlargement is about 4,000 diameters.

II

The Neuron

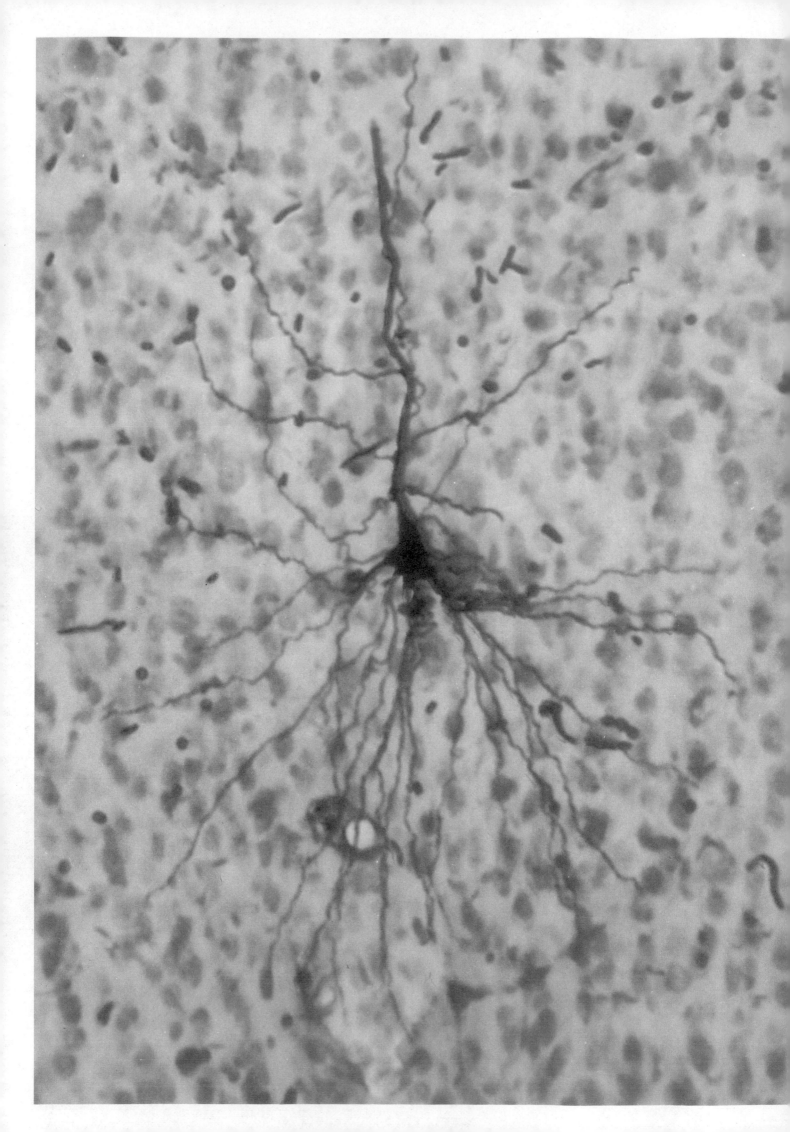

The Neuron

BY CHARLES F. STEVENS

It is the individual nerve cell, the building block of the brain. It transmits nerve impulses over a single long fiber (the axon) and receives them over numerous short fibers (the dendrites)

Neurons, or nerve cells, are the building blocks of the brain. Although they have the same genes, the same general organization and the same biochemical apparatus as other cells, they also have unique features that make the brain function in a very different way from, say, the liver. The important specializations of the neuron include a distinctive cell shape, an outer membrane capable of generating nerve impulses, and a unique structure, the synapse, for transferring information from one neuron to the next.

The human brain is thought to consist of 10^{11} neurons, about the same number as the stars in our galaxy. No two neurons are identical in form. Nevertheless, their forms generally fall into only a few broad categories, and most neurons share certain structural features that make it possible to distinguish three regions of the cell: the cell body, the dendrites and the axon. The cell body contains the nucleus of the neuron and the biochemical machinery for synthesizing enzymes and other molecules essential to the life of the cell. Usually the cell body is roughly spherical or pyramid-shaped. The dendrites are delicate tube-like extensions that tend to branch repeatedly and form a bushy tree around the cell body. They provide the main physical surface on which the neuron receives incoming signals. The axon extends away from the cell body and provides the pathway over which signals can travel from the cell body for long distances to other parts of the brain and

the nervous system. The axon differs from the dendrites both in structure and in the properties of its outer membrane. Most axons are longer and thinner than dendrites and exhibit a different branching pattern: whereas the branches of dendrites tend to cluster near the cell body, the branches of axons tend to arise at the end of the fiber where the axon communicates with other neurons.

The functioning of the brain depends on the flow of information through elaborate circuits consisting of networks of neurons. Information is transferred from one cell to another at specialized points of contact: the synapses. A typical neuron may have anywhere from 1,000 to 10,000 synapses and may receive information from something like 1,000 other neurons. Although synapses are most often made between the axon of one cell and the dendrite of another, there are other kinds of synaptic junction: between axon and axon, between dendrite and dendrite and between axon and cell body.

At a synapse the axon usually enlarges to form a terminal button, which is the information-delivering part of the junction. The terminal button contains tiny spherical structures called synaptic vesicles, each of which can hold several thousand molecules of chemical transmitter. On the arrival of a nerve impulse at the terminal button, some of the vesicles discharge their contents into the narrow cleft that separates the button from the membrane of another cell's dendrite, which is designed to receive

the chemical message. Hence information is relayed from one neuron to another by means of a transmitter. The "firing" of a neuron—the generation of nerve impulses—reflects the activation of hundreds of synapses by impinging neurons. Some synapses are excitatory in that they tend to promote firing, whereas others are inhibitory and so are capable of canceling signals that otherwise would excite a neuron to fire.

Although neurons are the building blocks of the brain, they are not the only kind of cell in it. For example, oxygen and nutrients are supplied by a dense network of blood vessels. There is also a need for connective tissue, particularly at the surface of the brain. A major class of cells in the central nervous system is the glial cells, or glia. The glia occupy essentially all the space in the nervous system not taken up by the neurons themselves. Although the function of the glia is not fully understood, they provide structural and metabolic support for the delicate meshwork of the neurons.

One other kind of cell, the Schwann cell, is ubiquitous in the nervous system. All axons appear to be jacketed by Schwann cells. In some cases the Schwann cells simply enclose the axon in a thin layer. In many cases, however, the Schwann cell wraps itself around the axon in the course of embryonic development, giving rise to the multiple dense layers of insulation known as myelin. The myelin sheath is interrupted every millimeter or so along the axon by narrow gaps called the nodes of Ranvier. In axons that are sheathed in this way the nerve impulse travels by jumping from node to node, where the extracellular fluid can make direct contact with the cell membrane. The myelin sheath seems to have evolved as a means of conserving the neuron's metabolic energy. In general myelinated nerve fibers conduct nerve impulses faster than unmyelinated fibers.

Neurons can work as they do because their outer membranes have special

NEURON FROM A CAT'S VISUAL CORTEX has been labeled in the photomicrograph on the opposite page by injection with the enzyme horseradish peroxidase. The cell bodies in the background are counterstained with a magenta dye. All the fibers extending from the cell body are dendrites, which receive information from other neurons. The fiber that transmits information, the axon, is much finer and not readily visible at this magnification. The thickest fiber, extending vertically upward, is known as the apical dendrite, only a small portion of which falls within this section. At this magnification (about 500 diameters) the complete apical dendrite would be about 75 centimeters long. (It can be traced through adjacent sections.) The activity of this particular cell was recorded in the living animal and was found to respond optimally to a light-dark border rotated about 60 degrees from the vertical. The neuron is classified as a pyramidal cell because of its form. It is one of two major types in cortex of mammals. Micrograph was made by Charles Gilbert and Torsten N. Wiesel of Harvard Medical School.

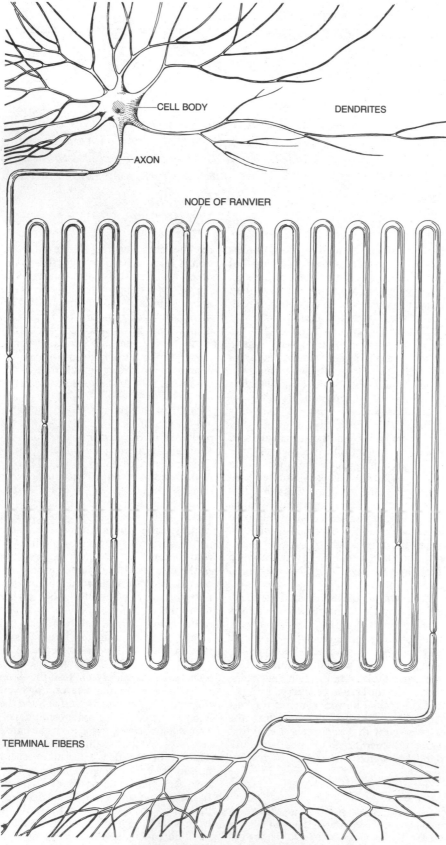

CELL BODY

DENDRITES

AXON

NODE OF RANVIER

TERMINAL FIBERS

TYPICAL NEURON of a vertebrate animal can carry nerve impulses for a considerable distance. The neuron depicted here, with its various parts drawn to scale, is enlarged 250 times. The nerve impulses originate in the cell body and are propagated along the axon, which may have one or more branches. This axon, which is folded for diagrammatic purposes, would be a centimeter long at actual size. Some axons are more than a meter long. The axon's terminal branches form synapses with as many as 1,000 other neurons. Most synapses join the axon terminals of one neuron with the dendrites forming a "tree" around the cell body of another neuron. Thus the dendrites surrounding the neuron in the diagram might receive incoming signals from tens, hundreds or even thousands of other neurons. Many axons, such as this one, are insulated by a myelin sheath interrupted at intervals by the regions known as nodes of Ranvier.

properties. Along the axon the membrane is specialized to propagate an electrical impulse. At the terminal of the axon the membrane releases transmitters, and on the dendrites it reponds to transmitters. In addition the membrane mediates the recognition of other cells in embryonic development, so that each cell finds its proper place in the network of 10^{11} cells. Much recent investigation therefore focuses on the membrane properties responsible for the nerve impulse, for synaptic transmission, for cell-cell recognition and for structural contacts between cells.

The neuron membrane, like the outer membrane of all cells, is about five nanometers thick and consists of two layers of lipid molecules arranged with their hydrophilic ends pointing toward the water on the inside and outside of the cell and with their hydrophobic ends pointing away from the water to form the interior of the membrane. The lipid parts of the membrane are about the same for all kinds of cells. What makes one cell membrane different from another are various specific proteins that are associated with the membrane in one way or another. Proteins that are actually embedded in the lipid bilayer are termed intrinsic proteins. Other proteins, the peripheral membrane proteins, are attached to the membrane surface but do not form an integral part of its structure. Because the membrane lipid is fluid even the intrinsic proteins are often free to move by diffusion from place to place. In some instances, however, the proteins are firmly fastened down by a substructure.

The membrane proteins of all cells fall into five classes: pumps, channels, receptors, enzymes and structural proteins. Pumps expend metabolic energy to move ions and other molecules against concentration gradients in order to maintain appropriate concentrations of these molecules within the cell. Because charged molecules do not pass through the lipid bilayer itself cells have evolved channel proteins that provide selective pathways through which specific ions can diffuse. Cell membranes must recognize and attach many types of molecules. Receptor proteins fulfill these functions by providing binding sites with great specificity and high affinity. Enzymes are placed in or on the membrane to facilitate chemical reactions at the membrane surface. Finally, structural proteins both interconnect cells to form organs and help to maintain subcellular structure. These five classes of membrane proteins are not necessarily mutually exclusive. For example, a particular protein might simultaneously be a receptor, an enzyme and a pump.

Membrane proteins are the key to understanding neuron function and therefore brain function. Because they play such a central role in modern views of the neuron, I shall organize my discussion around a description of an ion pump, various types of channel and some other proteins that taken together endow neurons with their unique properties. The general idea will be to summarize the important characteristics of the membrane proteins and to explain how these characteristics account for the nerve impulse and other complex features of neuron function.

Like all cells the neuron is able to maintain within itself a fluid whose composition differs markedly from that of the fluid outside it. The difference is particularly striking with regard to the concentration of the ions of sodium and potassium. The external medium is about 10 times richer in sodium than the internal one, and the internal medium is about 10 times richer in potassium than the external one. Both sodium and potassium leak through pores in the cell membrane, so that a pump must operate continuously to exchange sodium ions that have entered the cell for potassium ions outside it. The pumping is accomplished by an intrinsic membrane protein called the sodium-potassium adenosine triphosphatase pump, or more often simply the sodium pump.

The protein molecule (or complex of protein subunits) of the sodium pump has a molecular weight of about 275,000 daltons and measures roughly six by eight nanometers, or slightly more than the thickness of the cell membrane. Each sodium pump can harness the energy stored in the phosphate bond of adenosine triphosphate (ATP) to exchange three sodium ions on the inside of the cell for two potassium ions on the outside. Operating at the maximum rate, each pump can transport across the membrane some 200 sodium ions and 130 potassium ions per second. The actual rate, however, is adjusted to meet the needs of the cell. Most neurons have between 100 and 200 sodium pumps per square micrometer of membrane surface, but in some parts of their surface the density is as much as 10 times higher. A typical small neuron has perhaps a million sodium pumps with a capacity to move about 200 million sodium ions per second. It is the transmembrane gradients of sodium and potassium ions that enable the neuron to propagate nerve impulses.

Membrane proteins that serve as channels are essential for many aspects of neuron function, particularly for the nerve impulse and synaptic transmission. As an introduction to the role played by channels in the electrical activity of the brain I shall briefly describe the mechanism of the nerve impulse and then return to a more systematic survey of channel properties.

Since the concentration of sodium and potassium ions on one side of the cell membrane differs from that on the

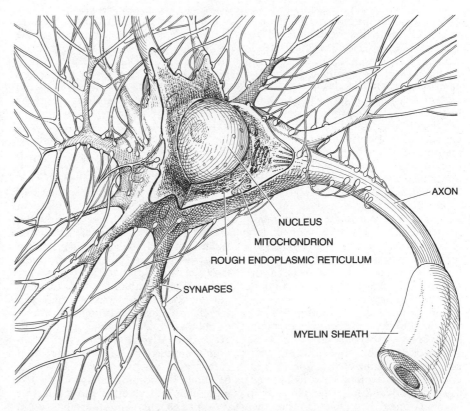

CELL BODY OF A NEURON incorporates the genetic material and complex metabolic apparatus common to all cells. Unlike most other cells, however, neurons do not divide after embryonic development; an organism's original supply must serve a lifetime. Projecting from the cell body are several dendrites and a single axon. The cell body and dendrites are covered by synapses, knoblike structures where information is received from other neurons. Mitochondria provide the cell with energy. Proteins are synthesized on the endoplasmic reticulum. A transport system moves proteins and other substances from cell body to sites where they are needed.

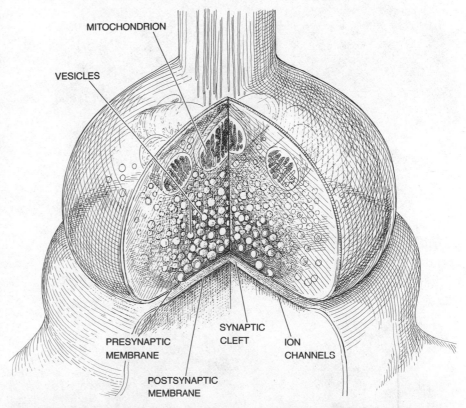

SYNAPSE is the relay point where information is conveyed by chemical transmitters from neuron to neuron. A synapse consists of two parts: the knoblike tip of an axon terminal and the receptor region on the surface of another neuron. The membranes are separated by a synaptic cleft some 200 nanometers across. Molecules of chemical transmitter, stored in vesicles in the axon terminal, are released into the cleft by arriving nerve impulses. Transmitter changes electrical state of the receiving neuron, making it either more likely or less likely to fire an impulse.

other side, the interior of the axon is about 70 millivolts negative with respect to the exterior. In their classic studies of nerve-impulse transmission in the giant axon of the squid a quarter of a century ago, A. L. Hodgkin, A. F. Huxley and Bernhard Katz of Britain demonstrated that the propagation of the nerve impulse coincides with sudden changes in the permeability of the axon membrane to sodium and potassium ions. When a nerve impulse starts at the origin of the axon, having been triggered in most cases by the cell body in response to dendritic synapses, the voltage difference across the axon membrane is locally lowered. Immediately ahead of the electrically altered region (in the direction in which the nerve impulse is propagated) channels in the membrane open and let sodium ions pour into the axon.

The process is self-reinforcing: the flow of sodium ions through the membrane opens more channels and makes it easier for other ions to follow. The sodium ions that enter change the internal potential of the membrane from negative to positive. Soon after the sodium channels open they close, and another group of channels open that let potassi-

um ions flow out. This outflow restores the voltage inside the axon to its resting value of −70 millivolts. The sharp positive and then negative charge, which shows up as a "spike" on an oscilloscope, is known as the action potential and is the electrical manifestation of the nerve impulse. The wave of voltage sweeps along until it reaches the end of the axon much as a flame travels along the fuse of a firecracker.

This brief description of the nerve impulse illustrates the importance of channels for the electrical activity of neurons and underscores two fundamental properties of channels: selectivity and gating. I shall discuss these two properties in turn. Channels are selectively permeable and selectivities vary widely. For example, one type of channel lets sodium ions pass through and largely excludes potassium ions, whereas another type of channel does the reverse. The selectivity, however, is seldom absolute. One type of channel that is fairly nonselective allows the passage of about 85 sodium ions for every 100 potassium ions; another more selective type passes only about seven sodium ions for every 100 potassium ions. The

first type, known as the acetylcholine-activated channel, has a pore about .8 nanometer in diameter that is filled with water. The second type, known as the potassium channel, has a much smaller opening and contains less water.

The sodium ion is about 30 percent smaller than the potassium ion. The exact molecular structure that enables the larger ion to pass through the cell membrane more readily than the smaller one is not known. The general principles that underlie the discrimination, however, are understood. They involve interactions between ions and parts of the channel structure in conjunction with a particular ordering of water molecules within the pore.

The gating mechanism that regulates the opening and closing of membrane channels takes two main forms. One type of channel, mentioned above in the description of the nerve impulse, opens and closes in response to voltage differences across the cell membrane; it is therefore said to be voltage-gated. A second type of channel is chemically gated. Such channels respond only slightly if at all to voltage changes but open when a particular molecule—a transmitter—binds to a receptor region

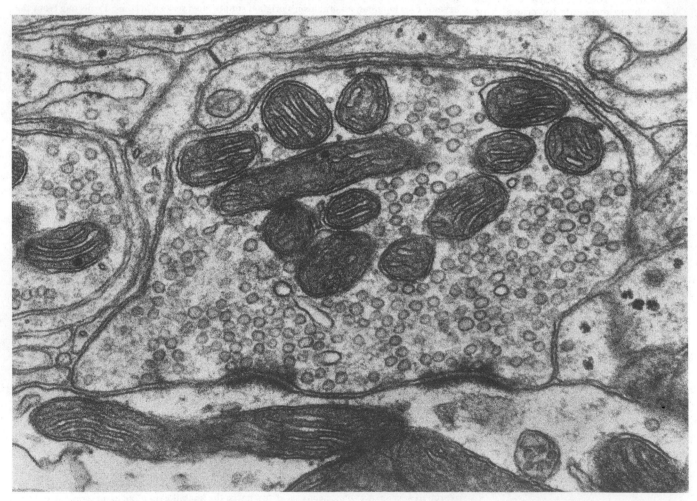

SYNAPTIC TERMINAL occupies most of this electron micrograph made by John E. Heuser of the University of California School of Medicine in San Francisco and Thomas S. Reese of the National Institutes of Health. The cleft separating the presynaptic membrane **from the postsynaptic one undulates across the lower part of the picture. The large dark structures are mitochondria. The many round bodies are vesicles that hold transmitter. The fuzzy dark thickenings along the cleft are thought to be principal sites of transmitter release.**

on the channel protein. Chemically gated channels are found in the receptive membranes of synapses and are responsible for translating the chemical signals produced by axon terminals into ion permeability changes during synaptic transmission. It is customary to name chemically gated channels according to their normal transmitter. Hence one speaks of acetylcholine-activated channels or GABA-activated channels. (GABA is gamma-aminobutyric acid.) Voltage-gated channels are generally named for the ion that passes through the channel most readily.

Proteins commonly change their shape as they function. Such alterations in shape, known as conformational changes, are dramatic for the contractile proteins responsible for cell motion, but they are no less important in many enzymes and other proteins. Conformational changes in channel proteins form the basis for gating as they serve to open and close the channel by slight movements of critically placed portions of the molecule that unblock and block the pore.

When either voltage-gated or chemically gated channels open and allow ions to pass, one can measure the resulting electric current. Quite recently it has become possible in a few instances to record the current flowing through a single channel, so that the opening and closing can be directly detected. One finds that the length of time a channel stays open varies randomly because the opening and closing of the channel represents a change in the conformation of the protein molecule embedded in the membrane. The random nature of the gating process arises from the haphazard collision of water molecules and other molecules with the structural elements of the channel.

In addition to ion pumps and channels neurons depend on other classes of membrane proteins for carrying out essential nervous-system functions. One of the important proteins is the enzyme adenylate cyclase, which helps to regulate the intracellular substance cyclic adenosine monophosphate (cyclic AMP). Cyclic nucleotides such as cyclic AMP take part in cell functions whose mechanisms are not yet understood in detail. The membrane enzyme adenylate cyclase appears to have two chief subunits, one catalytic and the other regulatory. The catalytic subunit promotes the formation of cyclic AMP. Various regulatory subunits, which are thought to be physically distinct from the catalytic one, can bind specific molecules (including transmitters that open and close channels) in order to control intracellular levels of cyclic AMP. The various types of regulatory subunit are named according to the molecule that normally binds to them; one, for example, is called serotonin-activated ade-

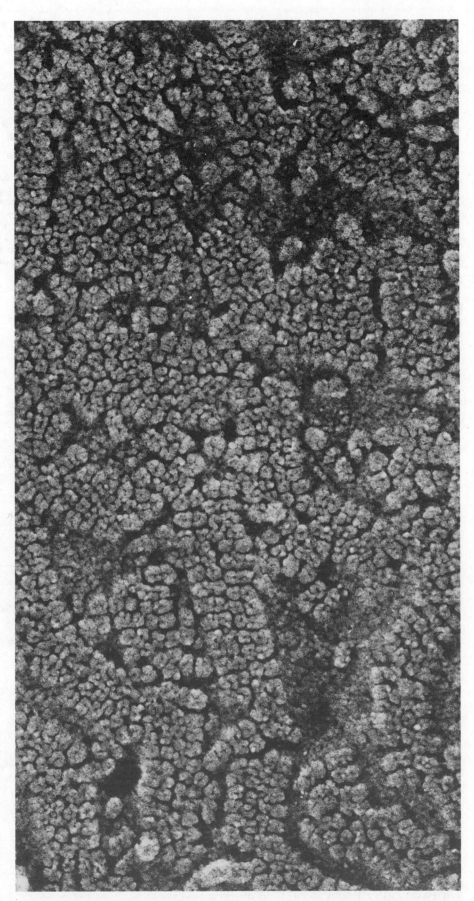

ACETYLCHOLINE-ACTIVATED CHANNELS are densely packed in the postsynaptic membrane of a cell in the electric organ of a torpedo, a fish that can administer an electric shock. This electron micrograph shows the platinum-plated replica of a membrane that had been frozen and etched. The size of the platinum particles limits the resolution to features larger than about two nanometers. According to recent evidence the channel protein molecule, which measures 8.5 nanometers across, consists of five subunits surrounding a channel whose narrowest dimension is .8 nanometer. The micrograph was made by Heuser and S. R. Salpeter.

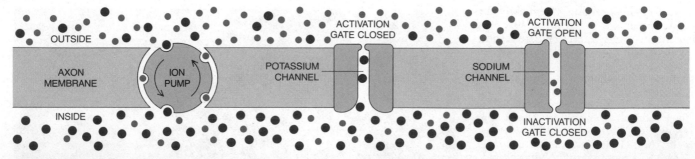

AXON MEMBRANE separates fluids that differ greatly in their content of sodium ions (*colored dots*) and potassium ions (*black dots*). The exterior fluid is about 10 times richer in sodium ions than in potassium ions; in the interior fluid the ratio is the reverse. The membrane is penetrated by proteins that act as selective channels for preferentially passing either sodium or potassium ions. In the resting state, when no nerve impulse is being transmitted, the two types of channel are closed and an ion pump maintains the ionic disequilibrium by pumping out sodium ions in exchange for potassium ions. The interior of the axon is normally about 70 millivolts negative with respect to the exterior. If this voltage difference is reduced by the arrival of a nerve impulse, the sodium channel opens, allowing sodium ions to flow into the axon. An instant later the sodium channel closes and the potassium channel opens, allowing an outflow of potassium ions. The sequential opening and closing of the two kinds of channel effects the propagation of the nerve impulse, which is illustrated below.

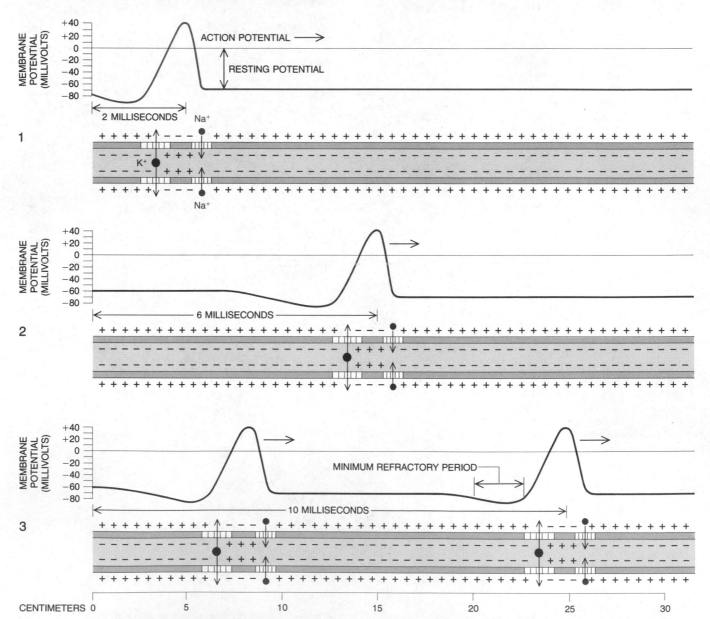

PROPAGATION OF NERVE IMPULSE along the axon coincides with a localized inflow of sodium ions (Na^+) followed by an outflow of potassium ions (K^+) through channels that are "gated," or controlled, by voltage changes across the axon membrane. The electrical event that sends a nerve impulse traveling down the axon normally originates in the cell body. The impulse begins with a slight depolarization, or reduction in the negative potential, across the membrane of the axon where it leaves the cell body. The slight voltage shift opens some of the sodium channels, shifting the voltage still further. The inflow of sodium ions accelerates until the inner surface of the membrane is locally positive. The voltage reversal closes the sodium channel and opens the potassium channel. The outflow of potassium ions quickly restores the negative potential. The voltage reversal, known as the action potential, propagates itself down the axon (*1, 2*). After a brief refractory period a second impulse can follow (*3*). The impulse-propagation speed is that measured in the giant axon of the squid.

nylate cyclase. Adenylate cyclase and related membrane enzymes are known to serve a number of regulatory functions in neurons, and the precise mechanisms of these actions are now under active investigation.

In the course of the embryonic development of the nervous system a cell must be able to recognize other cells so that the growth of each cell will proceed in the right direction and give rise to the right connections. The process of cell-cell recognition and the maintenance of the structure arrived at by such recognition depend on special classes of membrane proteins that are associated with unusual carbohydrates. The study of the protein-carbohydrate complexes associated with cell recognition is still at an early stage.

The intrinsic membrane proteins I have been describing are neither distributed uniformly over the cell surface nor all present in equal amounts in each neuron. The density and the type of protein are governed by the needs of the cell and differ among types of neuron and from one region of a neuron to another. Thus the density of channels of a particular type ranges from zero up to about 10,000 per square micrometer. Axons generally have no chemically gated channels, whereas in postsynaptic membranes the density of such channels is limited only by the packing of the channel molecules. Similarly, dendritic membranes typically have few voltage-gated channels, whereas in axon membranes the density can reach 1,000 channels per square micrometer in certain locations.

The intrinsic membrane proteins are synthesized primarily in the body of the neuron and are stored in the membrane in small vesicles. Neurons have a special transport system for moving such vesicles from their site of synthesis to their site of function. The transport system seems to move the vesicles along in small jumps with the aid of contractile proteins. On reaching their destination the proteins are inserted into the surface membrane, where they function until they are removed and degraded within the cell. Precisely how the cell decides where to put which membrane protein is not known. Equally unknown is the mechanism that regulates the synthesis, insertion and destruction of the membrane proteins. The metabolism of membrane proteins constitutes one of cell biology's central problems.

How do the properties of the various membrane proteins I have been discussing relate to neuron function? To approach this question let us now return to the nerve impulse and examine more closely the molecular properties that underlie its triggering and propagation. As we have seen, the interior of the neuron is about 70 millivolts negative with respect to the exterior. This "resting po-

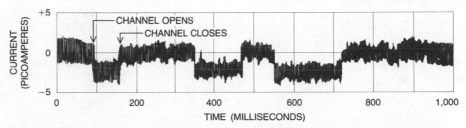

RESPONSE OF A SINGLE MEMBRANE CHANNEL to the transmitter compound acetylcholine is revealed by a recently developed technique that has been applied by Erwin Neher and Joseph H. Steinbach of the Yale University School of Medicine. Acetylcholine-activated channels, which are present in postsynaptic membranes, allow the passage of roughly equal numbers of sodium and potassium ions. The record shows the flow of current through a single channel in the postsynaptic membrane of a frog muscle activated by the compound suberyldicholine, which mimics action of acetylcholine but keeps channels open longer. Experiment shows that channels open on an all-or-none basis and stay open for random lengths of time.

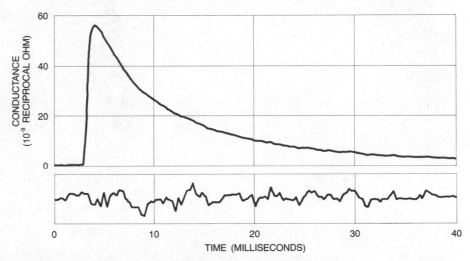

SODIUM CHANNELS IN AN AXON also operate in simple open-or-shut manner as well as independently of one another, according to investigations conducted by Frederick J. Sigworth of the Yale University School of Medicine. During the propagation of a nerve impulse about 10,000 channels normally open in a myelin-free region of the axon membrane, namely a node of Ranvier. The upper trace depicts the sodium permeability at such a node as a function of time. The lower trace, recorded at a 12-fold amplification of the upper one, shows fluctuations in permeability around the average due to the random opening and closing of channels.

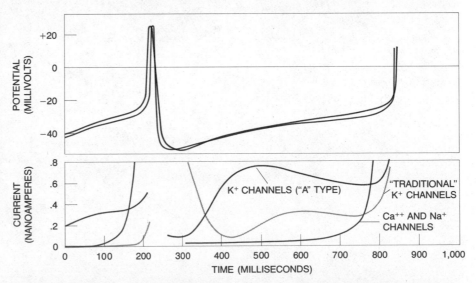

NERVE IMPULSES IN BODIES OF NEURONS require the coordinated opening and closing of five types of channel permeable to various kinds of ion (sodium, potassium or calcium). The contribution of the different channels to the nerve impulse can be represented by simultaneous nonlinear differential equations. The upper pair of curves represent an actual recording of voltage changes as a function of time in the body of a neuron (*black*) and changes computed from equations (*color*). The lower curves depict the current carried by the principal types of channel as a function of time. A complicated interaction of channel types is required to achieve a train of nerve impulses. The study on which curves are based was carried out by John A. Connor at the University of Illinois and by the author at the Yale University School of Medicine.

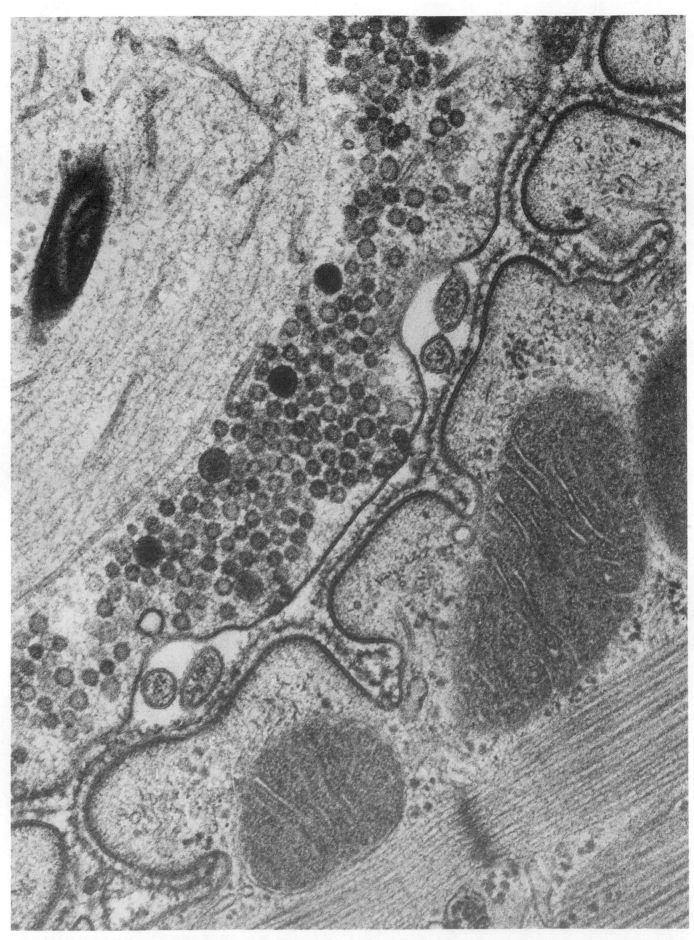

FROG NEUROMUSCULAR JUNCTION appears in this electron micrograph made by Heuser. The synaptic cleft separates the axon at the upper left from the muscle cell at the lower right. Synaptic vesicles cluster along the presynaptic membrane, with two synaptic contacts visible near the center. Postsynaptic membrane of the muscle cell exhibits a feature that is not seen at other synapses: the membrane forms postjunctional folds opposite each contact. Freeze-fracture replicas of presynaptic membrane are shown on opposite page.

tential" is a consequence of the ionic disequilibrium brought about by the sodium pump and by the presence in the cell membrane of a class of permanently open channels selectively permeable to potassium ions. The pump ejects sodium ions in exchange for potassium ions, making the inside of the cell about 10 times richer in potassium ions than the outside. The potassium channels in the membrane allow the potassium ions immediately adjacent to the membrane to flow outward quite freely. The permeability of the membrane to sodium ions is low in the resting condition, so that there is almost no counterflow of sodium ions from the exterior to the interior even though the external medium is tenfold richer in sodium ions than the internal medium. The potassium flow therefore gives rise to a net deficit of positive charges on the inner surface of the cell membrane and an excess of positive charges on the outer surface. The result is the voltage difference of 70 millivolts, with the interior being negative.

The propagation of the nerve impulse depends on the presence in the neuron membrane of voltage-gated sodium channels whose opening and closing is responsible for the action potential. What are the characteristics of these important channel molecules? Although the sodium channel has not yet been well characterized chemically, it is a protein with a molecular weight probably in the range of 250,000 to 300,000 daltons. The pore of the channel measures about .4 by .6 nanometer, a space through which sodium ions can pass in association with a water molecule. The channel has many charged groups critically placed on its surface. These charges give the channel a large electric dipole moment that varies in direction and magnitude when the molecular conformation of the channel changes as the channel goes from a closed state to an open one.

Because the surface membrane of the cell is so thin the difference of 70 millivolts across the resting membrane gives rise to a large electric field, on the order of 100 kilovolts per centimeter. In the same way that magnetic dipoles tend to align themselves with the lines of force in a magnetic field, the electric dipoles in the sodium-channel protein tend to align themselves with the membrane electric field. Changes in the strength of the membrane field can therefore drive the channel from the closed conformation to the open one. As the inner surface of the membrane is made more positive by the entering vanguard of sodium ions the sodium channels tend to spend an increasing fraction of their time in the open conformation. The process in which the channels are opened by a change in the membrane voltage is known as sodium-channel activation.

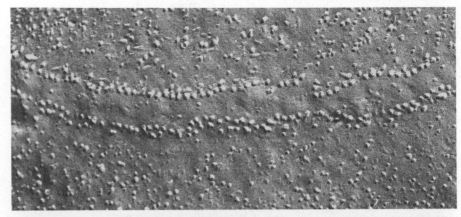

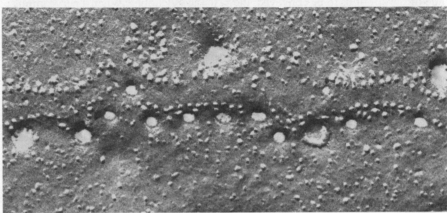

FREEZE-FRACTURE REPLICAS of the presynaptic membrane of the frog neuromuscular junction were made by Heuser. The upper micrograph shows the membrane three milliseconds after the muscle had been stimulated. Running across the axon membrane is a double row of particles: membrane proteins that may be calcium channels or structural proteins to which vesicles attach. The lower micrograph shows the membrane five milliseconds after stimulation. The stimulation has caused synaptic vesicles to fuse with presynaptic membrane and form pits.

The process is terminated by a phenomenon called sodium inactivation. Voltage differences across the membrane that cause sodium channels to open also drive them into a special closed conformation different from the conformation characteristic of the channel's resting state. The second closed conformation, called the inactivated state, develops more slowly than the activation process, so that channels remain open briefly before they are closed by inactivation. The channels remain in the inactivated state for some milliseconds and then return to the normal resting state.

The complete cycle of activation and inactivation normally involves the opening and closing of thousands of sodium channels. How can one tell whether the increase in overall membrane permeability reflects the opening and closing of a number of channels in an all-or-none manner or whether it reflects the operation of channels that have individually graded permeabilities? The question has been partly answered by a new technique that relates fluctuations in membrane permeability to the inherently probabilistic nature of conformational changes in the channel proteins. One can trigger repeated episodes of channel opening and calculate the average permeability at a particular time and also the exact permeability on a given trial. The exact permeability fluctuates 10 percent or so around a mean value. Analysis of the fluctuations shows that the sodium channels open in an all-or-none manner and that each channel opening increases the conductance of the membrane by 8×10^{-12} reciprocal ohms. One of the principal challenges in understanding the neuron is the development of a complete theory that will describe the behavior of the sodium channels and relate it to the molecular structure of the channel protein.

As I noted briefly above, axons also have voltage-gated potassium channels that help to terminate the nerve impulse by letting potassium ions flow out of the axon, thereby counteracting the inward flow of sodium ions. In the cell body of the neuron the situation is still more complex, because there the membrane is traversed by five types of channel. The different channels open at different rates, stay open for various intervals and are preferentially permeable to different species of ions (sodium, potassium or calcium).

The presence of the five types of channel in the cell body of the neuron, compared with only two in the axon, gives rise to a more complex mode of nerve-impulse generation. If an axon is presented with a maintained stimulus, it generates only a single impulse at the onset of the stimulus. Cell bodies, however, generate a train of impulses with a frequency that reflects the intensity of the stimulus.

Neurons are able to generate nerve impulses over a wide range of frequencies, from one or fewer per second to several hundred per second. All nerve impulses have the same amplitude, so that the information they carry is represented by the number of impulses generated per unit of time, a system known as frequency coding. The larger the magnitude of the stimulus to be conveyed, the faster the rate of firing.

When a nerve impulse has traveled the length of the axon and has arrived at a terminal button, one of a variety of transmitters is released from the presynaptic membrane. The transmitter diffuses to the postsynaptic membrane, where it induces the opening of chemically gated channels. Ions flowing through the open channels bring about the voltage changes known as postsynaptic potentials.

Most of what is known about synaptic mechanisms comes from experiments on a particular synapse: the neuromuscular junction that controls the contraction of muscles in the frog. The axon of the frog neuron runs for several hundred micrometers along the surface of the muscle cell, making several hundred synaptic contacts spaced about a micrometer apart. At each presynaptic region the characteristic synaptic vesicles can be recognized readily.

Each of the synaptic vesicles contains some 10,000 molecules of the transmitter acetylcholine. When a nerve impulse reaches the synapse, a train of events is set in motion that culminates in the fusion of a vesicle with the presynaptic membrane and the resulting release of acetylcholine into the cleft between the presynaptic and the postsynaptic membranes, a process termed exocytosis. The fused vesicle is subsequently reclaimed from the presynaptic membrane and is quickly refilled with acetylcholine for future release.

Many details of the events leading to exocytosis have recently been elucidated. The fusion of vesicles to the presynaptic membrane is evidently triggered by a rapid but transient increase in the concentration of calcium in the terminal button of the axon. The arrival of a nerve impulse at the terminal opens calcium channels that are voltage-gated and allows calcium to flow into the terminal. The subsequent rise in calcium concentration is brief, however, because the terminal contains a special apparatus that rapidly sequesters free calcium and returns its concentration to the normal very low level. The brief spike in the free-calcium level leads to the fusion of transmitter-filled vesicles with the presynaptic membrane, but the precise mechanism of this important process is not yet known.

Interesting details of the structure of the terminal membrane have been revealed by the freeze-fracture technique, a method that splits the layers of the bilayer membrane and exposes the intrinsic membrane proteins for examination by electron microscopy. In the frog neuromuscular junction a double row of large membrane proteins runs the width of each synapse. Synaptic vesicles become attached on or near the proteins. Only these vesicles then fuse to the membrane and release their transmitter; other vesicles seem to be held in reserve some distance away. The fusion of vesicles is a random process and occurs independently for each vesicle.

In less than 100 microseconds acetylcholine released from fused vesicles diffuses across the synaptic cleft and binds to the acetylcholine receptor: an intrinsic membrane protein embedded in the postsynaptic membrane. The receptor is also a channel protein that is chemically gated by the presence of acetylcholine. When two acetylcholine molecules attach themselves to the channel, they lower the energy state of the open conformation of the protein and thereby increase the probability that the channel will open. The open state of the channel is a random event with an average lifetime of about a millisecond. Each packet of 10,000 acetylcholine molecules effects the opening of some 2,000 channels.

During the brief period that a channel is open about 20,000 sodium ions and a roughly equal number of potassium ions pass through it. As a result of this ionic flow the voltage difference between the two sides of the membrane tends to approach zero. How close it approaches to zero depends on how many channels open and how long they stay open. The acetylcholine released by a typical nerve impulse produces a postsynaptic potential, or voltage change, that lasts for only about five milliseconds. Because postsynaptic potentials are produced by chemically gated chan-

TRANSMITTER IS DISCHARGED into the synaptic cleft at the synaptic junctions between neurons by vesicles that open up after they fuse with the axon's presynaptic membrane, a process called exocytosis. This electron micrograph made by Heuser has caught the vesicles in the terminal of an axon in the act of discharging acetylcholine into the neuromuscular junction of a frog. The structures that appear in the micrograph are enlarged some 115,000 diameters.

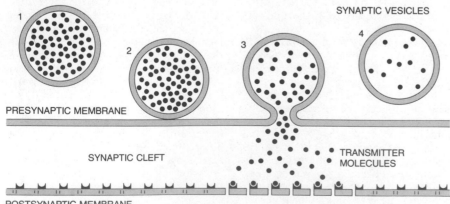

SYNAPTIC VESICLES are clustered near the presynaptic membrane. The diagram shows the probable steps in exocytosis. Filled vesicles move up to synaptic cleft, fuse with the membrane, discharge their contents and are reclaimed, re-formed and refilled with transmitter.

nels rather than by voltage-gated ones they have properties quite different from those of the nerve impulse. They are usually smaller in amplitude, longer in duration and graded in size depending on the quantity of transmitter released and hence on the number of channels that open.

Different types of chemically gated channels exhibit different selectivities. Some resemble the acetylcholine channel, which passes sodium and potassium ions with little selectivity. Others are highly selective. The voltage change that results at a particular synapse depends on the selectivity of the channels that are opened. If positive ions move into the cell, the voltage change is in the positive direction. Such positive-going voltage channels tend to open voltage-gated channels and to generate nerve impulses, and so they are known as excitatory postsynaptic potentials. If positive ions (usually potassium) move out of the cell, the voltage change is in the negative direction, which tends to close voltage-gated channels. Such postsynaptic potentials oppose the production of nerve impulses, and so they are termed inhibitory. Excitatory and inhibitory postsynaptic potentials are both common in the brain.

Brain synapses differ from neuromuscular-junction synapses in several ways. Whereas at the neuromuscular junction the action of acetylcholine is always excitatory, in the brain the action of the same substance is excitatory at some synapses and inhibitory at others. And whereas acetylcholine is the usual transmitter at neuromuscular junctions, the brain synapses have channels gated by a large variety of transmitters. A particular synaptic ending, however, releases only one type of transmitter, and channels gated by that transmitter are present in the corresponding postsynaptic membrane. In contrast with neuromuscular channels activated by acetylcholine, which stay open for about a millisecond, some types of brain synapses have channels that stay open for less than a millisecond and others have channels that remain open for hundreds of milliseconds. A final major difference is that whereas the axon makes hundreds of synaptic contacts with the muscle cell at the frog's neuromuscular junction, axons in the brain usually make only one or two synaptic contacts on a given neuron. As might be expected, such different functional properties are correlated with significant differences in structure.

As we have seen, the intensity of a stimulus is coded in the frequency of nerve impulses. Decoding at the synapse is accomplished by two processes: temporal summation and spatial summation. In temporal summation each postsynaptic potential adds to the cumulative total of its predecessors to yield a voltage change whose average amplitude reflects the frequency of incoming nerve impulses. In other words, a neuron that is firing rapidly releases more transmitter molecules at its terminal junctions than a neuron that is firing less rapidly. The more transmitter molecules that are released in a given time, the more channels that are opened in the postsynaptic membrane and therefore the larger the postsynaptic potential is. Spatial summation is an equivalent process except that it reflects the integration of nerve impulses arriving from all the neurons that may be in synaptic contact with a given neuron. The grand voltage change derived by temporal and spatial summation is encoded as nerve-impulse frequency for transmission to other cells "downstream" in the nerve network.

I have described what is usually regarded as the normal flow of information in neural circuits, in which postsynaptic voltage changes are encoded as nerve-impulse frequency and transmitted over the axon to other neurons. In recent years, however, a number of instances have been discovered where a postsynaptic potential is not converted into a nerve impulse. For example, the voltage change due to a postsynaptic potential can directly cause the release of transmitter from a neighboring site that lacks a nerve impulse. Such direct influences are thought to come into play in synapses between dendrites and also in certain reciprocal circuits where one dendrite makes a synaptic contact on a second dendrite, which in turn makes a synaptic contact back on the first dendrite. Such direct feedback seems to be quite common in the brain, but its implications for information processing remain to be worked out.

Much current investigation of the neuron focuses on the membrane proteins that endow the cell's bilayer membrane, which is otherwise featureless, with the special properties brain function depends on. With regard to channel proteins there are many unanswered questions about the mechanisms of gating, selectivity and regulation. Within the next five or 10 years it should be possible to relate the physical processes of gating and selectivity to the molecular structure of the channels. The basis of channel regulation is less well understood but is now coming under intensive investigation. It seems that hormones and other substances play a role in channel regulation that is now becoming appreciated. The central problems at synaptic junctions involve exocytosis and other activities related to the metabolism and release of transmitters. One can expect increasing attention to be focused on the role of the surface membrane in the growth and development of neurons and their synaptic connections, the remarkable process that establishes the integration of the nervous system.

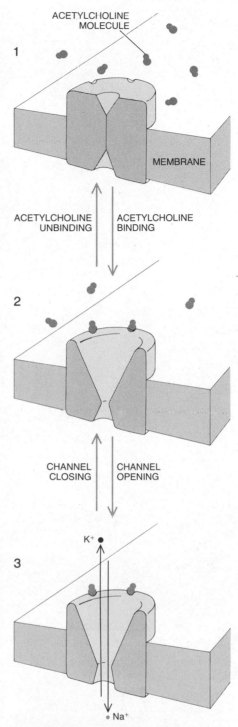

ACETYLCHOLINE CHANNEL in a postsynaptic membrane is opened by acetylcholine molecules' discharging into the synaptic cleft. The drawing shows the acetylcholine receptor at the frog neuromuscular junction. Two acetylcholine molecules bind rapidly to the resting closed channel to form a receptor-acetylcholine complex (*1, 2*). The complex undergoes a change in its conformation that opens the channel to the passage of sodium and potassium ions (*3*). The time required for conformational change in the complex limits the speed of the reaction. The channel remains open for about a millisecond on the average and then reverts to the receptor-acetylcholine complex. While it is open the channel passes about 20,000 sodium ions and an equal number of potassium ions. The acetylcholine rapidly dissociates and is destroyed by the enzyme acetylcholine esterase. Acetylcholine receptor appears in mircograph on page 19.

III

Small Systems
of Neurons

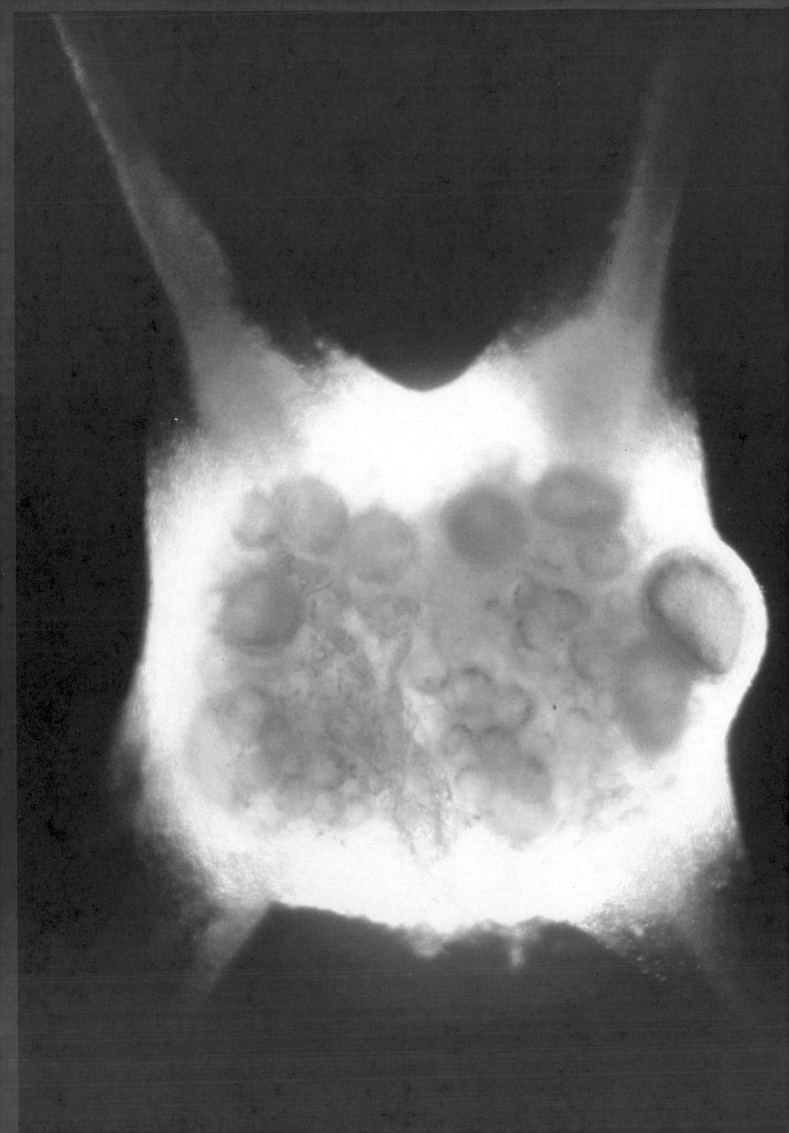

Small Systems of Neurons

BY ERIC R. KANDEL

*Such systems are the elementary units of mental function.
Studies of simple animals such as the large snail Aplysia
show that small systems of neurons are capable of
forms of learning and memory*

Many neurobiologists believe that the unique character of individual human beings, their disposition to feel, think, learn and remember, will ultimately be shown to reside in the precise patterns of synaptic interconnections between the neurons of the brain. Since it is difficult to examine patterns of interconnections in the human brain, a major concern of neurobiology has been to develop animal models that are useful for studying how interacting systems of neurons give rise to behavior. Networks of neurons that mediate complete behavioral acts allow one to explore a hierarchy of interrelated questions: To what degree do the properties of different neurons vary? What determines the patterns of interconnections between neurons? How do different patterns of interconnections generate different forms of behavior? Can the interconnected neurons that control a certain kind of behavior be modified by learning? If they can, what are the mechanisms whereby memory is stored?

Among the many functions that emerge from the interactions of neurons, the most interesting are the functions concerned with learning (the ability to modify behavior in response to experience) and with memory (the ability to store that modification over a period of time). Learning and memory are perhaps the most distinctive features of the mental processes of advanced animals, and these features reach their highest form in man. In fact, human beings are what they are in good measure because of what they have learned. It is therefore of theoretical importance, for the understanding of learning and for the study of behavioral evolution, to determine at what phylogenetic level of neuronal and behavioral organization one can begin to recognize aspects of the learning and

memory processes that characterize human behavior. This determination is also of practical importance. The difficulty in studying the cellular mechanisms of memory in the brain of man or other mammals arises because such brains are immensely complex. For the human brain ethical issues also preclude this kind of study. It would therefore be congenial scientifically to be able to examine these processes effectively in simple systems.

It could be argued that the study of memory and learning as it relates to man cannot be pursued effectively in simple neuronal systems. The organization of the human brain seems so complex that trying to study human learning in a reduced form in simple neuronal systems is bound to fail. Man has intellectual abilities, a highly developed language and an ability for abstract thinking, which are not found in simpler animals and may require qualitatively different types of neuronal organization. Although such arguments have value, the critical question is not whether there is something special about the human brain. There clearly is. The question is rather what the human brain and human behavior have in common with the brain and the behavior of simpler animals. Where there are points of similarity they may involve common principles of brain organization that could profitably be studied in simple neural systems.

The answer to the question of similarity is clear. Ethologists such as Konrad Lorenz, Nikolaas Tinbergen and Karl von Frisch have shown that human beings share many common behavioral patterns with simpler animals, including elementary perception and motor coordination. The capacity to learn, in particular, is widespread; it has evolved in many invertebrate animals and in all

vertebrates. The similarity of some of the learning processes suggests that the neuronal mechanisms for a given learning process may have features in common across phylogeny. For example, there appear to be no fundamental differences in structure, chemistry or function between the neurons and synapses in man and those of a squid, a snail or a leech. Consequently a complete and rigorous analysis of learning in such an invertebrate is likely to reveal mechanisms of general significance.

Simple invertebrates are attractive for such investigation because their nervous systems consist of between 10,000 and 100,000 cells, compared with the many billions in more complex animals. The cells are collected into the discrete groups called ganglia, and each ganglion usually consists of between 500 and 1,500 neurons. This numerical simplification has made it possible to relate the function of individual cells directly to behavior. The result is a number of important findings that lead to a new way of looking at the relation between the brain and behavior.

The first major question that students of simple systems of neurons might examine is whether the various neurons of a region of the nervous system differ from one another. This question, which is central to an understanding of how behavior is mediated by the nervous system, was in dispute until recently. Some neurobiologists argued that the neurons of a brain are sufficiently similar in their properties to be regarded as identical units having interconnections of roughly equal value.

These arguments have now been strongly challenged, particularly by studies of invertebrates showing that many neurons can be individually identified and are invariant in every member of the species. The concept that neurons are unique was proposed as early as 1912 by the German biologist Richard Goldschmidt on the basis of his study of the nervous system of a primitive worm, the intestinal parasite *Ascaris*. The brain

GROUP OF NEURONS appears in the photomicrograph on the opposite page, which shows the dorsal surface of the abdominal ganglion of the snail *Aplysia*. The magnification is 100 diameters. A particularly large, dark brown neuron can be seen at the right side of the micrograph. It is the cell identified as R2 in the map of the abdominal ganglion of *Aplysia* on page 31.

of this worm consists of several ganglia. When Goldschmidt examined the ganglia, he found they contained exactly 162 cells. The number never varied from animal to animal, and each cell always occupied a characteristic position. In spite of this clear-cut result Goldschmidt's work went largely unheeded.

More than 50 years later two groups at the Harvard Medical School returned to the problem independently. Masanori Otsuka, Edward A. Kravitz and David D. Potter, working with the lobster, and Wesley T. Frazier, Irving Kupfermann, Rafiq M. Waziri, Richard E. Coggeshall and I, working with the large marine snail *Aplysia,* found a similar but less complete invariance in the more complex nervous systems of these higher invertebrates. A comparable invariance was soon found in a variety of invertebrates, including the leech, the crayfish, the locust, the cricket and a number of snails. Here I shall limit myself to considering studies of *Aplysia,* particularly studies of a single ganglion: the abdominal ganglion. Similar findings have also emerged from the studies of other invertebrates.

In the abdominal ganglion of *Aplysia* neurons vary in size, position, shape, pigmentation, firing patterns and the chemical substances by which they transmit information to other cells. On the basis of such differences it is possible to recognize and name specific cells (R1, L1, R15 and so on). The firing patterns illustrate some of the differences. Certain cells are normally "silent" and others are spontaneously active. Among the active ones some fire regular action potentials, or nerve impulses, and others fire in recurrent brief bursts or trains. The different firing patterns have now

been shown to result from differences in the types of ionic currents generated by the membrane of the cell body of the neurons. The cell-body membrane is quite different from the membrane of the axon, the long fiber of the neuron. When the membrane of the axon is active, it typically produces only an inflow of sodium ions and a delayed outflow of potassium ions, whereas the membrane of the cell body can produce six or seven distinct ionic currents that can flow in various combinations.

Whether or not most cells in the mammalian nervous system are also unique individuals is not yet known. The studies in the sensory systems of mammals reviewed by David Hubel and Torsten Wiesel in this book, however, have revealed fascinating and important differences between neighboring neurons [see "Brain Mechanisms of Vision," by David H. Hubel and Torsten N. Wiesel, page 84]. Studies of the development of the vertebrate brain reviewed by Maxwell Cowan lead to a similar conclusion [see "The Development of the Brain," by W. Maxwell Cowan, page 56].

The finding that neurons are invariant leads to further questions. Are the synaptic connections between cells also invariant? Does a given identified cell always connect to exactly the same follower cell and not to others? A number of investigators have examined these questions in invertebrate animals and have found that cells indeed always make the same kinds of connections to other cells. The invariance applies not only to the connections but also to the "sign," or functional expression, of the connections, that is, whether they are excitatory or inhibitory.

Therefore Frazier, James E. Blan-

kenship, Howard Wachtel and I next worked with identified cells to examine the rules that determine the functional expression of connections between cells. A single neuron has many branches and makes many connections. We asked: Are all the connections of a neuron specialized for inhibition or excitation, or can the firing of a neuron produce different actions at different branches? What determines whether a connection is excitatory or inhibitory? Is the sign of the synaptic action determined by the chemical structure of the transmitter substance released by the presynaptic neuron, or is the nature of the postsynaptic receptor the determining factor? Does the neuron release the same transmitter from all its terminals?

One way to explore these questions is to look at the different connections made by a cell. The first cell we examined gave a clear answer: it mediated different actions through its various connections. The cell excited some follower cells, inhibited others and (perhaps most unexpectedly) made a dual connection, which was both excitatory and inhibitory, to a third kind of cell. Moreover, it always excited precisely the same cells, always inhibited another specific group of cells and always made a dual connection with a third group. Its synaptic action could be accounted for by one transmitter substance: acetylcholine. The reaction of this substance with different types of receptors on the various follower cells determined whether the synaptic action would be excitatory or inhibitory.

The receptors determined the sign of the synaptic action by controlling different ionic channels in the membrane: primarily sodium for excitation and chloride for inhibition. The cells that received the dual connection had two types of receptor for the same transmitter, one receptor that controlled a sodium channel and another that controlled a chloride channel. The functional expression of chemical synaptic transmission is therefore determined by the types of receptor the follower cell has at a given postsynaptic site. (Similar results have been obtained by JacSue Kehoe of the École Normale in Paris, who has gone on to analyze in detail the properties of the various species of receptors to acetylcholine.) Thus, as was first suggested by Ladislav Tauc and Hersch Gerschenfeld of the Institute Marey in Paris, the chemical transmitter is only permissive; the instructive component of synaptic transmission is the nature of the receptor and the ionic channels it interacts with. This principle has proved to be fairly general. It applies to the neurons of vertebrates and invertebrates and to neurons utilizing various transmitters: acetylcholine, gamma-aminobutyric acid (GABA), serotonin, dopamine and histamine. (The principle

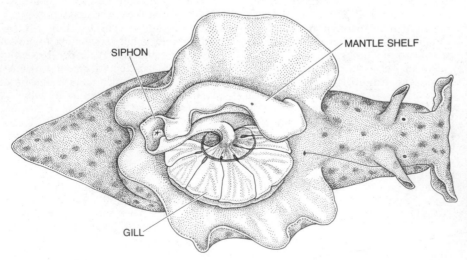

SIPHON

MANTLE SHELF

GILL

GILL-WITHDRAWAL REFLEX of *Aplysia* results when the siphon or the mantle shelf is somehow stimulated. The animal then retracts the gill to the position that is indicated in color.

also applies to the actions of certain peptide hormones on neurons, a subject to which I shall return.)

The discovery in invertebrate ganglia of identifiable cells that make precise connections with one another has led to the working out of the "wiring diagram" of various behavioral circuits and has therefore made possible an exact study of the causal relation of specific neurons to behavior. The term behavior refers to the observable actions of an organism. These range from complex acts such as talking or walking to simple acts such as the movement of a body part or a change in heart rate. Types of behavior that have been at least partly worked out in leeches, crayfishes and snails include feeding, various locomotor patterns and a variety of escape and defensive reactions.

The first finding to emerge from these studies is that individual cells exert a control over behavior that is specific and sometimes surprisingly powerful. The point can be illustrated by comparing the neural control of the heart in *Aplysia* with that in human beings.

The human heart beats spontaneously. Its intrinsic rhythm is neuronally modulated by the inhibitory action of cholinergic neurons (acetylcholine is the transmitter substance) with their axons in the vagus nerve and the excitatory action of noradrenergic neurons with their axons in the accelerator nerve. The modulation involves several thousand neurons. In *Aplysia* the heart also beats spontaneously; it is neuronally modulated by the inhibitory action of cholinergic neurons and the excitatory action of serotonergic neurons, but the modulation is accomplished by only four cells! Two cells excite the heart (only the "major excitor" cell is really important) and two inhibit it. Three other cells give rise to a constriction of the blood vessels and thereby control the animal's blood pressure.

Since individual cells connect invariably to the same follower cells and can mediate actions that have a different sign, certain cells at a critical point in the nervous system are in a position to control an entire behavioral sequence. As early as 1938 C. A. G. Wiersma, working with the crayfish at the California Institute of Technology, had appreciated the importance of single cells in behavior and had called them "command cells." Such cells have now been found in a variety of animals. A few of them have proved to be dual-action neurons. Hence John Koester, Earl M. Mayeri and I, working with *Aplysia* at the New York University School of Medicine, found that the dual-action neuron described above is a command cell for the neural circuit controlling the circulation. This one cell increases the rate and output of the heart by exciting the

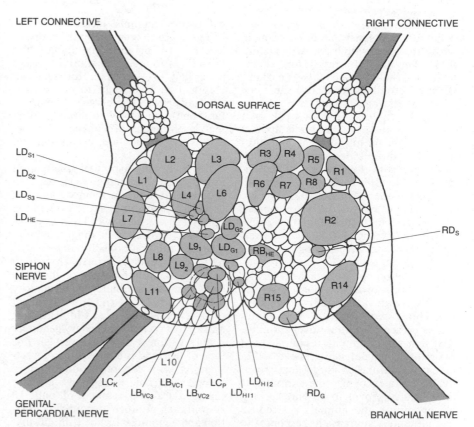

MAP OF ABDOMINAL GANGLION in *Aplysia californica* shows the location of the identified neurons, which have been labeled L or R (for left or right hemiganglion) and assigned a number. Neurons that are members of a cluster, consisting of cells with similar properties, are further identified by a cluster letter (LD) and a subscript representing the behavioral function of the neuron, such as HE for heart excitor and G1 and G2 for two gill motor neurons.

major cell that excites the heart while inhibiting the cells that inhibit the heart and the cells that constrict the major blood vessels. As a result of the increased activity of this one cell the heart beats faster and pumps more blood.

This is only a simple example of the behavioral functions of a command cell. In the crayfish and even in a more complex animal, the goldfish, a single impulse in a single command neuron causes the animal to flee from threatened danger. Recently Vernon Mountcastle of the Johns Hopkins University School of Medicine has suggested in this context that small groups of cells may serve similar command functions in the primate brain to control purposeful voluntary movements.

Hence a functional purpose of dual-action cells is to bring about a constellation of different physiological effects. A similar constellation can be achieved by the action of neuroendocrine cells, neurons that release hormones (the chemical substances that are usually carried in the bloodstream to act at distant sites). The abdominal ganglion of *Aplysia* contains two clusters of neuroendocrine cells, which are called bag cells because each cluster is bag-shaped. Kupfermann, working in our division at the Columbia University College of Physicians and Surgeons, has shown, as have

Stephen Arch of Reed College and Felix Strumwasser and his colleagues at Cal Tech, that the bag cells release a polypeptide hormone that controls egg laying. Mayeri has found that this hormone has long-lasting actions on various cells in the abdominal ganglion, exciting some and inhibiting others.

One of the cells excited by this hormone is the dual-action command cell that controls the heart rate. As a result the heart speeds up to provide the extra flow of blood to the tissues that the animal requires during egg laying. Thus superimposed on a precise pattern of connections that provide short-range interaction of neurons is an equally precise pattern of long-range interactions achieved by the hormones released by neuroendocrine cells. The precise effect of each hormone seems to be determined, as synaptic effects are, by the nature of the receptors on the target cells.

The finding that behavior is mediated by invariant cells interconnecting in precise and invariant ways might suggest that simple animals differ from more complex ones in having stereotyped and fixed repertories of activity. It is not so. Studies in different invertebrates have shown that behavior in simple animals is quite capable of being modified by learning.

We have explored this subject most

fully in one of *Aplysia*'s simplest kinds of behavior: a defensive reflex action in which the gill is withdrawn after a stimulus. The gill is in a respiratory chamber called the mantle cavity. The chamber is covered by a protective sheet, the mantle shelf, that terminates in a fleshy spout, the siphon. When a weak or a moderately intense stimulus is applied to the siphon, the gill contracts and withdraws into the mantle cavity. This reflex is analogous to the withdrawal responses found in almost all higher animals, such as the one in which a human being jerks a hand away from a hot object. *Aplysia* and the other animals exhibit two forms of learning with such reflexes: habituation and sensitization.

Habituation is a decrease in the strength of a behavioral response that occurs when an initially novel stimulus is presented repeatedly. When an animal is presented with a novel stimulus, it at first responds with a combination of orienting and defensive reflexes. With repeated stimulation the animal readily learns to recognize the stimulus. If the stimulus proves to be unrewarding or innocuous, the animal will reduce and ultimately suppress its responses to it. Although habituation is remarkably simple, it is probably the most widespread of all forms of learning. Through

habituation animals, including human beings, learn to ignore stimuli that have lost novelty or meaning; habituation frees them to attend to stimuli that are rewarding or significant for survival. Habituation is thought to be the first learning process to emerge in human infants and is commonly utilized to study the development of intellectual processes such as attention, perception and memory.

An interesting aspect of habituation in vertebrates is that it gives rise to both short- and long-term memory and has therefore been employed to explore the relation between the two. Thomas J. Carew, Harold M. Pinsker and I found that a similar relation holds for *Aplysia*. After a single training session of from 10 to 15 tactile stimuli to the siphon the withdrawal reflex habituates. The memory for the stimulus is short-lived; partial recovery can be detected within an hour and almost complete recovery generally occurs within a day. Recovery in this type of learning is equivalent to forgetting. As with the repetition of more complex learning tasks, however, four repeated training sessions of only 10 stimuli each produce profound habituation and a memory for the stimulus that lasts for weeks.

The first question that Vincent Castellucci, Kupfermann, Pinsker and I asked

was: What are the loci and mechanisms of short-term habituation? The neural circuit controlling gill withdrawal is quite simple. A stimulus to the skin of the siphon activates the 24 sensory neurons there; they make direct connections to six motor cells in the gill, and the motor cells connect directly to the muscle. The sensory neurons also excite several interneurons, which are interposed neurons.

By examining these cells during habituation we found that short-term habituation involved a change in the strength of the connection made by the sensory neurons on their central target cells: the interneurons and the motor neurons. This localization was most fortunate, because now we could examine what happened during habituation simply by analyzing the changes in two cells, the presynaptic sensory neuron and the postsynaptic motor neuron, and in the single set of connections between them.

The strength of a connection can be studied by recording the synaptic action produced in the motor cells by an individual sensory neuron. It is possible to simulate the habituation training session of from 10 to 15 stimuli by stimulating a sensory neuron following the exact time sequence used for the intact animal. The stimulus can be adjusted so that it generates a single action potential. The first time the neuron is caused to fire an action potential it produces a highly effective synaptic action, which is manifested as a large excitatory postsynaptic potential in the motor cell. The subsequent action potentials initiated in the sensory neuron during a training session give rise to progressively smaller excitatory postsynaptic potentials. This depression in the effectiveness of the connection parallels and accounts for the behavioral habituation. As with the behavior, the synaptic depression resulting from a single training session persists for more than an hour. Following a second training session there is a more pronounced depression of the synaptic potential, and further training sessions can depress the synaptic potential completely.

What causes the changes in the strength of the synaptic connection? Do they involve a change in the presynaptic sensory neuron, reflecting a decrease in the release of the transmitter substance, or a change in the postsynaptic cell, reflecting a decrease in the sensitivity of the receptors to the chemical transmitter? The questions can be answered by analyzing changes in the amplitude of the synaptic potential in terms of its quantal components.

As was first shown by José del Castillo and Bernhard Katz at University College London, transmitter is released not as single molecules but as "quanta," or multimolecular packets. Each packet contains roughly the same amount

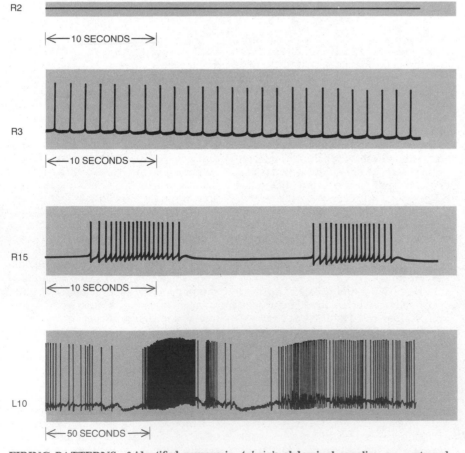

R2

|←—— 10 SECONDS ——→|

R3

|←—— 10 SECONDS ——→|

R15

|←—— 10 SECONDS ——→|

L10

|←—— 50 SECONDS ——→|

FIRING PATTERNS of identified neurons in *Aplysia*'s abdominal ganglion are portrayed. R2 is normally silent, R3 has a regular beating rhythm, R15 a regular bursting rhythm and L10 an irregular bursting rhythm. L10 is a command cell that controls other cells in the system.

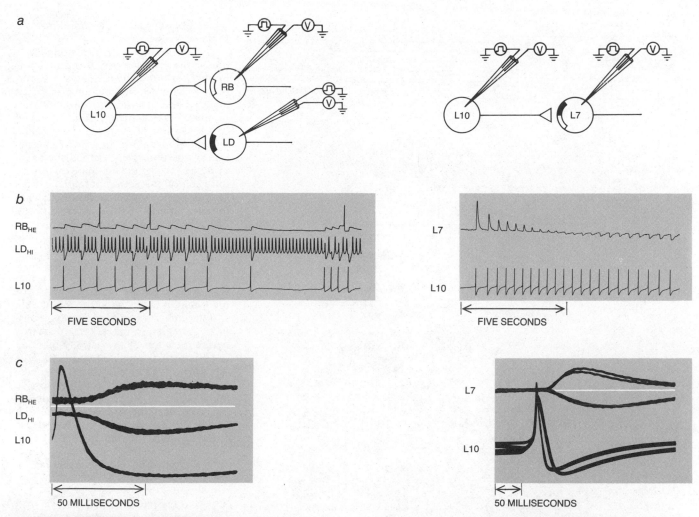

INVARIANCE OF CONNECTIONS between cell L10 and some of its follower cells was ascertained (a) by an arrangement in which double-barrel microelectrodes for recording and passing current were inserted in L10, which is a presynaptic neuron, and three of its follower cells. L10 produces excitation (white) in RB, inhibition (black) in LD and both excitation and inhibition in L7. The respective firing patterns are shown at b. Several superposed sweeps (at the left in c) illustrate the brief but constant latency between an impulse in the presynaptic neuron and the response of two follower cells. Superposed traces from L10 and L7 (at the right in c) show that effect is excitatory when L10 fires initially, as indicated by tall and narrow impulses, and inhibitory when it fires repeatedly, as shown by short and broad impulses.

of transmitter (several thousand molecules). The quanta are thought to be stored in subcellular organelles called synaptic vesicles that are seen in abundance at synaptic endings examined with the electron microscope. Since the number of transmitter molecules in each quantum does not ordinarily change, the number of quanta released by each action potential is a fairly reliable index of the total amount of transmitter released. Each quantum in turn produces a miniature excitatory postsynaptic potential of characteristic size in the postsynaptic cell. The size is an indication of how sensitive the postsynaptic receptors are to the several thousand molecules of transmitter released by each packet.

Castellucci and I, working with *Aplysia*, found that the decrease in the amplitude of the synaptic action potential with habituation was paralleled by a decrease in the number of chemical quanta released. In contrast, the size of the miniature postsynaptic potential did not change, indicating that there was no

change in the sensitivity of the postsynaptic receptor. The results show that the site of short-term habituation is the presynaptic terminals of the sensory neurons and that the mechanism of habituation is a progressive decrease in the amount of transmitter released by the sensory-neuron terminals onto their central target cells. Studies in the crayfish by Robert S. Zucker of the University of California at Berkeley and by Franklin B. Krasne of the University of California at Los Angeles and in the cat by Paul B. Farel and Richard F. Thompson of the University of California at Irvine indicate that this mechanism may be quite general.

What is responsible for the decrease in the number of quanta released by each action potential? The number is largely determined by the concentration of free calcium in the presynaptic terminal. Calcium is one of three kinds of ion involved in the generation of each action potential in the terminal. The depolarizing upstroke of the action potential is produced mainly by the inflow of so-

dium ions into the terminal, but it also involves a lesser and delayed flow of calcium ions. The repolarizing downstroke is largely produced by the outflow of potassium ions. The inflow of calcium is essential for the release of transmitter. Calcium is thought to enable the synaptic vesicles to bind to release sites in the presynaptic terminals. This binding is a critical step preliminary to the release of transmitter from the vesicles (the process termed exocytosis). It therefore seems possible that the amount of calcium coming into the terminals with each action potential is not fixed but is variable and that the amount might be modulated by habituation.

The best way to examine changes in the flow of calcium into terminals would be to record from the terminals directly. We have been unable to do so because the terminals are very small. Because the properties of the calcium channels of the cell body resemble those of the terminals, however, one of our graduate students, Marc Klein, set about examining the change in the calcium current of

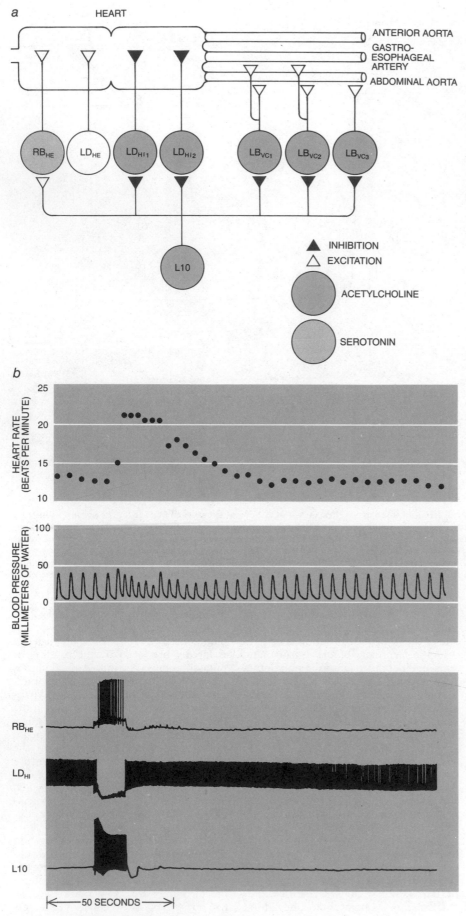

a HEART

ANTERIOR AORTA
GASTRO-ESOPHAGEAL ARTERY
ABDOMINAL AORTA

RB$_{HE}$ LD$_{HE}$ LD$_{HI1}$ LD$_{HI2}$ LB$_{VC1}$ LB$_{VC2}$ LB$_{VC3}$

L10

▲ INHIBITION
△ EXCITATION

ACETYLCHOLINE

SEROTONIN

b

HEART RATE (BEATS PER MINUTE)

25
20
15
10

BLOOD PRESSURE (MILLIMETERS OF WATER)

100
50
0

RB$_{HE}$

LD$_{HI}$

L10

|← 50 SECONDS →|

BEHAVIORAL CONTROL exerted by the single neuron L10 is shown by its effect on cardiovascular motor neurons of *Aplysia*. L10 is known to make synaptic connections (*a*) with six of the cells (LD$_{HE}$ has not yet been examined for this synaptic connection); the color of each cell indicates what chemical transmitter it utilizes. It can be seen (*b*) that activity in L10 increases the animal's heart rate and blood pressure by exciting RB$_{HE}$ and inhibiting LD$_{HI}$.

the cell body that accompanies the synaptic depression.

The calcium current turns on slowly during the action potential and so is normally overlapped by the potassium current. To unmask the calcium current we exposed the ganglion to tetraethylammonium (TEA), an agent that selectively blocks some of the delayed potassium current. By blocking the repolarizing action of the potassium current the agent produces a significant increase in the duration of the action potential. Much of this prolongation is due to the unopposed action of the calcium current. The duration of the action potential prolonged by TEA is a good assay for changes in calcium current.

We next examined the release of transmitter by the terminals of the sensory neurons, as measured by the size of the synaptic potential in the motor cell, and the changes recorded simultaneously in the calcium current, as measured by the duration of the action potential. We found that repeated stimulation of the sensory neuron at rates that produce habituation led to a progressive decrease in the duration of the calcium component of the action potential that paralleled the decrease in the release of transmitter. Spontaneous recovery of the synaptic potential and of the behavior were accompanied by an increase in the calcium current.

What we have learned so far about the mechanisms of short-term habituation indicates that this type of learning involves a modulation in the strength of a previously existing synaptic connection. The strength of the connection is determined by the amount of transmitter released, which is in turn controlled by the degree to which an action potential in the presynaptic terminal can activate the calcium current. The storage of the memory for short-term habituation therefore resides in the persistence, over minutes and hours, of the depression in the calcium current in the presynaptic terminal.

What are the limits of this change? How much can the effectiveness of a given synapse change as a result of learning, and how long can such changes endure? I have mentioned that repeated training sessions can completely depress the synaptic connections between the sensory and the motor cells. Can this condition be maintained? Can long-term habituation give rise to a complete and prolonged inactivation of a previously functioning synapse?

These questions bear on the longstanding debate among students of learning about the relation of short- and long-term memory. The commonly accepted idea is that the two kinds of memory involve different memory processes. This idea is based, however, on rather indirect evidence.

Castellucci, Carew and I set out to

examine the hypothesis more directly by comparing the effectiveness of the connections made by the population of sensory neurons on an identified gill motor cell, L7, in four groups of *Aplysia:* untrained animals that served as controls, and groups examined respectively one day, one week and three weeks after long-term habituation training. We found that in the control animals about 90 percent of the sensory neurons made extremely effective connections to L7, whereas in the animals examined one day and one week after long-term habituation the figure was 30 percent. Even in the three-week group only about 60 percent of the cells made detectable connections to L7. Here, then, are previously effective synaptic connections that become inactive and remain that way for more than a week as a result of a simple learning experience.

Hence whereas short-term habituation involves a transient decrease in synaptic efficacy, long-term habituation produces a more prolonged and profound change, leading to a functional disruption of most of the previously effective connections. The data are interesting for three reasons: (1) they provide direct evidence that a specific instance of long-term memory can be explained by a long-term change in synaptic effectiveness; (2) they show that surprisingly little training is needed to produce a profound change in synaptic transmission at synapses critically involved in learning, and (3) they make clear that short- and long-term habituation can share a common neuronal locus, namely the synapses the sensory neurons make on the motor neurons. Short- and long-term habituation also involve aspects of the same cellular mechanism: a depression of excitatory transmission. One now needs to determine whether the long-term synaptic depression is presynaptic and whether it involves an inactivation of the calcium current. If it does, it would support on a more fundamental level the notion that short- and long-term memory can involve a single memory trace.

Sensitization is a slightly more complex form of learning that can be seen in the gill-withdrawal reflex. It is the prolonged enhancement of an animal's preexisting response to a stimulus as a result of the presentation of a second stimulus that is noxious. Whereas habituation requires an animal to learn to ignore a particular stimulus because its consequences are trivial, sensitization requires the animal to learn to attend to a stimulus because it is accompanied by potentially painful or dangerous consequences. Therefore when an *Aplysia* is presented with a noxious stimulus

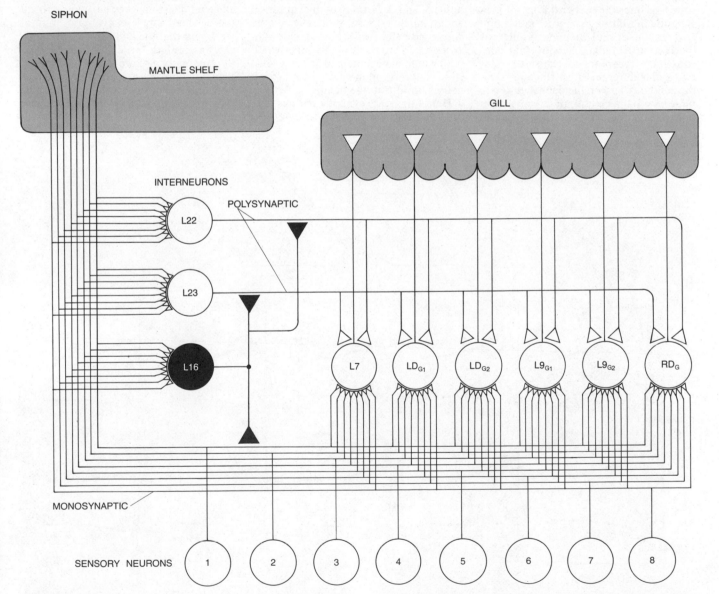

NEURAL CIRCUITRY of a behavioral reflex of *Aplysia*, the gill-withdrawal reflex, is depicted schematically. In the reflex action the animal withdraws its gill when a fleshy spout (the siphon) on a protective sheet (the mantle shelf) is stimulated in some way. The skin of the siphon is innervated by about 24 sensory neurons; the diagram has been simplified to focus on only eight of them. The sensory neurons make monosynaptic, or direct, connections to six identified gill motor neurons, which are shown in the row beginning with L7, and to at least one inhibitory cell (L16) and two interposed excitatory interneurons (L22 and L23), which make synapses with motor neurons.

to the head, the gill-withdrawal reflex response to a repeated stimulus to the siphon is greatly enhanced. As with habituation, sensitization can last from minutes to days and weeks, depending on the amount of training. Here I shall focus only on the short-term form.

Castellucci and I found that sensitization entails an alteration of synaptic transmission at the same locus that is involved in habituation: the synapses made by the sensory neurons on their central target cells. Our physiological studies and subsequent morphological studies by Craig Bailey, Mary C. Chen and Robert Hawkins indicate that the neurons mediating sensitization end near the synaptic terminals of the sensory neurons and enhance the release of transmitter by increasing the number of quanta turned loose by each action potential in the sensory neuron. The process is therefore called presynaptic facilitation. It is interesting because it illustrates (as does the earlier finding of presynaptic inhibition in another system by Joseph Dudel and Stephen Kuffler of the Harvard Medical School) that neurons have receptors to transmitters at two quite different sites. Receptors on the cell body and on the dendrites determine whether a cell should fire an action potential, and receptors on the synaptic

terminals determine how much transmitter each action potential will release.

The same locus—the presynaptic terminals of the sensory neurons—can therefore be regulated in opposite ways by opposing forms of learning. It can be depressed as a result of the intrinsic activity within the neuron that occurs with habituation, and it can be facilitated by sensitization as a result of the activity of other neurons that synapse on the terminals. These findings at the level of the single cell support the observation at the behavioral level that habituation and sensitization are independent and opposing forms of learning.

This finding raises an interesting question. Sensitization can enhance a normal reflex response, but can it counteract the profound depression in the reflex produced by long-term habituation? If it can, does it restore the completely inactivated synaptic connections produced by long-term habituation? Carew, Castellucci and I examined this question and found that sensitization reversed the depressed behavior. Moreover, the synapses that were functionally inactivated (and would have remained so for weeks) were restored within an hour by a sensitizing stimulus to the head.

Hence there are synaptic pathways in the brain that are determined by devel-

opmental processes but that, being predisposed to learning, can be functionally inactivated and reactivated by experience! In fact, at these modifiable synapses a rather modest amount of training or experience is necessary to produce profound changes. If the finding were applicable to the human brain, it would imply that even during simple social experiences, as when two people speak with each other, the action of the neuronal machinery in one person's brain is capable of having a direct and perhaps long-lasting effect on the modifiable synaptic connections in the brain of the other.

Short-term sensitization is particularly attractive from an experimental point of view because it promises to be amenable to biochemical analysis. As a first step Hawkins, Castellucci and I have identified specific cells in the abdominal ganglion of *Aplysia* that produce presynaptic facilitation. By injecting an electron-dense marker substance to fill the cell and label its synaptic endings we found that the endings contain vesicles resembling those found in *Aplysia* by Ludmiela Shkolnik and James H. Schwartz in a neuron whose transmitter had previously been established to be serotonin. Consistent with the possible serotonergic nature of this cell, Marcel-

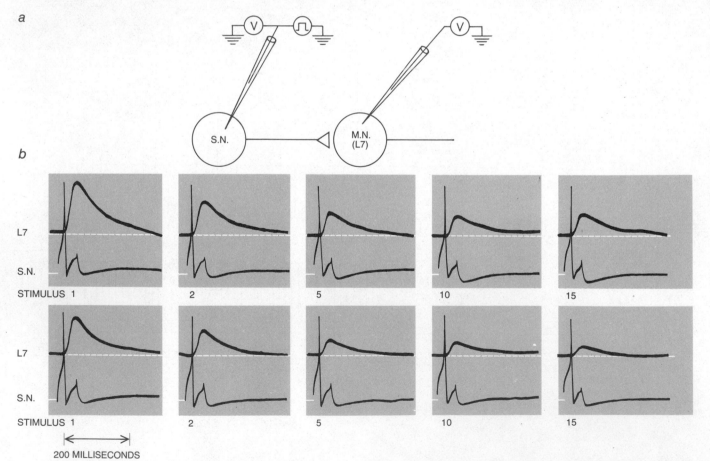

HABITUATION PROCESS, in which an animal's response to a stimulus gradually declines if the stimulus proves to be unimportant, is an elementary form of learning and memory that can be seen at the level of the single motor neuron. Here a sensory neuron (*S.N.*) from *Aplysia* that synapses on motor neuron L7 has been set up (*a*) so that the sensory neuron can be stimulated every 10 seconds. Selected records from two consecutive training sessions of 15 stimuli, separated by 15 minutes, show that the response of L7 declines and vanishes.

lo Brunelli, Castellucci, Tom Tomosky-Sykes and I found that serotonin enhanced the monosynaptic connection between the sensory neuron and the motor cell L7, whereas other likely transmitters did not.

We next uncovered an interesting link between serotonin and the intracellular messenger cyclic adenosine monophosphate (cyclic AMP). It has been known since the classic work of Earl W. Sutherland, Jr., and his colleagues at Vanderbilt University that most peptide hormones do not enter the target cell but instead act on a receptor on the cell surface to stimulate an enzyme called adenylate cyclase that catalyzes the conversion in the cell of adenosine triphosphate (ATP) into cyclic AMP, which then acts as a "second messenger" (the hormone is the first messenger) at several points inside the cell to initiate a set of appropriate changes in function.

Howard Cedar, Schwartz and I found that strong and prolonged stimulation of the pathway from the head that mediates sensitization in *Aplysia* gave rise to a synaptically mediated increase in cyclic AMP in the entire ganglion. Cedar and Schwartz and Irwin Levitan and Samuel Barondes also found that they could generate a prolonged increase in cyclic AMP by incubating the ganglion with serotonin. To explore the relation between serotonin and cyclic AMP, Brunelli, Castellucci and I injected cyclic AMP intracellularly into the cell body of the sensory neuron and found that it also produced presynaptic facilitation, whereas injection of 5'-AMP (the breakdown product of cyclic AMP) or still another second messenger, cyclic GMP, did not.

Since habituation involves a decrease in calcium current, it was attractive to think that cyclic AMP might exert its facilitating actions by increasing the calcium current. As I have mentioned, the calcium current is normally masked by the potassium current. Klein and I therefore examined action potentials in the sensory neurons with the potassium current reduced by TEA. Stimulating the pathway from the head that mediates sensitization or a single facilitating neuron enhanced the calcium current, as was evident in the increased duration of the action potential in TEA, and the enhancement persisted for 15 minutes or longer. The increase in calcium current paralleled the enhanced transmitter release, and both synaptic changes in turn paralleled the increase in the reflex response to a sensitizing stimulus.

The enhancement of the calcium current, as it is seen in the prolongation of the calcium component of the action potential after stimulation of the sensitizing pathway, could be produced by extracellular application of either serotonin or two substances that increase the intracellular level of cyclic AMP by in-

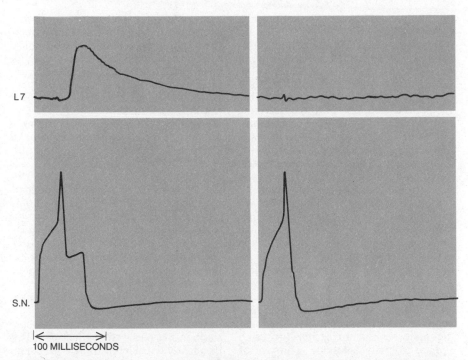

|← 100 MILLISECONDS →|

LONG-TERM HABITUATION is revealed in a comparison of synaptic connections between a sensory neuron (*S.N.*) and the motor neuron L7 in untrained *Aplysia* (*left*), which served as controls, and in *Aplysia* that had received long-term habituation training (*right*). In the control animals an impulse in the sensory neuron is followed by a large excitatory synaptic response from the motor neuron. In the trained animals the synaptic connection is almost undetectable.

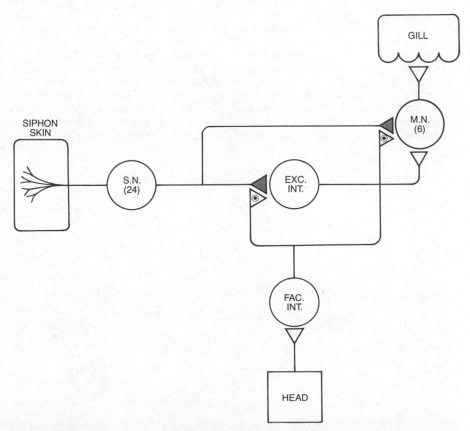

SENSITIZATION is a form of learning and memory in which the response to a stimulus is enhanced because of another and more noxious stimulus. Here gill-withdrawal reflex of *Aplysia* is intensified because of a noxious stimulus to the head. This stimulus activates neurons that excite facilitating interneurons, which end on the synaptic terminals of the sensory neurons. Those neurons are plastic, that is, capable of changing the effectiveness of their synapse. The transmitter of the facilitating interneurons, thought to be serotonin (*circled dots*), modulates the release of sensory-neuron transmitter to the excitatory interneurons and motor neurons.

hibiting phosphodiesterase, the enzyme that breaks down cyclic AMP. Similar effects were observed after direct intracellular injection of cyclic AMP, but not of 5'-AMP.

On the basis of these results Klein and I have proposed that stimulation of the facilitating neurons of the sensitizing pathway leads to the release of serotonin, which activates a serotonin-sensitive enzyme (adenylate cyclase) in the membrane of the sensory-neuron terminal. The resulting increase in cyclic AMP in the terminal leads to a greater activation of the calcium current either directly by activation of the calcium channel or indirectly by a decrease in an opposing potassium current. With each action potential the influx of calcium rises and more transmitter is released.

The availability of large cells whose electrical properties and interconnections can be thoroughly studied was the major initial attraction for using *Aplysia* to study behavior. The size of these cells might now prove to be an even greater advantage for exploring the subcellular and biochemical mechanisms of learning on the one hand and possible changes in membrane structure on the other. For example, it will be interesting to see more precisely how the increase in the level of cyclic AMP during sensitization is linked to the activation of a calcium current, because the linkage could provide the first step toward a molecular understanding of this simple form of short-term learning.

A number of mechanisms come to mind. The channels through which ions traverse the neuronal membranes are thought to consist of protein molecules. An obvious possibility is therefore that

cyclic AMP activates one or more protein kinases, enzymes that Paul Greengard of the Yale University School of Medicine has suggested may provide a common molecular mechanism for mediating the various actions of cyclic AMP within the cell. Protein kinases are enzymes that phosphorylate proteins, that is, they link a phosphoryl group to a side chain of the amino acids serine or threonine in the protein molecule, thereby changing the charge and configuration of proteins and altering their function, activating some and inactivating others. Phosphorylation could serve as an effective mechanism for the regulation of memory. One way sensitization might work is that the calcium-channel protein becomes activated (or the opposing potassium-channel protein becomes inactivated) when it is phosphorylated by a protein kinase that is dependent on cyclic AMP.

Sensitization holds an interesting position in the hierarchy of learning. It is frequently considered to be a precursor form of classical conditioning. In both sensitization and classical conditioning a reflex response to a stimulus is enhanced as a result of the activation of another pathway. Sensitization differs from conditioning in being nonassociative; the sensitizing stimulus is effective in enhancing reflex responsiveness whether or not it is paired in time with the reflex stimulus. Several types of associative learning have now been demonstrated in mollusks by Alan Gelperin of Princeton University, by George Mpitsos and Stephen Collins of Case Western Reserve University and by Terry Crow and Daniel L. Alkon of the National Institutes of Health. Recently Terry Walters, Carew and I have

obtained evidence for associative conditioning in *Aplysia*. We may therefore soon be in a position to analyze precisely how the mechanisms of sensitization relate to those of associative learning.

Another direction that research can now take is to examine the relation between the initial development of the neural circuit in the embryo and its later modification by learning. Both development and learning involve functional changes in the nervous system: changes in the effectiveness of synapses and in other properties of neurons. How are such changes related? Are the mechanisms of learning based on those of developmental plasticity, or do completely new processes specialized for learning emerge later?

Whatever the answers to these intriguing questions may be, the surprising and heartening thing that has emerged from the study of invertebrate animals is that one can now pinpoint and observe at the cellular level, and perhaps ultimately at the molecular level, simple aspects of memory and learning. Although certain higher mental activities are characteristic of the complex brains of higher animals, it is now clear that elementary aspects of what are regarded as mental processes can be found in the activity of just a very few neurons. It will therefore be interesting both philosophically and technically to see to what degree complex forms of mentation can be explained in terms of simpler components and mechanisms. To the extent that such reductionist explanations are possible it will also be important to determine how the units of this elementary alphabet of mentation are combined to yield the language of much more complex mental processes.

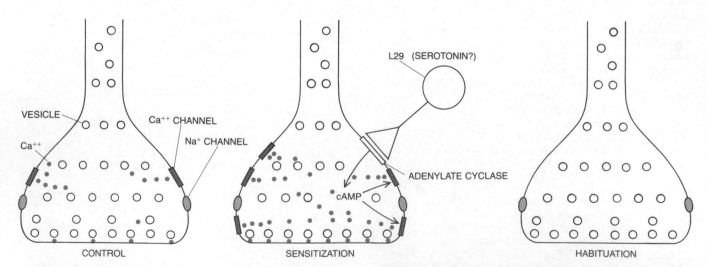

SHORT-TERM SENSITIZATION AND HABITUATION at the level of the single sensory neuron are modeled, beginning with what happens in a control situation (*left*) in which a cell fires before either sensitization or habituation has set in. A nerve impulse in the terminal membrane of the neuron opens up a number of channels for calcium ions (Ca^{++}) in parallel with the sodium channels (Na^+). Sensitization is produced by cell group L29 (perhaps more) that are believed to release the transmitter serotonin. It acts on an adenylate cyclase, an enzyme that catalyzes the synthesis of cyclic adenosine monophosphate (cyclic AMP) in the neuron terminals. The cyclic AMP increases the influx of calcium ions, perhaps by making more calcium channels available. The calcium causes a greater binding of transmitter-bearing vesicles to release sites, increasing the probability that the neuron will release transmitter. In habituation repeated impulses in the terminals could decrease the number of open calcium channels, depressing the calcium influx and inactivating the synapse.

IV

The Organization
of the Brain

The Organization of the Brain

BY WALLE J. H. NAUTA AND MICHAEL FEIRTAG

The brain and spinal cord of mammals, including man, consist of some billions of neurons, and a single neuron may connect with thousands of others. How is this enormous three-dimensional network organized?

We see two broadside approaches to the presentation of neuroanatomy. The first one is heroic: it affirms that the brain is the embodiment of thinking and feeling and wanting, of learning and memory and of that curious sense that human beings share, a sense of the future. Then one contemplates this mystery made flesh. Certain parts of the brain, most notably the cerebral cortex, are wonderfully organized; others are startling in their seeming disarray. Yet even the most highly ordered structures, with neurons and their various interconnections aligned as if on circuit boards, resist our present understanding.

The other approach is more matter-of-fact. The brain plainly has divisions, because the appropriate staining techniques reveal aggregations of neurons embedded in a feltwork of their filamentous extensions. Moreover, in other places the tissue is composed primarily of the long nerve-cell fibers—the axons—that subserve long-distance communications in the nervous system. The first kind of tissue is gray matter, the second is white matter.

One is of course tempted to assign a function to each district, as if the entire brain were something like a radio. Yet the essence of the central nervous system—the brain and the spinal cord—is a channeling of incoming sensory information to a multiplicity of structures and a convergence of information on the neurons that animate the effector tissues of the body: the muscles and the glands. The overall system therefore assumes properties beyond those to be discovered in a mere set of modules.

Consider the brain structure named the subthalamic nucleus. Its destruction in the human brain leads to the motor dysfunction known as hemiballism, in which the patient uncontrollably makes motions that resemble the throwing of a ball. Is the normal function of the intact subthalamic nucleus therefore the suppression of motions resembling the throwing of a ball? Of course not; the condition represents only the action of a central nervous system unbalanced by the absence of a subthalamic nucleus.

We mention these things to establish the limitations of any account of the anatomy of the brain. We shall give such an account here, but it will necessarily be somewhat shadowy. To suggest otherwise would simply not be frank.

Some preliminaries will be useful. In the early decades of this century George Parker of Yale University had been searching for the primeval reflex arc. Such arcs had been identified in vertebrate animals; they are pathways consisting of one or more neurons by which the excitatory event elicited by a sensory stimulus to some part of the body can be conducted to an effector tissue and thereby can entail a movement. In Parker's time reflex arcs were commonly taken to be the simplest pattern by which nature had organized cells into a nervous system; accordingly the nervous system was widely supposed to have originated when some organism came to have a cell, or chain of cells, that mediated between an environmental stimulus and the organism's responsive movement. Presumably it would one day be established that the evolution of the nervous system had brought forth, in ever more advanced organisms, an ever increasing number and complexity of such chains.

Parker's attention was drawn first to the epithelial layer of certain marine polyps and sea anemones, because it contained an occasional cell that stood out (when it was appropriately stained) as if it were a neuron. At the base of such a cell Parker could see the beginning of a filament, looking rather like an axon, that broke up into end branches as it approached a muscle fiber. He could not be certain that the two made contact, but he assumed that there was communication between them. Surely he was right, but the arrangement is quite primitive; its circuitry could be called a one-neuron nervous system, since the entire line of conduction consists of only a single cell. What such a nervous system will do in response to a stimulus is as predictable as what a doorbell will do when the button is pressed. What is plain about the human nervous system, however, is that the behavior it makes human beings capable of is least of all predictable.

Obviously something must intervene in the doorbell mechanism, and so Parker examined the situation in somewhat more complex organisms. In certain polyps and jellyfishes he found an array of neurons in the epithelial layer similar to the array he had found earlier. Under the epithelium, however, he now found additional neurons that together form a widely distributed plexus. The nervous system in this second group of organisms has thereby gained in sophistication: neurons in the epithelial layer make contact with a subepithelial net, and the cells of that net make contact in turn with contractile tissue in the depths of the organism. One may therefore speak of a two-neuron nervous system, in which sensory neurons (in these simple creatures the neurons at the body surface, in direct contact with the organism's ambient environment) communi-

ORDER AND DISORDER in the cellular organization of the brain are apparent in the photomicrographs on the opposite page. Both are of thin sections of cat brain that were stained with two procedures: the Golgi stain, which causes some neurons to stand out in black silhouette with all their processes revealed, and the Nissl stain, which renders every neuronal cell body blue. (Here the blue is purplish.) The Golgi method stains only 5 percent or fewer of the neurons, apparently at random; if all the neurons were stained, the tissue would appear completely black. The micrograph at the top of the page shows the dentate gyrus of the hippocampus. Each neuronal cell body is an elongated pyramid aligned with its neighbors and extending its fibers in a parallel array. Micrograph at the bottom is of the magnocellular reticular formation. Here neurons are organized as an irregular net. Magnification of micrographs is 48 diameters.

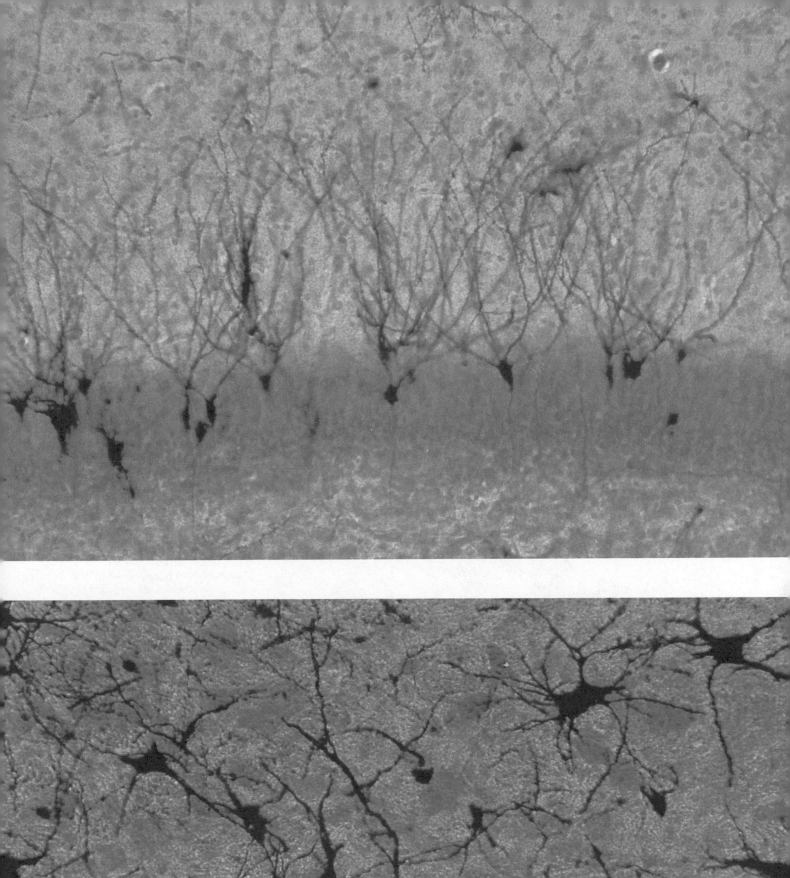

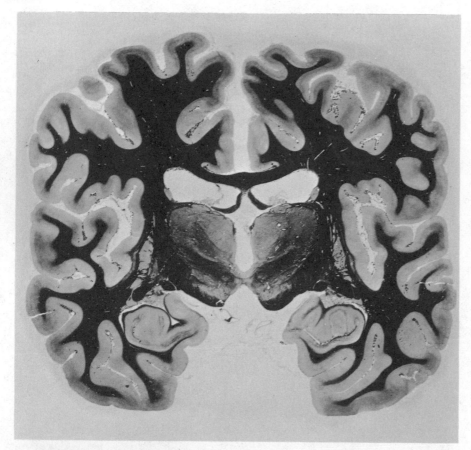

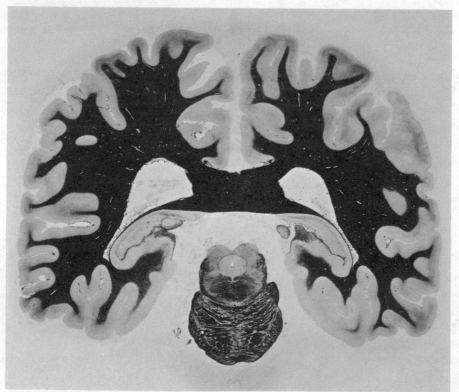

TWO SLICES through a fixed human brain perpendicular to its long axis reveal the complexity of the brain's internal anatomy. The thin slices were treated with a stain that selectively blackens the fatty myelin sheath of the nerve fibers. As a result the white matter appears black and the gray matter (which consists primarily of neuronal cell bodies) is more or less unstained. The empty spaces in the slices indicate the location of the ventricles: fluid-filled cisterns deep within the brain. The slice at the top (*a*) was made near the middle of the length of the brain and includes the cerebral cortex, the hippocampus and the thalamus. The slice at the bottom (*b*) was made more to the rear and includes a section through the brain stem. The location of the two slices and the identity of the structures shown are indicated on the opposite page. Specimens are from the collection of Professor Paul I. Yakovlev at the Harvard Medical School.

cate with motor neurons (neurons that make contact with effector cells, in this instance contractile cells and therefore in essence muscle fibers).

Is this not circuitry that remains extremely predictable? Perhaps not. Imagine that the motor neurons communicate with one another, so that the input to any one of them includes not only messages coming from the ambient environment by way of sensory neurons but also messages from neighboring motor neurons. Imagine further that some messages might be excitatory, making the motor neuron more likely to generate and transmit its own activity if other signals should arrive, and that other messages might be inhibitory. Under such circumstances there is a riddle to solve: predicting what a neuron will do in response to its various inputs seems to be a matter of algebraically summing the excitatory and inhibitory messages that converge on it.

Perhaps the two-neuron arrangement enables the jellyfish so favored by nature to be more unpredictable in its behavior than the anemone and other organisms with one-neuron nervous systems. Then, however, comes a further advance, and it too is found in very primitive organisms, such as certain other jellyfishes. In a way it is the final advance, because the nervous system of these latter jellyfishes and the nervous system of man both consist in essence of only three classes of neurons. In these jellyfishes, as in man, the sensory neurons as a rule no longer communicate directly with motor neurons. Between the two has developed a barrier of neurons that have interconnections not only with motor neurons but also with one another.

To be sure, this third and final step may already have been taken by all organisms that have a subepithelial nerve-cell plexus. In the foregoing account of a two-neuron nervous system all the cells composing that plexus were assumed to be motor neurons: cells that innervate effector tissues. In reality, however, only some of the many subepithelial cells may make such connections. The remainder may be positioned in the plexus in such a way that they receive input from the sensory neurons in the epithelium but can communicate only with others of their kind or with motor neurons, not with effector tissue. Neither sensory nor motoric, they are go-betweens in the path of sensory-to-motor conduction.

In short, here too are "intermediate neurons." Although a three-neuron organization is difficult to identify in a diffuse neuronal net, it is abundantly apparent at later stages in evolution; in animals more highly developed than a jellyfish the diffuse subepithelial nerve-cell plexus has been concentrated into either a segmental sequence of ganglia

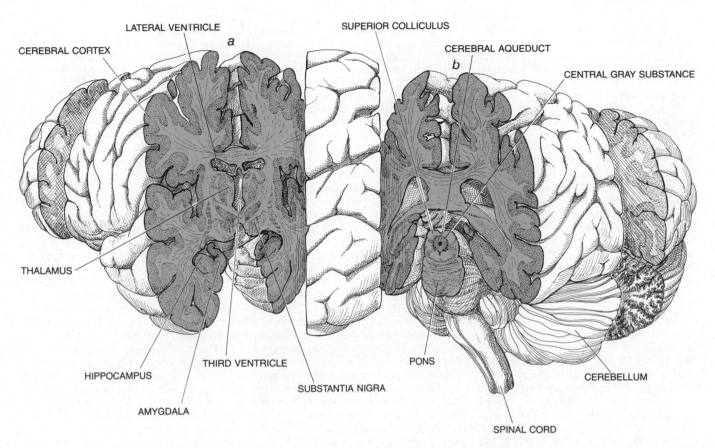

CEREBRAL CORTEX
LATERAL VENTRICLE
a
SUPERIOR COLLICULUS
CEREBRAL AQUEDUCT
b
CENTRAL GRAY SUBSTANCE
THALAMUS
HIPPOCAMPUS
AMYGDALA
THIRD VENTRICLE
SUBSTANTIA NIGRA
PONS
SPINAL CORD
CEREBELLUM

HUMAN BRAIN is cut in five sections and opened like a book for the purpose of correlating its external and internal anatomy. The two slices appearing on the opposite page are designated *a* and *b*. At the level of slice *b* the brain stem lies below the mass of the forebrain.

(aggregates of neurons) or a single unsegmented central nervous system. The crucial point is therefore the advent of "the great intermediate net": a barrier of intermediate neurons that interposes itself between the sensory neurons and the motor neurons early in the evolution of animal life.

Just how far the development of the great intermediate net has progressed to this day is best shown by some numbers. To begin with, how many neurons are there in the human central nervous system? One often hears that the answer is on the order of 10^{10}. This is an accounting of the intermediate and motor neurons, since it happens that the true sensory neurons lie not in the central nervous system but in ganglia that flank the brain and the spinal cord. It is an attractive number, easy to remember and easy to state. Yet there are classes of neurons so small and so densely crowded that it is difficult or impossible to judge their number. One such class is the granule cell. There are so many granule cells in just one part of the human brain—the cerebellum—that the estimate of 10^{10} neurons in the entire central nervous system becomes suspect. The total could easily be an order of magnitude, perhaps two orders of magnitude, higher.

Still, assume for a moment that the total is 10^{10}. How many of these cells are motor neurons? It appears that the answer cannot be many more than two or three million, which is a disconcertingly small number in view of the fact that only through motor neurons can the workings of the nervous system find expression in movement. Moreover, this answer suggests that an incredibly large number of influences must converge on the motor neurons; it suggests, in other words, that a typical motor neuron forms synapses with an enormous number of axons put out by an equally enormous number of neurons in the great intermediate net.

It is thought that a typical motor neuron in the human spinal cord has perhaps 10,000 synaptic contacts on its surface, of which about 2,000 are on the cell body and 8,000 are on its dendrites: its local branchings, as distinct from its single axon. This does not mean that 10,000 intermediate neurons impinge on one motor neuron; the intermediate neurons tend to make multiple synaptic contacts when they communicate with a cell. Even so, the average motor neuron must be heavily impinged on; a neuron count of 10^{10} in the central nervous system implies that for every motor neuron there are between 3,000 and 5,000 neurons of the great intermediate net.

One last conclusion must be drawn from the numbers we have quoted: the entire human brain and spinal cord are a great intermediate net, with the exception of a mere few million motor neurons. And when the great intermediate net comes to include 99.98 percent of all the neurons that make up the central nervous system, the term loses much of its meaning: it comes to represent the very complexity one must face in trying to comprehend the nervous system. The term remains useful only as a reminder that most of the brain's neurons are neither sensory nor motor. Strictly speaking, they are intercalated between the true sensory side of the organization and the true motoric side. They are the components of a computational network.

A second set of preliminaries concerns the gross anatomy of the central nervous system. In particular the brain and spinal cord of all vertebrate species first appear in the embryo as no more than a tube only one cell layer thick. The anterior part of this neural tube, ultimately to be enclosed within the cranium, soon shows a series of three swellings: the primary brain vesicles. These are the rhombencephalon, or hindbrain; the mesencephalon, or midbrain, and the prosencephalon, or forebrain. (The suffix -encephalon is from the Greek for "within the head.")

Of the three primary vesicles the prosencephalon is the most productive in terms of both further subdivision and further differentiation. The major event in its embryonic development is the formation of chambers on its left and right sides. These become the paired cerebral hemispheres, also called the telencephalon or endbrain, which in some species are of modest size but in others are enormous. Between the hemispheres lies the unpaired central component of the prosencephalon from which the hemispheres diverge. It is called the diencephalon, which literally means "between-brain."

Concurrent with these developments the prosencephalon grows a further pair of chambers: the optic vesicles. Even sightless animals have them, but in animals that can see they elongate toward the surface of the head and ultimately become the two retinas, connected to the base of the forebrain by their stalks, the optic nerves. Lastly the underside of the primary prosencephalon develops an unpaired midline chamber that differentiates to form the posterior lobe of the pituitary complex.

The bottom illustration on page 47 suggests the outcome of these embryonic unfoldings. It is a schematic diagram that by and large holds for all mammals, and it depicts the fully formed mammalian central nervous system broken down into several subdivisions. At the left is the spinal cord, greatly foreshortened in the illustration. To its right, without any abrupt transition, is the rhombencephalon, the lowermost division of the brain itself. Its dorsal part (the part nearest the back of the animal) is the appendage called the cerebellum.

Above the rhombencephalon is the mesencephalon, which in mammals includes two pairs of structures that together form a region of four hills known as the lamina quadrigemina, the tectum mesencephali or simply the tectum, meaning roof. The lower pair of structures are the inferior colliculi. The upper pair are the superior colliculi. Other than that the mesencephalon gives little reason to subdivide it, at least in the longitudinal direction. It is in fact a rather short stretch of the human brain.

Next is the central, unpaired division of the forebrain, namely the diencephalon. Its dorsal two-thirds is the thalamus. The rest is the hypothalamus. (Somewhat off to the side of the hypothalamus is a third district of the diencephalon, the subthalamus, whose most striking cell group, the subthalamic nucleus, we mentioned at the beginning. Its inclusion here would overcrowd the illustration.) The hypothalamus is characterized by the glandular appendage called the pituitary complex. It is also continuous in the forward direction with the septum, a structure that is best classified, in spite of its position, as being diencephalic.

The remaining subdivision of the forebrain is the telencephalon, the cerebral hemisphere. In the brain of a mammal it is by far the largest part, and in many mammalian species its shell, the cerebral mantle or cerebral cortex, is furrowed into the convolutions called gyri and the fissures called sulci. The mammalian cerebral cortex can be subdivided into several districts. At the base of the hemisphere a structure protrudes forward that is composed entirely of cortex, although it is cortex of a primitive cell architecture. Its swollen front end is the olfactory bulb and its shank is the olfactory peduncle; only the part immediately under the rest of the cerebral hemisphere is the olfactory cortex proper. A second great district of the mammalian cerebral cortex is found at the free edge of the cortex, where the cortical mantle rolls inward on itself to form a composite gyrus whose cross section is reminiscent of a rococo ornament. This remarkable structure is known as the hippocampus.

There remains even after the foregoing parcellation an expanse of the mammalian cerebral cortex that has enormous extent and structural complexity; in man and other primates it is estimated to contain no fewer than 70 percent of all the neurons in the central nervous system. This is the neocortex. It is the latest form of cortex to appear in evolution. We owe it to a branching; beyond the reptiles one strain of animals elaborated on the reptilian pattern and became the birds, while a more venturesome strain developed the neocortex as it became the mammals. From a strictly phylogenetic point of view birds are thus the logical end of the brain's traditional development and the mammals are deviants, since there are no birds in their ancestry. In one of the many radiations of mammalian evolution the primates appeared, an order in which the neocortex reaches its maximal development. We human beings are heir to all the consequences, perhaps including psychiatry.

In the depths of the mammalian cerebral hemisphere are several masses of gray matter. One is the amygdala, which lies under the olfactory cortex. Another is the corpus striatum, at the very core of the cerebral hemisphere. It consists in turn of two districts that are distinct in cell composition. The first of these is an inner zone called the pallidum or globus pallidus. The other is an outer district known as the striatum.

We turn now to the circuitry of the mammalian central nervous system. Let us begin with an identification of sensory neurons, such as those Parker found in the epithelial layer of jellyfishes. In vertebrates, however, the position of the sensory neurons is quite different. Only one known instance remains in which a vertebrate's sensory neuron is also a receptor at the surface of the body; only the olfactory epithelial cells, in the lining of the roof of the nasal cavity, are exposed to the external environment. All other sensory neurons in the body of a vertebrate are stationed well below the surface, in ganglia along the length of the spinal cord or in similar ganglia flanking the brain. (In vertebrates the term ganglion is reserved for a cluster of neurons outside the central nervous system.) Each sensory neuron has an axon that divides into two parts: one part enters the central nervous system and the other innervates structures of the periphery.

In the illustration on page 48 one of these cells—let us call it a primary sensory neuron—sends an axon into the spinal cord bearing reports of somatic sensory events such as a touch on the skin, the movement of a joint or the contraction of a muscle. These messages do not immediately reach motor neurons; the primary sensory neuron makes its first synaptic contacts with what are called intermediate neurons.

There is, however, an exception. It is the monosynaptic reflex arc, in which a side branch from a primary sensory fiber bridges over and makes direct synaptic contact on a motor neuron. At first this seems dismaying: only a few paragraphs above we noted that after the earliest stages of neural evolution motor neurons no longer were bothered with raw data. We suggested they were instead always given digests of information by neurons of the great intermediate net. A monosynaptic reflex might therefore seem to be a very primitive type of neural circuitry. On the other hand, it could be fairly new; perhaps only terrestrial animals have redeveloped it. Air and land, after all, are the cruelest of environments; for a mountain goat one misstep could be fatal. A fish, in contrast, can make any number of similar faux pas and not be harmed in any way. The fish is splendidly suspended; the force of gravity is not nearly so stringent and hostile. Hence it is terrestrial life, not aquatic, that seems to require a high-security reflex system for maintaining balance, and specifically a way in which a muscle can signal to the appropriate motor neurons (and only the appropriate ones) that it is being unduly stretched by the force of gravity.

Monosynaptic reflex arcs have never been found outside the realm of such corrections. Thus the short circuits between sensory input and motor output appear to be a small minority. The large majority of mammalian primary sensory fibers enter the great intermediate net and synapse with members of what we shall call a secondary sensory cell group: neurons first in line to receive primary sensory input. From there many pathways are directed more or less promptly toward motor neurons. They might collectively be called a local reflex channel, if it is kept in mind that "local" may be misleading because

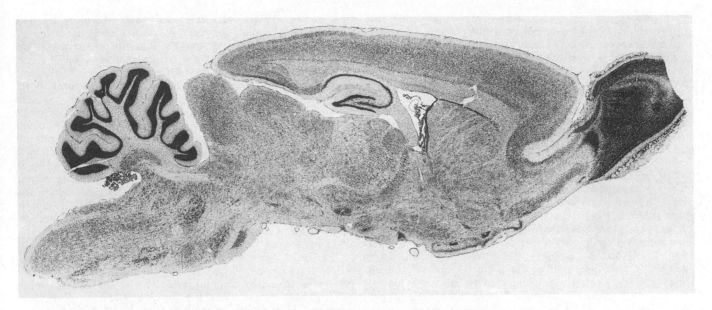

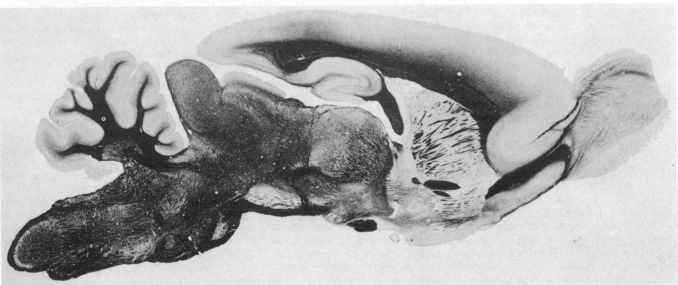

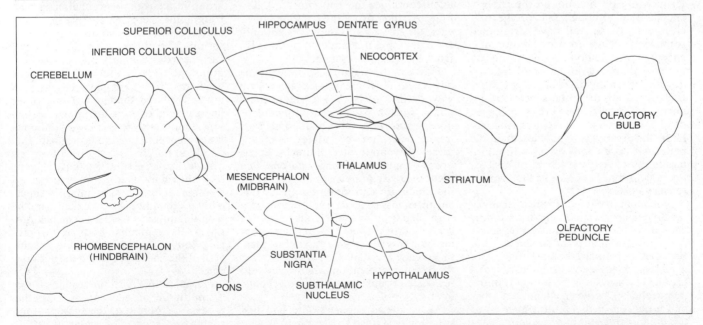

SUPERIOR COLLICULUS   HIPPOCAMPUS   DENTATE GYRUS

INFERIOR COLLICULUS   NEOCORTEX

CEREBELLUM

OLFACTORY
BULB

THALAMUS

MESENCEPHALON
(MIDBRAIN)   STRIATUM

RHOMBENCEPHALON
(HINDBRAIN)   SUBSTANTIA
NIGRA   OLFACTORY
PEDUNCLE

HYPOTHALAMUS

PONS   SUBTHALAMIC
NUCLEUS

TWO STAINING TECHNIQUES provide complementary views of the internal organization of the rat brain. The section at the top, made just off the midplane and parallel to it, was treated by the Nissl technique, which selectively stains cell bodies. Each dot in the micrograph therefore corresponds to an individual cell. The section in the middle was treated with the Loyez technique, which selectively stains myelinated fibers and leaves cell bodies unstained, selectively revealing the fiber pathways. Map indicates the various anatomical structures.

there are several reflexes that involve the entire length of the spinal cord but nonetheless are local because they remain within it. The first link in the local reflex channel is a cell of the secondary sensory cell group. Many such cells do not themselves make contact with a motor neuron; they synapse instead on yet other neurons of the great intermediate net, and it is only these latter neurons that finally complete the arc.

Other channels consist of axons not directed toward motor neurons. Take the cerebellar channel: from secondary sensory cell groups in the hindbrain and spinal cord there are many axons ascending directly to the cerebellum. The axon that does so in the illustration on page 48 originates in a secondary sensory cell group of the spinal cord and is therefore called a spinocerebellar fiber. ("Axon" and "fiber" are synonymous in neuroanatomical usage.) Many of these fibers together would compose a spinocerebellar tract or bundle.

A third channel is the lemniscal channel. The word lemniscus is Latin for ribbon, and it refers here to fiber bundles that originate in secondary sensory cell groups and ascend toward the forebrain, in particular toward the thalamus. In the illustration on page 48 one such bundle is shown ascending at the center of the spinal cord. Actually it ascends near the cord's lateral edge; the simple scheme of the illustration cannot be topographic. The bundle is called the spinothalamic tract, although only one of its three representative fibers is depicted as arriving at the thalamus. The other fibers accompany it for some distance and then crash-land, so to speak: both are shown terminating on neurons in the rhombencephalon, although one or the other might just as well have terminated somewhat farther forward, in the mesencephalon. The point is that of the spinothalamic fibers only a small fraction actually reach the thalamus. Even so the tract is named after the successful minority, which terminate in a specific part of the thalamus: the ventral nucleus. Here the fibers synapse with thalamic neurons whose axons travel without interruption to a specific field of neocortex, a field that is known as the somatic sensory cortex.

Note that the path from a primary sensory neuron to the neocortex in this case involves only two synaptic interruptions. The first is in the spinal cord, between a primary sensory fiber and a neuron in a secondary sensory cell group. The second interruption is in the diencephalon, between a lemniscal fiber and a neuron in the ventral nucleus of the thalamus. What happens in the neocortex, however, is a synaptic cataclysm. In the neocortex the response to an arriving signal initially involves hundreds or even thousands of neurons.

And acting through synaptic connections, the first neurons engaged by the signal will engage innumerable further neurons.

A two-synapse sensory conduction line to the neocortex might be called a through line, because two synapses appears to be a minimum in such systems. It might be also be called a closed or labeled line, because in general the sensory pathways of minimal interruption rigorously maintain the topography of the sensory periphery from which they come. A fingertip, for example, can detect two distinct stimuli when it is touched by the points of a pair of drafting dividers no more than two or three millimeters apart. This ability is called two-point discrimination. Its existence means that each of the compass points must stimulate paths of conduction that are independent enough to allow what might be called sensory resolution. Some cell in the somatic sensory cortex, if interrogated with a microelectrode, might reveal that its only interest is a square millimeter of skin on the index finger. One of its close neighbors might be the monitor of an adjoining square millimeter, and so on. In that way the topography of the body surface would be faithfully reproduced.

A conduction path diametrically opposed to one that is "labeled" would be one in which the line becomes involved in the conduction of topographically muddled messages from a given sensorium, or even messages from several different sensoria. This curious arrangement in fact exists: one of the spinothalamic dropouts in the illustration on page 48 ends in synaptic contact with a rhombencephalic neuron whose axon continues the line into the thalamus. At that extra interruption, however, the line accepts messages not only from the spinothalamic fiber but also from the auditory system.

How can the thalamus know what has happened when an impulse arrives by way of this system? The rhombencephalic neuron is called multimodal or nonspecific, and the conduction path might be called open-line: wherever there is a synaptic interruption the line is open to inputs from other neurons. The great majority of neurons in the core of the hindbrain and midbrain are of this curious nonspecific nature. They sit with their dendrites—their cellular hands—spread across several millimeters, hoping, it seems, to catch any kind of message. They are typical of what is called the reticular formation, where relatively few cell groups receive homogeneous inputs.

An electrical engineer who had this situation described to him might frown; he would say that one could never hope to get anything but noise from it. The situation nonetheless prevails in the brains of all vertebrates, including man.

Its existence would therefore seem to correspond to some particular need. At the moment it seems permissible to say that the reticular formation includes among its functions the production of a background of general arousal in the central nervous system and that the formation embodies a mechanism by which activity states throughout the central nervous system are regulated. Some of these regulations are diurnal; one state is sleep, another is wakefulness. Between the two there are a great many shadings of alertness and inattentiveness. All are expressions of one or another pattern of activity in the reticular formation.

Surely the electrical engineer would more happily contemplate a second somatic sensory lemniscus rising from the spinal cord. This is the medial lemniscus. It is far more tightly organized: almost all its fibers are labeled lines that ascend directly to the ventral nucleus of the thalamus from a pair of secondary sensory cell groups at the transition between the spinal cord and the hindbrain that are called the nuclei of the dorsal funiculus. The engineer would not be surprised to learn that two-point discrimination is represented far more prominently in the medial lemniscus than it is in the spinothalamic tract.

What of the other sensoria? The little organ that appears for diagrammatic convenience near the cerebellum in the illustration on page 49 is the organ of hearing. Within it cells that have a single cilium are found in a highly specialized epithelial complex called Corti's organ. They are innervated by primary sensory neurons whose centrally directed processes terminate on neurons of the cochlear nuclei, a secondary sensory cell group in the rhombencephalon specializing in the reception and processing of afflux exclusively from the auditory sensorium. The illustration shows only two such neurons; actually there are tens of thousands. From the cochlear nuclei originates the lateral lemniscus, ascending toward the thalamus. None of its fibers extend beyond the inferior colliculus. In this unbypassable way station in the mesencephalon axons originate that do attain the thalamus, where they terminate in the medial geniculate body. (Not shown in the illustration are several other auditory way stations, apparently more optional, associated with the lateral lemniscus itself.) The neurons of the medial geniculate body in turn project—send their axons—to the specific area of the neocortex called the auditory cortex.

Compare this with the visual system. A multitude of neurons in the retina process the output of the eye's photoreceptor apparatus. The axons of certain of these cells first form the optic nerve. Then comes a rechanneling of axons in which those entrained by the nasal half of each retina cross the midplane of the

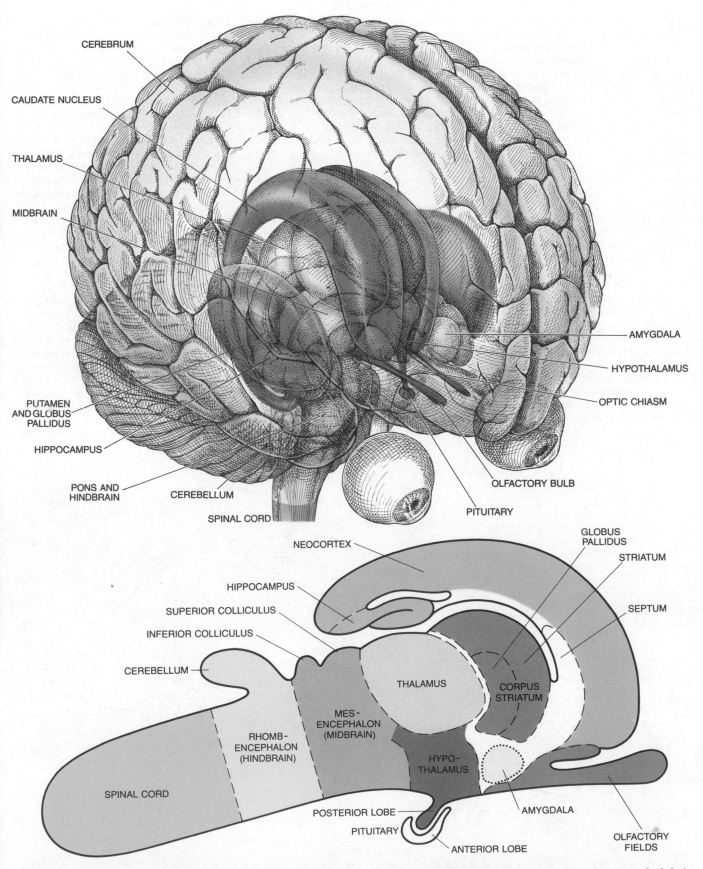

CEREBRUM

CAUDATE NUCLEUS

THALAMUS

MIDBRAIN

PUTAMEN AND GLOBUS PALLIDUS

HIPPOCAMPUS

PONS AND HINDBRAIN

CEREBELLUM

SPINAL CORD

AMYGDALA

HYPOTHALAMUS

OPTIC CHIASM

OLFACTORY BULB

PITUITARY

NEOCORTEX

GLOBUS PALLIDUS

STRIATUM

HIPPOCAMPUS

SUPERIOR COLLICULUS

INFERIOR COLLICULUS

CEREBELLUM

THALAMUS

CORPUS STRIATUM

SEPTUM

MES-ENCEPHALON (MIDBRAIN)

RHOMB-ENCEPHALON (HINDBRAIN)

HYPO-THALAMUS

SPINAL CORD

POSTERIOR LOBE

PITUITARY

ANTERIOR LOBE

AMYGDALA

OLFACTORY FIELDS

BRAIN AND SPINAL CORD of human beings and other mammals can be subdivided into smaller regions according to gross appearance, embryology or cellular organization. At the top a human brain has been drawn so that its internal structures are visible through "transparent" outer layers of the cerebrum. At the bottom a generalized mammalian brain is shown in a highly schematic view, a convention adopted in the rest of the illustrations for this article. Corresponding structures in the realistic and schematic models are the same color. The most general way of dividing the brain is into hindbrain, midbrain and forebrain. The hindbrain includes the cerebellum. The midbrain includes the two elevations known as the inferior and superior colliculi. The forebrain is more complex. Its outer part is the cerebral hemisphere, the surface of which is the convoluted sheet of the cerebral cortex, which incorporates the hippocampus, the neocortex and the olfactory fields. Within the hemisphere are the amygdala and corpus striatum; the latter includes the globus pallidus and the striatum, which includes the caudate nucleus and putamen. The rest of the forebrain is the diencephalon: the upper two-thirds comprises the thalamus (which has numerous subdivisions) and the lower third the hypothalamus (which connects to pituitary complex).

head to join those entrained by the lateral half of the other eye's retina. The result is the optic tract. Each optic tract distributes its constituent axons to two great terminal areas. One is the superior colliculus, but in all primates the more important area, at least in terms of the number of axons, is the lateral geniculate body of the thalamus. The neurons of that group of cells project in turn to the neocortex, specifically to an area at the posterior pole of the cerebral hemisphere that is known as the visual cortex.

Note that whereas no auditory fiber can reach its thalamic way station without synaptic interruption, most visual fibers (in primates) can. It should be added, however, that many of the neurons in the superior colliculus that receive visual fibers send their own axons into the thalamus, not to the lateral geniculate body but to the nucleus lateralis posterior. The neurons of this latter cell group in turn project to the neocortex. They project, however, not to the area in which axons entrained by the lateral geniculate body terminate but to a nearby cortical region that is distinct from the visual cortex. The visual system apparently has two channels ascending to the cerebral cortex.

The olfactory system breaks all the laws that seem to govern the organization of other sensory mechanisms. It is, as we have noted, the only system known in which the primary sensory neurons lie at the body surface. There is no transducing element, as there is in, say, Corti's organ; the olfactory epithelial cell itself is buffeted by the external environment. From such a neuron a very thin axon projects to the olfactory bulb, whose neurons in turn give rise to axons that terminate in synaptic contact on cells in the olfactory cortex.

We now have traced the fibers of four sensoria: the somatic sensorium and the sensoria of hearing, vision and olfaction. A number of conclusions may by now have begun to emerge. For one thing, the thalamus appears to be a crucial way station, a final checkpoint, before messages from all the sensoria (except, it seems, olfaction) are allowed entrance to higher stations of the brain. It is tempting to call any such interruption a relay, but what happens at these breaks in neural circuitry can be far more than what happens in an athletic relay where each runner hands a baton to the next and the baton arrives unmodified at the end of the course. In the central nervous system the "relay" is en-

tirely different. At each synaptic interruption in a sensory pathway the input is transformed: the code in which the message arrived is fundamentally changed. Presumably the data could not be understood at higher levels; translation is needed, and the synaptic relays are better spoken of as processing stations.

Then there is the conclusion that the cerebral cortex is an end station of the sensory conduction pathways. The neuroanatomist is highly satisfied when he can trace the visual system, for example, from the retina to the lateral geniculate body and from there to the visual cortex. The problem with any further tracing is the complexity of the cerebral cortex, with its 70 percent of all the neurons in the human central nervous system. What are they doing with their input? Two observations might be offered.

First, the thalamocortical projections are reciprocated: the visual cortex projects back to the lateral geniculate body, from which it received its input; the auditory cortex projects back to the medial geniculate body, and the somatic sensory cortex projects back to the ventral nucleus. This reciprocity undoubtedly signifies that the functional state of the cortex can influence the manner in which the sensory way stations of the

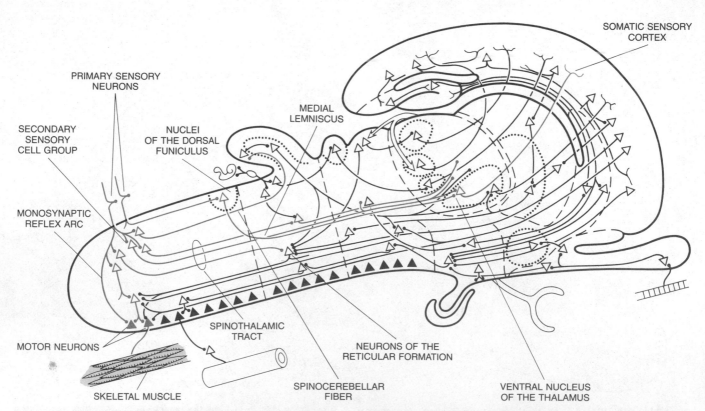

SOMATIC SENSORY INFORMATION such as skin sensation is transmitted along several spinal pathways. At the left side of the diagram a representative pair of primary sensory neurons deliver signals from peripheral sensory receptors into the spinal cord. One path branches immediately to motor neurons (*solid triangles*), whose fibers lead outward to the skeletal musculature. All the other paths lead initially to secondary sensory cell groups, either in the same region of the spinal cord or at the top of the cord in the nuclei of the dorsal funiculus. A pathway called the medial lemniscus travels upward from the nuclei of the dorsal funiculus to the ventral nucleus of the thalamus, which in turn projects to the somatic sensory area of the cortex. A second pathway called the spinothalamic tract travels upward to the forebrain from the secondary cell groups throughout the length of the spinal cord, sending out fibers en route. A small fraction of the spinothalamic-tract fibers ultimately reach the ventral nucleus. The secondary cell groups also send fibers to the cerebellum.

thalamus screen the cortically directed flow of information.

Second, the visual, auditory and somatic sensory areas embody only a first cortical step in the sensory processing. Out from these primary sensory fields come fibers that synaptically affect adjoining areas that cannot unreservedly be called sensory; they are a block away, so to speak, from the arriving input. And out from these areas come fibers that terminate in areas still farther away from the primary sensory fields. The areas of the neocortex at various removes from the primary fields are called association areas, and in man they represent by far the largest fraction of the cortical expanse: visual cortex, auditory cortex and somatic sensory cortex together account for only about a fourth of the total. More advanced stages of processing presumably are embodied in association cortex. For example, there are places where the auditory and the visual converge. It is now known that the march of neural processing through the neocortex typically involves a sequence of association areas, and that a destination of the march seems invariably to be the hippocampus or the amygdala, or both.

In 1870 Gustav Theodor Fritsch and Eduard Hitzig published a report that electric current of minimal strength, applied to an area of the neocortex immediately in front of what is called the central sulcus, would elicit twitchings of skeletal (as opposed to visceral) musculature on the side of the body opposite the site of stimulation. Often it was the hand or foot that moved. This discovery, perhaps the first suggestion of a functional compartmentalization in the cerebral cortex, aroused an enduring interest in the organization of those parts of the brain involved in effector (or motor) functions. After all, here was a motor cortex: a circumscribed place at the highest level of the brain that plainly was implicated in bodily movement. Perhaps a purely motoric organization could now be dissected out, so to speak, throughout the brain and spinal cord.

So began the quest for the "motor system," a vague term designating not only the motor neurons governing the skeletal musculature but also the neural channels that converge on motor neurons. The quest continues to this day, and one may fairly ask whether it can ever be completed. Consider area 19, a band of neocortex distinct in cell architecture from neighboring zones and situated not far from the visual cortex. When area 19 is stimulated electrically in an experimental animal, the eyes of the animal turn in unison to the contra-

lateral side, that is, the gaze moves to an alignment directed away from the side of the brain receiving the electric current. It is therefore tempting to call area 19 a "motor" area. To do so, however, would be arbitrary, because from another point of view area 19 is sensory: it is known to reprocess information that has passed through the visual cortex. A similar example is associated with the auditory sensorium: there is a locus designated area 22, near the auditory cortex proper, where electrical stimulation will again cause the animal to turn its eyes to the contralateral side. Yet area 22 stands in synaptic relation to the auditory cortex much as area 19 does to the visual cortex.

The lesson is that no line can be drawn between a sensory side and a motor side in the organization of the brain. To put it another way, all neural structures are involved in the programming and guidance of an organism's behavior. Surely that is in essence the function of the nervous system, and the reason evolution has favored its development. Of course, some structures lie within the great intermediate net in a way that encourages their identification as sensory; the lateral geniculate body of the thalamus is an example. To other structures, situated not too many synapses away from motor neurons, one is tempted to apply the

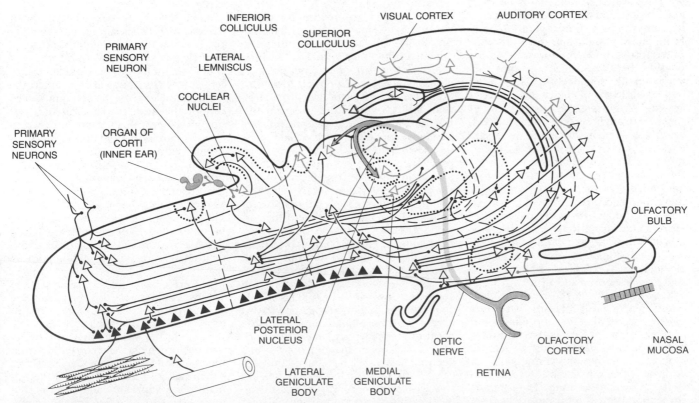

THREE SENSORIA (hearing, vision and olfaction) send their information to the cerebral cortex in different ways. The pathways for hearing pass successively through the cochlear nuclei of the hindbrain, the inferior colliculus of the midbrain and the medial geniculate body of the thalamus before they reach the auditory area of the cerebral cortex. The pathways for vision begin in the retina (which is actually a part of the brain) and then enter two different channels: one traveling by way of the lateral geniculate body in the thalamus to the visual cortex, the other projecting by way of the superior colliculus in the midbrain to a way station in the thalamus and then to a cortical area near the visual cortex. In the olfactory system the receptor neurons in the nasal mucosa project without the mediation of the thalamus to the olfactory bulb, which is a part of the cerebral cortex. The olfactory bulb then projects in turn to the olfactory cortex proper.

label motor. That, however, is the only way in which either of these labels can reasonably be employed. Accordingly it may be best to explore the motor aspects of the central nervous system by beginning at the level of the motor neuron, which is unequivocally a part of the motor system by anyone's definition, and then attempting to trace into the brain the lines that play on it. Be aware, though, that following this strategy means moving upstream: against the prevailing direction of neural traffic.

The first step "upward" from the motor neuron is in general a short one, since the strongest force acting to guide a typical motor neuron seems to emanate from a pool of cells that usually are smaller and usually are nearby. Let us call the sum of all motor neurons and their guiding neuronal pools the "lower motor system," and let us divide this system into functional subunits, each called a "local motor apparatus," that correspond to the parts of the body: the arms, the legs, the eyes and so on. Each local motor apparatus is, it seems, a kind of file room in which blueprints, each one representing a possible movement of a particular body part, are stored. The brain, with its descending fiber systems, reaches down and selects the appropriate blueprint.

What, then, are the sources of the descending systems? What influences the local motor apparatus? Motor neurons lie within the spinal cord and the hindbrain and the midbrain; there are none in the forebrain. Here, however, we can consider only the projections that converge on the spinal cord. They originate at all levels of the central nervous system. Within the cord itself many of them originate in secondary sensory cell groups, or even, in the case of monosynaptic reflex arcs, as the collaterals of certain primary sensory fibers. Within the rhombencephalon the projections originate mainly in the inner two-thirds of the rhombencephalic reticular formation, a district known as the magnocellular reticular formation in recognition of its content of large and very large neuronal cell bodies. Within the mesencephalon the projections originate in the superior colliculus and also in a large cell mass called the red nucleus. Generally speaking, all three of these fiber systems descending into the spinal cord (reticulospinal, tectospinal and rubrospinal tracts by name) must be seen as bearing information—commands, if you wish—that may have antecedents in wide regions of the brain. The superior colliculus receives input not only from the optic nerve but also from large areas of the cerebral cortex, including the visual cortex and much else. The red nucleus receives input primarily from the cerebellum and the motor cortex.

As for the reticular formation, it is particularly notable as a place of convergence for information of widespread origin. We suggested this above, of course, when we were speaking of ascending systems; it also applies here, in a context of descent. A neuron that represents it appears in the illustration on page 51; it is modeled on neurons whose electrical activity was recorded by Giuseppe Moruzzi of the University of Pisa and others. It lies in the rhombencephalic reticular formation, and it will respond, it seems, to inputs from a secondary sensory cell group in the spinal cord. A flash of light, however, may also provoke it, because a report of that event could conceivably reach the reticular formation by a descending path originating in the superior colliculus. Further still, the cell may respond to a message from the cerebellum, or from the neocortex, or from the mesencephalic reticular formation. In short, a large number of heterogeneous inputs converge on the cell. Clearly the reticular formation must integrate this vast variety of neural afflux, ascending and descending in the brain, and then it may dispatch impulses over reticulospinal fibers that terminate on spinal intermediate neurons, or even, although infrequently, on motor neurons directly. Perhaps the reader will hear again the outcry of the electrical engineer that the reticular formation makes no engineering sense.

It now remains to superimpose on the encephalospinal systems of the hindbrain and midbrain the descending systems that have their origin in the forebrain. In the first place essentially all areas of the neocortex project to the striatum, the outer zone of the corpus striatum. The layout is a topographical one: the somatic sensory cortex projects to a striatal district distinct from that receiving the visual projection, or the auditory projection, or the projections from the association areas or from the motor cortex. From the striatum a massive projection converges on the globus pallidus (or pallidum), the inner division of the corpus striatum. There are many fewer neurons in the globus pallidus than there are in the striatum, so that this system must be seen as a kind of funneling.

From the globus pallidus the path continues downward in a fiber bundle called the ansa lenticularis, downward except for a curious exception: a large part of the ansa lenticularis curves back on itself and enters the upper part of the ventral nucleus. We have noted that this cell mass of the thalamus receives the two great somatic sensory lemnisci, the medial lemniscus and the spinothalamic tract, and that it projects to the somatic sensory cortex. Only the posterior part of the ventral nucleus, however, is a somatic sensory way station. The more forward part of the same cell group receives two large systems: the ansa lenticu-

ularis and the cerebellum's upward projection, the brachium conjunctivum. It too projects to neocortex, not to any sensory area but to the motor cortex.

Pathologies that disrupt this curious looping circuitry cause great havoc in bodily movements. One such pathology involves an input to the striatum that does not come from the cerebral cortex. It comes from a cell group in the midbrain whose neurons are pigmented; in man they are black even in unstained preparations. For that reason the cell group became known late in the 18th century as the substantia nigra, the black substance. Extensive loss of the black-pigmented neurons causes the disorder of movement known as Parkinsonism. It is characterized by a muscular rigidity that greatly hampers movement and is betrayed by, among other things, a masklike face. There is also a peculiar tremor, of low frequency and almost rotatory, that affects the arms and hands. The patient's first complaint, however, is typically that he has difficulty initiating the movements he intends to make. He may want to adjust his clothing, but somehow he cannot start.

The corpus striatum can therefore be considered an important influence on bodily movement. To speak more broadly it can be regarded as one among the large number of brain structures whose output seems channeled toward motor neurons. Yet the remarkable fact remains that the corpus striatum cannot directly affect such neurons, or even directly affect the neuronal pools that act as their gatekeepers. We have just seen that a part of its outgoing tract, the ansa lenticularis, turns upward and enters the ventral nucleus of the thalamus. The rest of the ansa lenticularis continues downward past this turning but goes no farther than the caudal limit of the midbrain, where a single neuron in the illustration [p.51] symbolizes a group of several thousand neurons composing the pedunculopontine nucleus. It is a part of the mesencephalic reticular formation. From here the descending path becomes vague. The reticular formation is a site of formidable difficulty in both anatomical and functional analysis.

The projections from the neocortex to the striatum are by no means the only corticofugal fibers. As we have noted, some of the neocortical outflow terminates in the various thalamic nuclei and reciprocates the projections from the thalamus to the neocortex. Some penetrates into the midbrain, to terminate in the superior colliculus, the red nucleus and the mesencephalic reticular formation. Still another contingent, arising from all parts of the neocortex, makes its synapses in the pons, a district of the hindbrain, which projects in turn to the cerebellum. The remaining corticofugal fibers, the ones that extend beyond the pons, originate mostly in the motor cortex. Some of them will reach no farther than the rhombencephalic reticular formation; others will attain all levels of the spinal cord.

These latter fibers, which compose the corticospinal tract, are particularly noteworthy. It is remarkable in itself that they travel from the cortex to the spinal cord, since fibers descending from the corpus striatum get no farther than the midbrain. It also is remarkable that an estimated 5 percent of the corticospinal fibers synapse directly on motor neurons. That is a formidable bypass; these fibers not only enter the spinal cord but also avoid the neuronal pools of the local motor apparatus. It turns out that they synapse preferentially on the motor neurons that animate the musculature of the extremities. Doubtless the existence of the corticospinal tract accounts for the observation that of all the areas of the cerebral cortex the motor cortex needs the least electrical stimulation to elicit experimental bodily movement. The explanation is that of all the areas of the cerebral cortex the motor cortex lies the fewest synapses away from motor neurons.

The motor system almost defies examination from the standpoint of volitional behavior, as opposed to nonvolitional. Consider a humiliating experience common among tennis players. The player makes a brilliant return and feels elated. Then he decides it was simply a fluke; the next time a tennis ball rushes at him with a similar trajectory he will probably hit it badly. It is true that a difficult volitional movement has been performed successfully, but does the person who performed it deserve any credit?

In spite of the enigma of volitional control, the subjective experience of volition has given a name to the motor system that innervates skeletal musculature: it is the voluntary, or somatic, nervous system, as distinguished from the involuntary, or autonomic, nervous system that innervates glands and the smooth musculature of the viscera. A misunderstanding is implicit in this latter nomenclature, however, just as surely as one was implicit in the former. It has to do with the term "autonomic," which means "self-governing." The autonomic nervous system is not self-governing at all. Its functions are integrated with voluntary movements no less than with motivations and affects. In short, its roots are in the brain: one's experiences from moment to moment dictate not only the contractions of one's skeletal muscles but also large functional shifts in the body's internal organs. The term autonomic has nonetheless won out in the English-speaking world. Other languages use other terms. In German one speaks of *das viszerale Nervensystem,* in French of *le système nerveux végétatif.*

The autonomic periphery is suggested in the illustration on page 52 by a tube-like hollow organ, perhaps the intestinal tract or the urinary bladder or a bronchus or an artery; all are in essence tubelike structures whose width is determined by one or more coatings of smooth musculature. The motor innervation of such muscle tissue (or of gland) employs two neurons. The first neuron lies within the central nervous system. It entrains a rather thin axon that synapses in the periphery on a second neuron, which is often situated in a ganglion. The second neuron in turn sends its axon to terminate in the visceral effector tissue.

Within the brain neurons that specifically affect the activity of the autonomic nervous system appear to be concentrated in the hypothalamus. The evidence is clear: When the hypothalamus of almost any animal, emphatically including man, is suddenly destroyed, its possessor dies, with upheavals in what Claude Bernard called the internal milieu, a term embracing tissue fluids and organ functions, as determined by blood

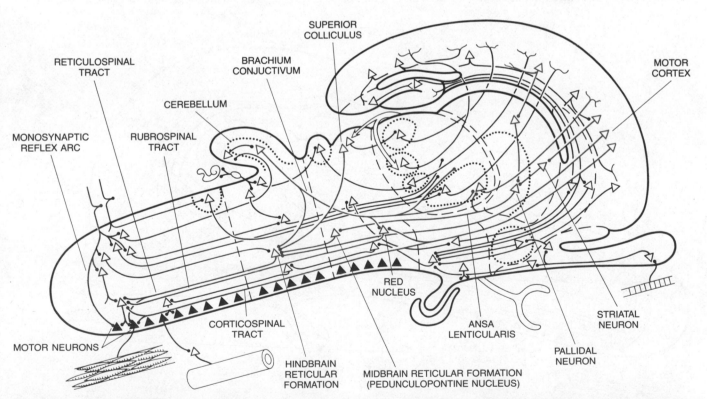

MOTOR NEURONS of the brain and spinal cord (*solid triangles*) receive information from highly convergent channels. Here motor neurons are shown receiving input from a primary sensory neuron, from a secondary sensory cell group in the spinal cord, from the reticular formation of the brain stem, from the red nucleus of the midbrain and from the motor cortex of the forebrain. The red nucleus and the reticular formation receive inputs from a variety of sources. One example of convergence on the motor neurons is particularly striking: the entire neocortex, which includes auditory, visual, somatic sensory and motor fields and other fields as well, sends projections to the corpus striatum. This cell mass projects its fibers in turn to the reticular formation, which ultimately acts on motor neurons. A second pathway from the corpus striatum serves as a feedback loop: it sends its fibers to a part of the thalamus that projects back again to the motor cortex.

pressure, heart rate, respiration rate and so on. Neurosurgeons obliged to operate near the hypothalamus therefore are always concerned lest the structure be so much as buffeted. Indeed, patients have died of hyperthermia (an acute rise in body temperature) after otherwise successful brain surgery in which caution about injuring the hypothalamus seems to have been exemplary. On the other hand, when a massive lesion of the hypothalamus develops slowly, perhaps in the form of a slow-growing tumor, there may be no dramatic effects at all. It is as if there were a chain of command in the autonomic nervous system, or, as Bernard put it, an automatism of levels: when the hypothalamus is slowly incapacitated, regions of the brain below the hypothalamus can keep the internal milieu stable, albeit within narrow limits.

All of this accords well with what is known about the autonomic circuitry. Fibers passing without interruption from the hypothalamus to the autonomic motor neurons of the spinal cord's gray matter have recently been found, but they seem to constitute a small minority of the outgoing hypothalamic fibers; the hypothalamus has nothing like a corticospinal tract to carry its downflowing output. Instead it appears in large measure to project no farther than the midbrain, where neurons of the reticular formation take over. In

fact, the pathways descending to autonomic motor neurons typically are interrupted at numerous levels. At each such interruption various further instructions can enter the descending conduction lines. It is appropriate that this should be the case. Life depends on the innervation of the viscera; in a way all the rest is biological luxury. And vital systems ought to be organized on the principle that no single excitation should greatly affect their workings. Indeed, the convergence of information on motor neurons may be as characteristic of the autonomic nervous system as it is of the somatic.

So much for the descending neural influences that ultimately act on the effector tissues of the viscera. What acts to set these influences? More specifically, what projects to the hypothalamus? The illustration below shows an input that originates in a cell of the mesencephalic reticular formation, a cell whose own input derives from a fiber of the spinothalamic tract. The supposition is that in such fashion the hypothalamus may monitor the state of the internal milieu. Beyond that the search for input to the hypothalamus leads one deep into a realm of brain tissue implicated in affect and motivation, a realm in which epileptic seizures, for example, include among their signs a change in mood, sometimes to anguish or an unreasoning fear. This should not be surprising. Af-

ter all, affect and motivation find observable expression in visceral and endocrine changes.

There can be little doubt, then, that the major influence exerted on the hypothalamus from the cerebral hemisphere derives from the hippocampus and the amygdala. They share this influence with few other parts of the cerebral hemisphere. For that reason a collective reference to hippocampus and amygdala is justified: they are the two principal components of what is called the limbic system. In the illustration below note the presence of a two-way fiber system that curves along the edge of the neocortex from the hippocampus to the hypothalamus. The bundle is the fornix. It marks the free edge of the cerebral mantle. In both the cat and the monkey approximately two-thirds of the bundle's fibers leaving the hippocampus extend into the hypothalamus directly. The remaining third establish their synapses in the septum, from which, as the illustration shows, the lines are extended, again to the hypothalamus.

We have noted that the hippocampus is a destination for sequential projections that span the neocortical sheet. It therefore becomes apparent in the tracing of visceral motor governance, as it did in the tracing of somatic, that when the tracing is done countercurrent, against the direction of impulse

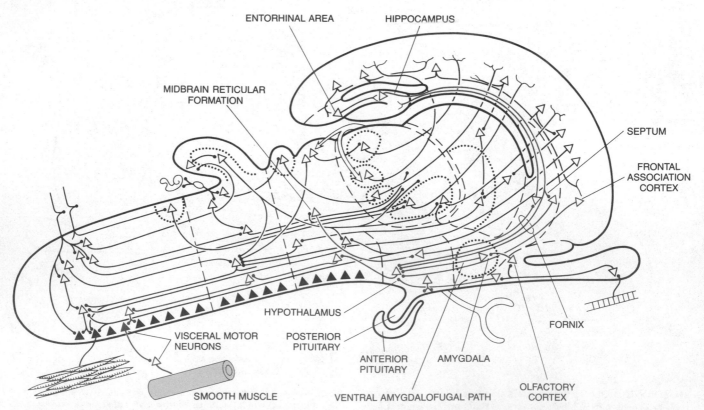

LOOPING CIRCUITS center on the hypothalamus, which regulates the activities of glands and smooth muscle (such as the involuntary muscle of the viscera) through the autonomic nervous system and the pituitary complex. The hypothalamus receives projections from the hippocampus and the amygdala, which are the principal components of what is known as the limbic system. Input to the hypothalamus also derives from the reticular formation. A further source of input is the frontal cortex, in the most forward part of the cerebral hemispheres. The limbic system is the destination for pathways from the cerebral cortex, including direct projections from olfactory cortex.

transmission, one implicates ever greater portions of the great intermediate net. Of course, there is a difference. From a given area of neocortex, say the primary visual cortex, the road to the hippocampus must pass, with interruption, through a series of intermediate neocortical fields. The end of the neocortical road is the entorhinal area, a region of the cerebral cortex adjoining the hippocampus and intermediate in structure between it and neocortex. From here a final link completes the fiber pathways to the hippocampus. In contrast, the road to the striatum from any neocortical field whatsoever is an uninterrupted projection.

Consider next the amygdala. Although its cell architecture is quite different from that of the hippocampus, it too directs its outflow in large part to the hypothalamus. For its part the amygdala is the recipient of fibers from a district of neocortex synaptically remote from any primary sensory field. It is also, however, the recipient of fibers that originate in the olfactory cortex; indeed, so is the entorhinal area. Moreover, a part of the amygdala receives fibers from the olfactory bulb. In olfaction, therefore, the transmission of sensory data to the limbic system is remarkably direct. Why should this be so? Why should olfaction, among all the sensoria, be privileged?

One conceivable answer lies in the probability that the olfactory sensorium constitutes the earliest appearance in evolution of a capacity for sensory apprehension at a distance; it is perhaps the earliest system whereby free-ranging organisms could track sources of food and identify members of their own species and members of others. Perhaps the olfactory system, having arrived earliest, made some rather direct connections. A second conceivable answer, which does not negate the first, is that the visual recognition of an object (to take only one example) calls for complicated processing: in its highest form it requires that the arriving sensory data be made to yield a representation free from the circumstances of viewing angle, distance and illumination. How else could the object be recognized, that is, matched with past experience? Even at its simplest, say the recognition of a stripe (as by one fish viewing the flank of another) or of a moving dot (as by a frog viewing a fly), it requires the preservation well into the neural processing of topological relations in the input to the sensory sheet: the retina. Olfaction, in contrast, functions simply as a discriminator of intensity gradients. In short, olfaction as a guide to life-supporting behavior lacks much of the computational difficulty, if you will, that is inherent in vision and other sensoria.

To be sure, arguments such as these may not seem entirely convincing. If the limbic system requires of the visual, the auditory and the somatic sensoria a neocortical march, and therefore a cascading re-representation of data that originally were sensory, then why not, to an equal degree, the striatum? And why, moreover, does the striatum receive input both from the primary sensory fields and from the various association areas, in which the primary cortical data undergo successive transformations? Perhaps the heart of the difficulty is the mystery of any brain structure whose input derives, one way or another, from all (or most of) the neocortical expanse. To glibly characterize such input seems impossible, and so it is beyond us to imagine what the structure that gets it is doing with it. Yet we are presented by the central nervous system with several such structures: the limbic system, the striatum, the pons (and through it the cerebellum) and the superior colliculus.

Our survey of the mammalian central nervous system is here at its end. Its shortcomings are necessarily many. In the first place it could do little justice to the true complexity of the circuitry; if all the known systems of conduction had been mentioned, the illustrations for the article might have been rendered a hopeless tangle. For example, we left out the pons, even though that structure receives massive projections from all parts of the neocortex and sends a massive projection to the cerebellum. The lines representing those projections would have cut across several ascending and descending systems in the hindbrain.

In the second place we could make few distinctions between projections comprising millions of fibers and those comprising only a fraction of that number. It happens, for example, that the spinothalamic fibers attaining the ventral nucleus of the thalamus may number no more than a few hundred in primates, whereas the medial lemniscus has a million fibers, maybe more. Then too we could give no indication of which projections cross the midplane to the opposite side of the central nervous system and which have destinations on the same side as their origin. The central nervous system, like the rest of the body, is bilaterally symmetrical. Such distinctions play a crucial role in clinical diagnosis.

Most important, in addressing only the connectedness of the brain—that is to say, only the origins and destinations of the various fiber systems—we can evoke no more than a rough sketch of neuroanatomy: the three-dimensional architecture of the tissues stationed inside the cranium and down the core of the vertebral column. We have thereby neglected a view that has tantalized men for millenniums: the very appearance of the brain.

V

The Development
of the Brain

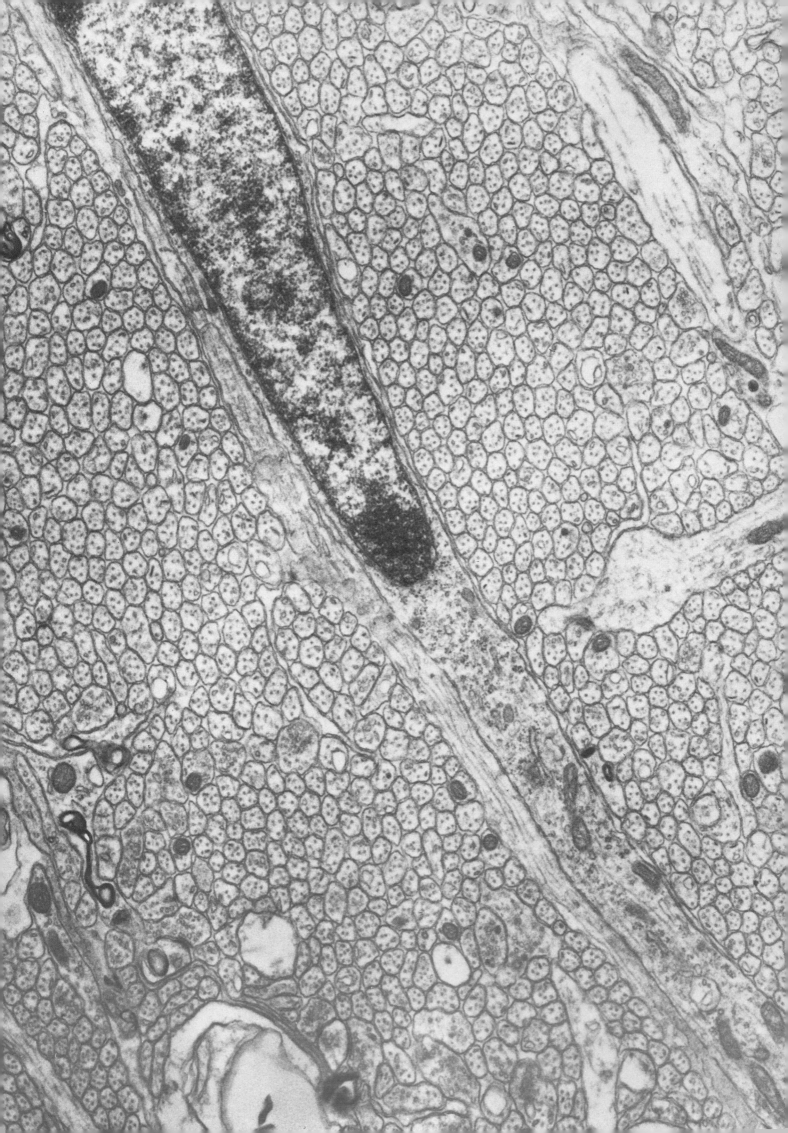

The Development of the Brain

BY W. MAXWELL COWAN

As the human brain develops in utero it gains neurons at the rate of hundreds of thousands a minute. One problem of neurobiology is how the neurons find their place and make the right connections

The gross changes that take place during the embryonic and fetal development of the brain have been known for almost a century, but comparatively little is known about the underlying cellular events that give rise to the particular parts of the brain and their interconnections. What is clear is that the nervous system originates as a flat sheet of cells on the dorsal surface of the developing embryo (the neural plate), that this tissue subsequently folds into an elongated hollow structure (the neural tube) and that from the head end of the tube three prominent swellings emerge, prefiguring the three main parts of the brain (the forebrain, the midbrain and the hindbrain).

It is not on these changes in the external form of the developing brain, however, that the attention of developmental neurobiologists has focused in recent years. More interesting questions intrude. How, for instance, are the various components that constitute the major parts of the nervous system generated? How do they come to occupy their definitive locations within the brain? How do the neurons and their supporting glial cells become differentiated? How do neurons in different parts of the brain establish connections with one another? In spite of a great deal of research effort it is still not possible to give a complete account of the development of any part of the brain, let alone of the brain as a whole. By determining what the main events in neural development are, however, one can begin to see how the critical issues are likely to be resolved.

Eight major stages can be identified in the development of any part of the brain. In the order of their appearance they are (1) the induction of the neural plate, (2) the localized proliferation of cells in different regions, (3) the migration of cells from the region in which they are generated to the places where they finally reside, (4) the aggregation of cells to form identifiable parts of the brain, (5) the differentiation of the immature neurons, (6) the formation of connections with other neurons, (7) the selective death of certain cells and (8) the elimination of some of the connections that were initially formed and the stabilization of others.

The process whereby some cells in the ectoderm, or outer layer, of the developing embryo become transformed into the specialized tissue from which the brain and spinal cord develop is called neural induction. It has been known since the 1920's that the critical event in neural induction is an interaction of the ectoderm and a part of the underlying layer of tissue called the mesoderm. The nature of this interaction remains to be elucidated, but there are good reasons for thinking that it involves the specific transfer of substances from the mesoderm to the ectoderm, and that as a result of that transfer the generalized tissue of the ectoderm becomes irreversibly committed to the formation of neural tissue. It is also clear that the sequential interaction of different parts of the ectoderm and the mesoderm results in the regional determination of the major parts of the future brain and spinal cord. The first part of the mesoderm to become associated with the ectoderm specifically induces forebrain structures, the next part leads to the formation of midbrain and hindbrain structures, and the last part to grow under the ectoderm is responsible for the later formation of the spinal cord.

Exactly how these regional determinations are brought about remains baffling. Experiments with disaggregated ectodermal and mesodermal cells from embryos of the appropriate age suggest that the critical element may be the relative concentration of two factors that are thought to be proteins with a low molecular weight. One of these, the neuralizing factor, seems to "prime" the ectoderm and to ensure its future neural character; the other, the mesodermalizing factor, appears in differing concentrations to determine the regional differences within the ectoderm.

Although a major effort was made in the 1930's and 1940's to isolate the putative inducing agents, it is clear in retrospect that much of the work was premature. Only in the past two decades has anything substantial been learned about the nature of gene induction generally, and it is still far from evident that the inductive mechanisms that have been identified in microorganisms operate in the same way in animal cells. There is another reason the problem of neural induction has proved to be so intractable. The only assay system suitable for the study of neural induction is ectoderm taken from embryos of the appropriate age, and since there is a limited period in development when the ectoderm is able to respond to the relevant inductive signals, it is necessary to work with extremely small amounts of tissue. Indeed, it is a tribute to the ingenuity and experimental skill of those who have addressed this problem that so much progress has already been made.

Once the major regions of the developing nervous system have been determined their potentialities become progressively limited as development pro-

MIGRATION OF A YOUNG NEURON from its birthplace deep in the cerebellum of a fetal monkey toward its final destination closer to the outer surface of the developing brain is captured in the electron micrograph on the opposite page, made by Pasko Rakic of the Yale University School of Medicine. The migrating neuron is the broader of the two diagonal bands running all the way across the micrograph from the top left to the bottom right; the dark, oblong object inside the upper part of this band is the nucleus of the nerve cell. The lighter, narrower band along the underside of the neuron is the elongated process of a glial cell, which serves both as a supporting structure and as a guide for the migrating neuron. The neuron travels through a dense neuropile, or feltwork of nerve fibers, which run in various directions. (Most of the circular structures in this view, for example, are the cross sections of axons that run more or less at right angles to the plane of the page.) Although the migrating neuron is therefore in contact with thousands of other cellular processes, it remains intimately associated with the glial cell along its entire length. This section of brain tissue is magnified about 25,000 diameters.

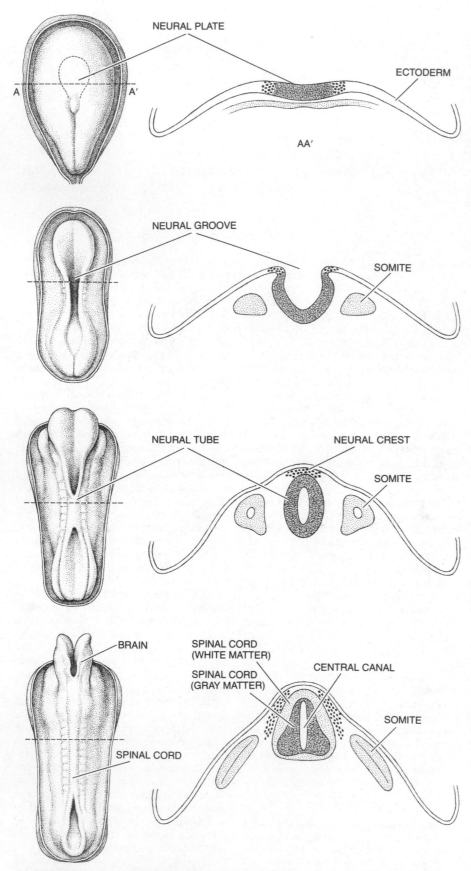

NEURAL PLATE

ECTODERM

A — A'

AA'

NEURAL GROOVE

SOMITE

NEURAL TUBE

NEURAL CREST

SOMITE

BRAIN

SPINAL CORD
(WHITE MATTER)

SPINAL CORD
(GRAY MATTER)

CENTRAL CANAL

SOMITE

SPINAL CORD

GENESIS OF THE NERVOUS SYSTEM from the ectoderm, or outer cell layer, of a human embryo during the third and fourth weeks after conception is represented in these four pairs of drawings, which show both an external view of the developing embryo (*left*) and a corresponding cross-sectional view at about the middle of the future spinal cord (*right*). The central nervous system begins as the neural plate, a flat sheet of ectodermal cells on the dorsal surface of the embryo. The plate subsequently folds into a hollow structure called the neural tube. The head end of the central canal widens to form the ventricles, or cavities, of the brain. The peripheral nervous system is derived largely from the cells of the neural crest and from motor-nerve fibers that leave the lower part of the brain at each segment of the future spinal cord.

ceeds. For example, the entire head end of the neural plate initially constitutes a forebrain-eye field from which both the forebrain and the neural part of the eye develop. If one removes a small piece of ectodermal tissue at this stage, the defect is quickly replaced by the proliferation of the neighboring cells, and the development of both the forebrain and the eye proceeds quite normally. If the same operation is done at a slightly later stage, there is a permanent defect in either the forebrain or the eye, depending on the location of the piece of tissue that was removed. In other words, at this later stage it is possible to identify a forebrain field that will give rise to definitive forebrain structures, and an eye field that will form only the neural part of the eye.

At still later stages specific regions of the forebrain become delimited within the overall forebrain field. With the aid of a variety of cell-marking techniques it has been possible to construct "fate maps" that define rather precisely the final distribution of the cells in each part of the early forebrain field [*see illustration on page 60*]. The factors that lead to this progressive blocking out of smaller and smaller units, giving rise to specific parts of the brain, are not known, but it is not unreasonable to suppose that when more is learned about cellular differentiation in general, the problem will be clarified.

From studies of the embryos of amphibians it appears that the number of cells in the neural plate is comparatively small (on the order of 125,000) and that this number does not change much during the formation of the neural tube. Once the neural tube has been closed off, however, cell proliferation proceeds at a brisk pace, and before long the simple layer of epithelial cells that formed the neural plate is transformed into a rather thick epithelial layer in which the cell nuclei reside at several levels. Microscopic examination of the cells, aided in some cases by the use of radioactively labeled thymidine, a specific DNA precursor, has established that all the cells in the wall of the neural tube are capable of proliferation and that the characteristic "pseudostratified" appearance of the epithelium is attributable to the fact that the nuclei of the cells are at different levels. The nuclei synthesize DNA while they lie in the depths of the epithelium, and then they migrate toward the ventricular surface and withdraw their peripheral processes before dividing. After mitosis (cell division) the daughter cells re-form their peripheral processes, and their nuclei return to the deeper part of the epithelium before reentering the mitotic cycle. The migration of the nuclei of proliferating neurons is characteristic of epithelial cells of this kind.

After the cells pass through a number

of such cycles (the number varies from region to region and from population to population within any one region) they apparently lose their capacity for synthesizing DNA, and they migrate out of the epithelium to form a second cellular layer adjacent to the ventricular zone. The cells that constitute this mantle, or intermediate, layer are young neurons, which never again divide, and glial-cell precursors, which retain their capacity for proliferation throughout life.

Although it is not known what turns the proliferative mechanism on and off in any region of the nervous system, it is clear that the relative times at which different populations of cells cease dividing is rigidly determined, and there is now a sizable body of evidence to suggest that this is a critical stage in the life of all neurons. Not only does the withdrawal of a cell from the mitotic cycle seem to trigger its subsequent migration into the intermediate layer but also the

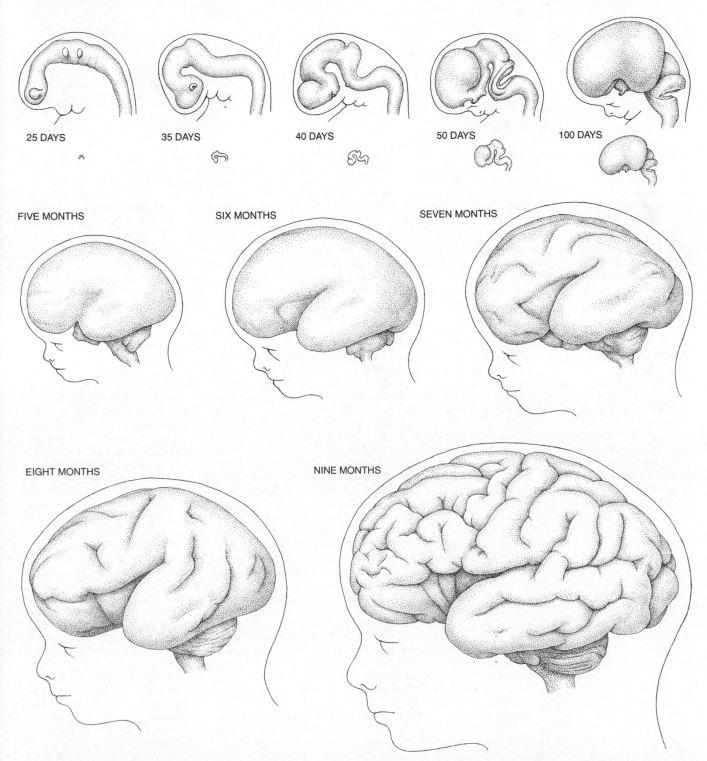

25 DAYS

35 DAYS

40 DAYS

50 DAYS

100 DAYS

FIVE MONTHS

SIX MONTHS

SEVEN MONTHS

EIGHT MONTHS

NINE MONTHS

DEVELOPING HUMAN BRAIN is viewed from the side in this sequence of drawings, which show a succession of embryonic and fetal stages. The drawings in the main sequence (*bottom*) are all reproduced at the same scale: approximately four-fifths life-size. The first five embryonic stages are also shown enlarged to an arbitrary common size to clarify their structural details (*top*). The three main parts of the brain (the forebrain, the midbrain and the hindbrain) originate as prominent swellings at the head end of the early neural tube. In human beings the cerebral hemispheres eventually overgrow the midbrain and the hindbrain and also partly obscure the cerebellum. The characteristic convolutions and invaginations of the brain's surface do not begin to appear until about the middle of pregnancy. Assuming that the fully developed human brain contains on the order of 100 billion neurons and that virtually no new neurons are added after birth, it can be calculated that neurons must be generated in the developing brain at an average rate of more than 250,000 per minute.

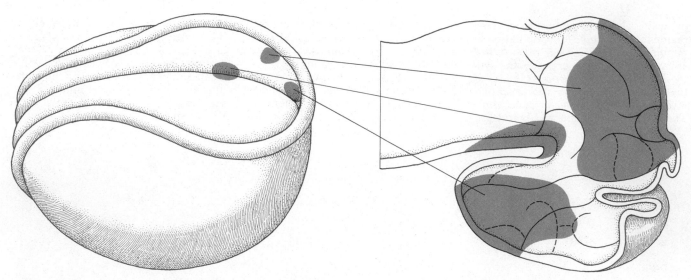

DERIVATION of each of the major regions of the brain can be traced by labeling different regions of the neural plate of an experimental animal at a very early embryonic stage with the aid of a variety of cell-marking techniques. In this demonstration of how such "fate maps" are constructed three regions have been marked on the neural plate of the early embryo of the axolotl, a large amphibian (*left*). The final positions of the cells in the marked regions are then plotted as they would be seen in a sagittal section of the brain at a later stage of embryonic development (*right*). This illustration is adapted from the work of D. C.-O. Jacobson of the University of Uppsala.

cell seems at the same time to acquire a definitive "address," in the sense that if its "birth date" (defined as the time when a cell loses its capacity for DNA synthesis) is known, it is possible to predict where the cell will finally reside. Furthermore, it seems in some cases that the pattern of connections the neuron will ultimately form is also determined at this time.

From experiments in which small amounts of radioactively labeled thymidine have been administered to embryos (or in the case of mammals to their pregnant mothers) investigators now know the birth dates of the cells in many parts of the brain for a number of different species. From these studies it is now possible to make several generalizations about the patterning of cell proliferation in the brain. First, the larger neurons, including most of the cells whose processes extend for considerable distances, such as the cells in the retina that project to the visual centers of the brain, are usually generated earlier than the smaller neurons, whose fibers are confined to the region of the cell body. Second, the sequence of cell proliferation is characteristic for each region of the brain. For example, in the cerebral cortex the first cells to withdraw from the proliferative cycle will in time come to occupy the deepest cortical layer, whereas those that are generated at successively later times form the progressively more superficial layers of the cortex.

On the other hand, in the neural retina (which is actually an extension of the brain) the sequence of cell proliferation is essentially the reverse; the first population of cells to be generated (the ganglion cells) migrates to the most superficial layer of the retina, and subsequent populations of cells occupy progressively deeper layers. In other regions of the

brain the sequences are more complex, but in each region it is evident that cells occupying similar positions are always generated at the same time; conversely, cells generated at different times invariably come to reside in different zones within the region. A third generalization that can be made is that in most parts of the brain the first supporting cells to be formed appear at about the same time as the first neurons, but as a rule the proliferation of glial cells continues for a much longer period.

The number of neurons initially formed in any region of the brain is determined by three factors. The first factor is the duration of the proliferative period as a whole; in the regions that have been studied to date, it has been found to range from a few days to several weeks. The second factor is the duration of the cell cycle; in young embryos it is usually on the order of a few hours, but as development progresses it may become as long as four or five days. The third factor is the number of precursor cells from which the neuronal population is derived.

A number of methods are now available for determining the duration of the proliferative period and the length of the cell cycle, but except in a few cases it is not possible to estimate the size of the precursor pool of cells. Part of the reason for this difficulty is that it is impossible at present to follow the fate of individual cells in the developing mammalian brain, as has been done in the much simpler nervous systems of certain invertebrates. In these organisms the embryos are often quite transparent, and individual cells can be followed through several mitotic divisions with the aid of a light microscope equipped with differential-interference optics. Alternatively, the precursor cells in such organisms

may be so large that they can be readily labeled by the intracellular injection of marker molecules such as horseradish peroxidase; if the marker is not degraded, it can be distributed to all the cell's progeny, at least over several cell generations.

Since most neurons are generated in or close to the ventricular lining of the neural tube and finally come to rest at some distance from this layer, they have to go through at least one phase of migration after withdrawing from the proliferative cycle. There are a few situations in which cells migrate away from the ventricular zone but continue to proliferate. This is usually observed in a special region found between the ventricular and the intermediate zone, known as the subventricular zone. This layer, which is particularly prominent in the forebrain, gives rise to many of the smaller neurons in some of the deep structures of the cerebral hemisphere (the basal ganglia), to certain small cortical neurons and to many of the glial cells in the cerebral cortex and the underlying white matter. In the hindbrain some of the cells in the corresponding subventricular region undergo a second migration under the surface of the developing cerebellum, where they set up a special proliferative zone known as the external granular layer. In the human brain proliferation in this layer continues for several weeks and gives rise to most of the interneurons in the cerebellar cortex, including the billions of granule cells that are a distinctive feature of the cerebellum. With these and a few other exceptions, most migrations of neurons involve the movement of postmitotic cells.

The process of neuronal migration appears in most cases to be amoeboid.

The migrating cells extend a leading process that attaches itself to some appropriate substrate; the nucleus flows or is drawn into the process, and the trailing process behind the nucleus is then withdrawn. It is a fairly slow procedure, the average rate of migration being on the order of a tenth of a millimeter per day. In a few cases the cell as a whole does not migrate. Instead it begins to form some of its processes at an early stage in its development, and later the cell body begins to move progressively farther away from the first processes, which remain essentially where they originated.

Since neurons often migrate over considerable distances, it would be interesting to know to what types of directional cue they respond. In particular, how do they know when to stop migrating and to begin aggregating with other neurons of the same kind? It has been known for some time that there are specialized glial cells within the developing brain whose cell bodies lie inside the ventricular zone and whose processes extend radially to the surface. Since these cells appear at an early stage of development and persist until some time after neuronal migration has ceased, it has been suggested that they might provide an appropriate scaffolding along which the migrating neurons might move. Certainly in electron micrographs of most parts of the developing brain the migrating cells are almost invariably found to be closely associated with the neighboring glial processes. This relation has led Pasko Rakic of the Yale University School of Medicine to postulate that migrating cells are directed to their definitive locations by such glial processes. In support of this view Rakic and Richard L. Sidman of the Children's Hospital Medical Center in Boston have noted that in one of the most striking genetic mutations affecting the cerebellum of the mouse the radial glial processes degenerate at a comparatively early stage; apparently as a result of this degeneration the migration of most of the granule cells is severely disrupted.

Considering the distances over which many neurons move in the course of development, it is perhaps not surprising that during their migration some cells are misdirected and end up in distinctly abnormal positions. Such neuronal misplacements (termed ectopias) have long been recognized by pathologists as a concomitant of certain gross disorders in brain development, but it is not generally appreciated that even during normal development a proportion of the migrating cells may respond inappropriately to the usual directional cues and end up in aberrant locations. Recent technical advances have made it possible to recognize cells of this kind in several situations, and it is significant that the majority of such misplaced neurons appear to be eliminated during the later

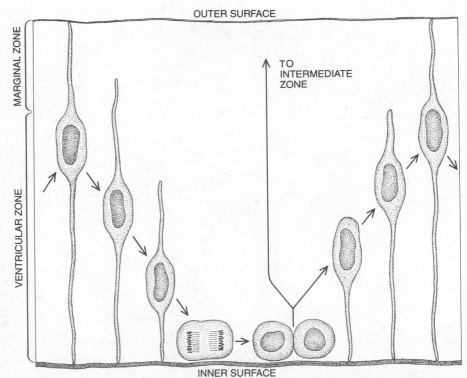

NUCLEI OF NERVE CELLS MIGRATE in the layer of epithelial tissue that forms the wall of the neural tube in the developing embryo, as this multistage schematic diagram shows. When the cells in this layer, called the neuroepithelium or ventricular zone, replicate their DNA, their nuclei migrate toward the inner surface of the epithelium, their peripheral processes become detached from the outermost layer and the cells become rounded before dividing. After mitosis (cell division) the daughter cells either extend a new process so that their nuclei can migrate back to the middle level of the epithelium, or (if the cells have stopped dividing) they migrate out of the epithelium to form part of the intermediate zone in the wall of the brain.

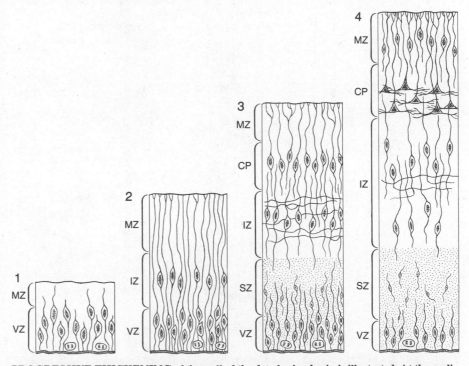

PROGRESSIVE THICKENING of the wall of the developing brain is illustrated. At the earliest stage (1) the wall consists only of a "pseudostratified" epithelium, in which the ventricular zone (VZ) contains the cell bodies and the marginal zone (MZ) contains only the extended outer cell processes. When some of the cells lose their capacity for synthesizing DNA and withdraw from the mitotic cycle (2), they form a second layer, the intermediate zone (IZ). In the forebrain the cells that pass through this zone aggregate to form the cortical plate (CP), the region in which the various layers of the cerebral cortex develop (3). At the latest stage (4) the original ventricular zone remains as the ependymal lining of the cerebral ventricles, and the comparatively cell-free region between this lining and the cortex becomes the subcortical white matter, through which nerve fibers enter and leave the cortex. Subventricular zone (SZ) is a second proliferative region in which many glial cells and some neurons in forebrain are generated.

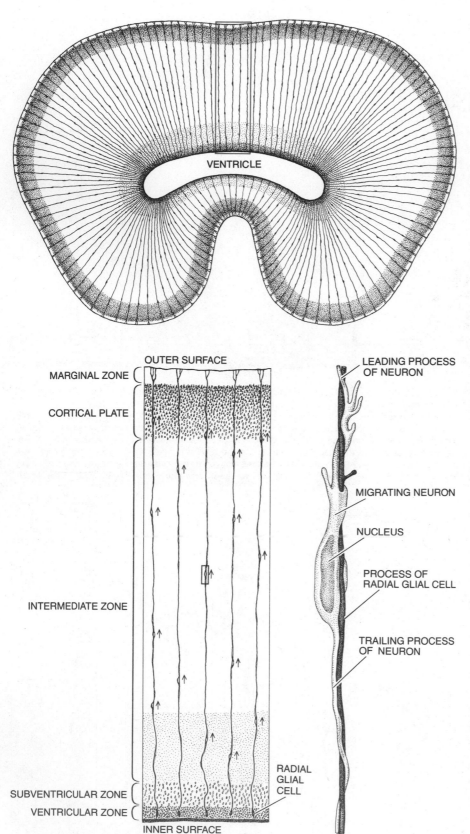

SPECIALIZED SUPPORTING CELLS, the radial glial cells, arise during the early stages of the development of the nervous system. These cells are distinguished by their extremely long processes, which span the entire thickness of the wall of the neural tube and its derivative structures. The drawing at the top shows how the radial glial cells look in a Golgi-stained preparation of a thick transverse section through the wall of the cerebral hemisphere of a fetal monkey. The cell bodies lie in the ventricular zone and their processes extend to the outer surface of the surrounding layers, where they appear to form expanded terminal attachments. An enlarged view of a segment of this transverse section is shown at the bottom left. The small portion of tissue inside the colored rectangle in this enlargement is further magnified in the detailed three-dimensional view at the bottom right, which is based on the microscopic studies of Rakic. This illustration reveals the close relation between the processes of the radial glial cells and the migrating neurons, a relation that is observed in the development of most parts of the brain.

stages of development. In one population of neurons that has been carefully studied from this point of view, about 3 percent of the cells have been found to migrate to some abnormal location; all but a handful of these misplaced neurons, however, degenerate during the later phase of naturally occurring cell death.

When the migrating neurons reach their definitive locations, they generally aggregate with other cells of a similar kind to form either cortical layers or nuclear masses. The tendency of developing cells of the same embryonic origin to selectively adhere to one another was first demonstrated more than 50 years ago, but it is only in the past decade that this subject has attracted the attention it deserves from neuroembryologists. Much of the initial stimulus for the more recent work stemmed from the search for the molecular mechanisms underlying the formation of specific connections between related groups of neurons. Unfortunately that problem has proved to be intractable, but much of the work that was done on it bears directly on the important issue of how discrete populations of neurons are formed in the developing brain.

Perhaps the most important finding to come out of these studies is that when cells from two or three regions of the developing nervous system are dissociated (usually mechanically or by mild chemical treatment), mixed together and then allowed to reaggregate in an appropriate medium, they tend to sort themselves out so that the cells from each region preferentially aggregate with other cells from the same region. This selective adhesiveness seems to be a general property of all living cells and is probably due to the appearance on their surfaces of specific classes of large molecules that serve both to "recognize" cells of the same kind and to bind the cells together. These molecules, which function as ligands between cells, appear to be highly specific for each major type of cell. Moreover, they appear to change in either number or distribution as development proceeds. At present workers in several laboratories are endeavoring to isolate and characterize these and other surface ligands, and it seems likely that this may be the first major problem in neural development to be successfully analyzed at the molecular level.

One special feature of cell aggregation in the developing nervous system is that in most regions of the brain the cells not only adhere to one another but also adopt some preferential orientation. For example, in the cerebral cortex the majority of the large pyramidal neurons are consistently aligned with their prominent apical dendrites directed toward the surface and their axons directed toward the underlying white matter. It is not evident how cells come to be aligned

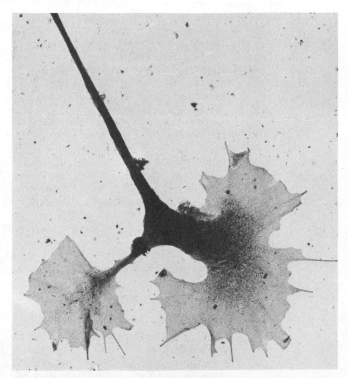 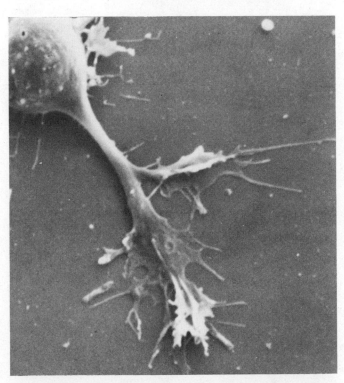

GROWTH CONES (expanded, highly motile structures found at the ends of growing neuronal processes) are seen in these two electron micrographs. The transmission electron micrograph at the left shows a pair of growth cones at the end of an axonlike process of a sympathetic ganglion cell from a rat. The cell had been dissociated and grown in tissue culture, and the process seen here had branched just a few minutes before the cell was fixed and prepared (without sectioning) for viewing in the electron microscope. The fine, fingerlike extensions are filopodia; the flattened veil-like sheets between them are lamellipodia. The scanning electron micrograph at the right shows a growing dendrite of a neuron obtained from the hippocampus of a fetal rat's brain. The growth cones in this surface view were formed after the neuron had been dissociated and grown in tissue culture for only two hours. Both pictures were made at the Washington University School of Medicine, the one at the left by J. Michael Cochran and Mary Bartlett Bunge, the one at the right by Steven R. Rothman.

in this way, but it seems likely that it is attributable either to the existence of different classes of cell-surface molecules specifically concerned with cell-cell orientation or to the selective redistribution of surface molecules responsible for the cell's initial aggregation.

One of the most striking features in the development of neurons is the progressive elaboration of their processes, but this is only one aspect of their differentiation. Equally important are their adoption of a particular mode of transmission (most neurons generate action potentials but some show only decremental transmission) and the selection of one or the other of two modes of interaction with other cells (either by the formation of conventional synapses to provide for the release of a chemical transmitter or by the formation of gap junctions to provide for electrical interactions of cells). Neurobiologists are only now beginning to learn something of these more covert aspects of neuronal differentiation, and it is becoming clear that neurons may be considerably more complex than had been imagined. For example, it has recently been shown that some neurons can switch from one chemical transmitter to another (specifically from norepinephrine to acetylcholine) under the influence of certain environmental factors, whereas others can show a change in the principal ion they

use for the propagation of nerve impulses at different developmental stages (changing, for instance, from calcium to sodium).

Rather more is known about the formation of neuronal processes. Most neurons in the brain of mammals are multipolar, with several tapering dendrites, which generally function as receptive processes, and a single axon, which serves as the cell's main effector process. Although some cells are known to form processes before they start migrating, the majority begin to generate processes only after reaching their final position. Exactly what stimulates the formation of processes is not clear. Studies in which immature neurons have been isolated and maintained in tissue culture reveal that processes are formed only when the cells are able to adhere to an appropriate substrate and that under these conditions the cells are often able to form a fairly normal complement of both dendrites and axons. In some cases, in spite of the highly artificial conditions in which the neurons are grown, the overall appearance of the dendrites that are formed closely resembles that seen in the intact brain, even though the cells are deprived of all contact with other neurons or even glial cells. Observations of this kind suggest that the information required for a neuron to generate its distinctive dendritic branching is genetically determined.

It is also evident, however, that during the normal development of the brain most neurons are subject to a variety of local mechanical influences that may modify their form. Certainly the number and distribution of the inputs the cells receive may critically affect their final shape. A striking example of this effect is seen in the cerebellum. The dendrites of the most distinctive class of neurons in the cerebellar cortex, the Purkinje cells, normally have a characteristic planar arrangement that is oriented at right angles to the axons of the granule cells that constitute their principal input; if for any reason the usual regular arrangement of the granule cells' axons is disrupted, the planar distribution of the dendrites of the Purkinje cells is correspondingly altered.

The actual mechanism by which the processes of a neuron are elongated is now quite well understood. Most processes bear distinctive structures at their growing ends called growth cones. These expanded, highly motile structures, which in the living state seem to be continually exploring their immediate environment, are the sites where most new material is added to the growing process. When a process branches, it almost always does so by the formation of a new growth cone. Although the evidence is largely indirect, there are reasons for thinking the growth cone has encoded within (or on) it the necessary

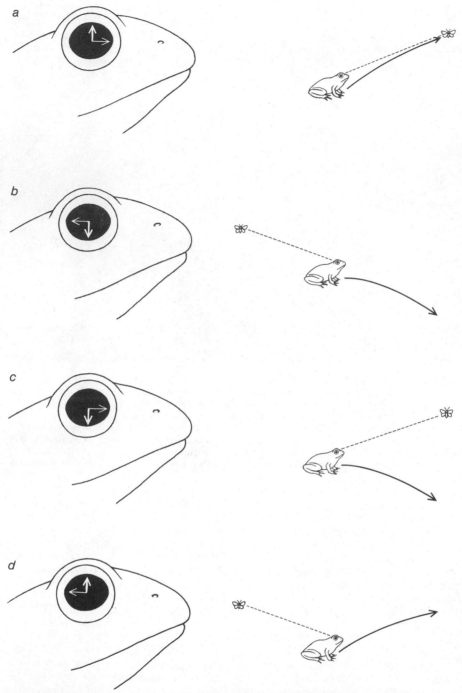

ONE EXPERIMENTAL APPROACH to the study of how neurons make specific patterns of connections in the developing brain involves manipulating the projection of the retina on the optic tectum of the midbrain. In this approach, pioneered by Roger W. Sperry of the California Institute of Technology, the eyes of adult frogs (or tadpoles at various stages in development) are rotated or transplanted. Later, when the optic nerve has regenerated (or when the tadpoles have grown into frogs and the axons of the retinal ganglion cells, which comprise the optic nerve, have made connections in the optic tectum), one can observe what effect the operation has had on the frogs' visual behavior; one can also map the retinal projection on the tectum electrophysiologically. This series of drawings, based on the work of Sperry, shows first the behavior of a control frog with its eyes in the normal positions (a). In experiment b the right eye had been rotated through 180 degrees; when the frog was tested some time after the optic nerve had regenerated, the frog's attempt to strike at a lure placed in its upper field of view was exactly 180 degrees in the wrong direction. In experiment c the left eye had been substituted for the right eye, inverting only the dorsoventral axis (thick arrow); in this case the frog directed its strike forward toward the lure, but in the direction of the lower visual field instead of the upper one. In experiment d a similar transplantation had been done, but this time inverting the eye only in the anteroposterior direction (thin arrow); the frog sensed that the lure was in the upper visual field, but it now struck forward instead of backward. The outcome of these experiments is consistent with the view that during regeneration the fibers of the optic nerve always grow back to the part of the optic tectum they originally innervated, and that during normal development they similarly "find their way" to their correct positions in the tectum. These findings are best explained by the hypothesis that both the retinal ganglion cells and their target neurons in the tectum have chemical characteristics that enable them to identify each other.

molecular features that enable it both to detect appropriate substrates along which to grow and to identify appropriate targets. Experiments in which neurons have been grown on a variety of artificial substrates indicate that most processes grow preferentially along surfaces of high adhesiveness.

One of the least well understood problems in the entire field of developmental neurobiology is how axons are able to find their way. It is particularly difficult to see how they do so when they may have to extend for considerable distances within the brain and at one or more points along their course deviate either to the right or to the left, cross to the opposite side of the brain and give off one or more branches before finally reaching their predetermined destination. In some systems it looks as if the axons simply grow under the influence of certain gradients that act along the major axes of the brain and spinal cord; in other systems the axons seem to be guided by their relation to their nearest neighbors. In many cases, however, it appears that the growing axon has encoded within it a sophisticated molecular mechanism that enables it to correctly respond to structural or chemical cues along its route.

Such directionally guided growth has recently been demonstrated by Rita Levi-Montalcini of the Laboratory of Cell Biology of the National Research Council in Rome. When she and her colleagues injected the protein known as nerve-growth factor into the brain of young rats, there was an abnormal growth of axons from sympathetic ganglion cells (peripheral neurons that lie alongside the vertebral column and are known to be sensitive to nerve-growth factor) into the spinal cord and up toward the brain, apparently along the route of diffusion of the injected nerve-growth factor. In this case the nerve-growth factor was acting not so much as a trophic, or growth-promoting, substance (as it usually does) but rather as a tropic, or direction-determining, substance, and the sympathetic nerve axons were responding chemotropically to its presence.

There are two other features of the growth of nerve processes that merit comment. The first is that most neurons seem to generate many more processes than are needed or than they are subsequently able to maintain. Hence most young neurons bear large numbers of short dendritelike processes, all but a few of which are later retracted as the cells mature. Similarly, most developing axons appear to make many more connections than are needed in the mature state, and commonly there is a phase of process elimination during which many (and in some cases all but one) of the initial group of connections are withdrawn. The second feature is that there is a strong tendency for axons to grow in close association with their neighbors, a phenomenon known as fasciculation. Recent work suggests that the tendency to fasciculate may be associated with the appearance along the length of most axons of surface ligands that enable them to join up and grow with other axons of a similar kind. In at least one instance it seems that because of this type of lateral association only the first axon in the group needs to develop a conventional growth cone; the other axons simply follow the leader.

Undoubtedly the most important unresolved issue in the development of the brain is the question of how neurons make specific patterns of connections. Earlier notions that most of the connectivity of the brain was functionally selected from a randomly generated set of connections are now seen to be untenable. Most of the connections seem to be precisely established at an early stage of development, and there is much evidence that the connections formed are specific not only for particular regions of the brain but also for particular neurons (and in some cases particular parts of the neurons) within these regions.

Several hypotheses have been put forward to explain how this remarkable precision is brought about. Some workers have argued that it can be simply explained on the basis that growing axons maintain the same topographical relation to one another as their parent cell bodies have. Others have suggested that the timing of events (in particular the time at which different groups of fibers reach their target regions) is critical. The one explanation that seems to fit all the observed phenomena is the chemoaffinity hypothesis, first formulated by Roger W. Sperry of the California Institute of Technology. According to this view most neurons (or more likely most small populations of neurons) become chemically differentiated at an early stage in their development depending on the positions they occupy, and this aspect of their differentiation is expressed in the form of distinguishing labels that enable the axons of the neurons to recognize either a matching label or a complementary one on the surface of their target neurons.

Although the problem is a general one affecting all parts of the nervous system, it has been most intensively studied in two systems: the innervation of the limb musculature by the relevant motor neurons in the spinal cord and the projection of the ganglion cells in the retina of the eye to their principal terminus in the brain of lower vertebrates, the optic tectum. Studies of muscle innervation indicate that under normal circumstances small populations of motor neurons, called motor-neuron pools, become segregated at an early stage in development, and that each motor-neuron pool

preferentially innervates a specific limb muscle, few errors being made in the process. Although the specificity of the innervation pattern is normally precise, it is not absolute. Hence if a supernumerary hindlimb from a donor chick embryo is transplanted alongside the normal hindlimb of a host embryo, the muscles in the supernumerary limb invariably become innervated by motorneuron pools that normally innervate either parts of the trunk or the limb-girdle musculature. The pattern of innervation is clearly aberrant, but the fact that the muscles in the transplanted limb are always innervated by the same populations of cells strongly suggests that even under these unusual conditions the axons of the motor neurons obey some (as yet unidentified) set of rules.

The retinotectal system has proved to be particularly advantageous for the analysis of the problem. In amphibians it is possible at the embryonic and larval stages to carry out a variety of experimental manipulations such as rotating the eye, making compound eyes with pieces of tissue obtained from different segments of two or more retinas and ablating or rotating parts of the tectum. Later, when the system is fully developed, it is quite easy to determine the connections formed by the retinal ganglion cells anatomically, electrophysiologically or behaviorally. Furthermore, in fishes and amphibians the optic nerve (which is formed by the axons of the retinal ganglion cells) is capable of regeneration after its fibers have been interrupted, so that it is possible to carry out many of the same kinds of experimental manipulation in juvenile or adult animals. Since there is now a vast body of literature on this system, only some of the major findings can be summarized here.

Perhaps the most important findings to have emerged from this work come from two main groups of experiments. In the first group of experiments an optic nerve was cut in frogs and salamanders, and the eye was rotated through 180 degrees. In the other experiments portions of the optic tectum of goldfish and frogs were excised and the excised portions were either rotated or transferred to another part of the tectum. In both groups of experiments the regenerating fibers of the optic nerve could be shown, either electrophysiologically or behaviorally, to have grown back to the same parts of the tectum as those they originally innervated. The simplest explanation for this finding is that the axons of the ganglion cells and their target neurons in the optic tectum are labeled in some way, and that the regenerating axons grow back until they "recognize" the appropriate labels on the neurons in the relevant part of the optic tectum.

It is difficult to refute the argument

that under such circumstances the fibers from different parts of the retina had earlier "imprinted" themselves on the related groups of tectal cells, and that the axons or the tectal neurons simply "remembered" their previous position. There is some evidence to suggest, however, that a similar mechanism may account for the initial development of the system. If the developing eye of a frog is rotated before a certain critical stage in development, the resulting projection of the retina on the tectum tends to be normal. If the rotation is done after the critical period, however, the retinal projection is invariably rotated to the same degree. Similarly, if the entire embryonic optic tectum is rotated by 180 degrees in the head-to-tail dimension (together with a portion of the forebrain that lies just in front of it), the retinal projection that is formed is again inverted.

These experiments suggest that there is a certain stage in the development of most neural centers during which they become topographically polarized in such a way that the constituent neurons acquire some determining characteristic that establishes the spatial organization of the projection as a whole. Marcus Jacobson of the University of Miami School of Medicine showed some years ago that in the clawed frog *Xenopus laevis* the retina becomes polarized in this way at about the time the first ganglion cells withdraw from the mitotic cycle. Although at this stage only about 1 percent of the ganglion cells are present, the entire future patterning of the retinal projection on the tectum seems to be established at the same time. It is not at all clear how neurons acquire positional information of this type or how it is expressed in the outgrowth of their processes. It appears, however, that the polarity-determining mechanisms are not confined to the nervous system but operate throughout the organism. R. Kevin Hunt of Johns Hopkins University and Jacobson have found that if a developing eye is transplanted into the flank of a larval frog before the period of axial specification and allowed to pass through the critical period in this abnormal position, then when it is retransplanted into the orbit, or eye socket, the ganglion cells form connections within the optic tectum that reflect the orientation of the eye during the period it was in the flank, rather than its position after it was replaced in the orbit.

When a growing axon reaches its appropriate target, whether it is another group of neurons or an effector tissue such as a collection of muscle or gland cells, it forms specialized functional contacts—synapses—with these cells. It is at such sites that information is transmitted from one cell to another, usually through the release of small quantities of an appropriate transmitter [see "The Chemistry of the Brain," by Leslie L. Iversen, page 70]. A large body of phe-

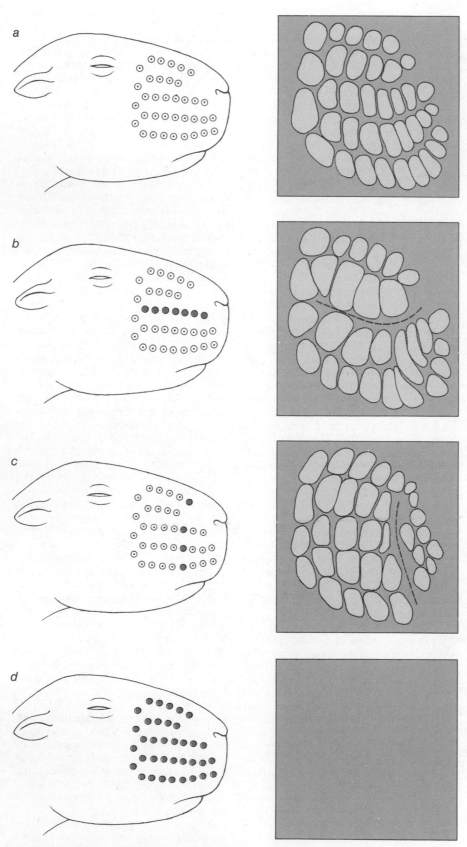

WHISKERS AND BARRELS in a young mouse are one of many systems that have been found to demonstrate the critical dependence of the developing nervous system on its inputs. The whiskers in this case are the sensory hairs on a mouse's snout; the barrels are specialized aggregations of neurons in the fourth layer of the mouse's cerebral cortex. Each barrel receives its input from a single whisker on the opposite side of the mouse's snout (a). If one row of whiskers is destroyed shortly after birth, the corresponding row of barrels in the cerebral cortex will later be found to be missing and the adjoining barrels to be enlarged (b, c). If all the whiskers are destroyed, the entire group of barrels will have disappeared (d). There must be a considerable degree of plasticity in the developing cortex, since the fibers that innervate the whiskers are not directly connected to the cortex but are linked to it through at least two synaptic relays. Illustration is based on work of Thomas A. Woolsey of Washington University School of Medicine.

nomenological evidence suggests that at synapses there is an important two-way transfer of substances essential for the survival and normal functioning of both the presynaptic and the postsynaptic cells. These substances, which are collectively referred to as trophic factors, are for the most part hypothetical; only one (nerve-growth factor) has been identified and chemically characterized. This substance, which was first identified by Viktor Hamburger and Levi-Montalcini at Washington University in the 1950's, has been found to be a protein that normally exists in the form of a pair of identical amino acid chains, each with a molecular weight of slightly more than 13,000 daltons.

Although the mode of action of nerve-growth factor has not yet been defined, it is known to be essential for the growth and survival of sympathetic ganglion cells, and during development it specifically promotes the outgrowth of processes from these and from certain spinal ganglion cells. In addition, as I have already noted, in some cases it may influence the directed outgrowth of sympathetic nerve fibers. Conversely, if an antibody to nerve-growth factor is administered to newborn mice, it leads to the destruction of the entire sympathetic nervous system. Even in adult animals nerve-growth factor appears to be continually supplied to sympathetic neurons by their target tissues, the protein being taken up by the terminal portions of their axons and transported back to the cell body. If the supply is interrupted by cutting the axons of the sympathetic neurons, their functional integrity is seriously disturbed and the synapses that end on the cells are promptly withdrawn. It seems probable that in the next few years several other substances of this kind will be isolated, and it may well be shown that most classes of neurons are dependent on a specific agent for their survival and for the directed growth of their processes.

It has become evident in recent years that the development of many structures and tissues is sculptured by highly programmed phases of cell death. This is true also of the developing brain. In many regions of the brain the number of neurons originally generated greatly exceeds the number of neurons that survive beyond the developmental period. In each region for which quantitative data are available it has been found that the number of neurons is adjusted during a phase of selective cell death that always occupies a predictable period (usually at about the time when the population of neurons as a whole is forming synaptic connections with its target tissue). It is not known whether this phenomenon operates in every part of the brain (it has been studied mainly in small groups of cells), but in those where it has been documented it involves between 15 and 85 percent of the initial neuronal population.

It seems, therefore, that in many parts of the brain the final size of the neuronal population is established in two stages: an early stage in which a comparatively large number of cells are generated, and a later stage in which the number of neurons is adjusted to match the size of the field they innervate. It is commonly assumed that the limiting factor determining the final number of cells is the number of functional contacts available to the axons of the developing neurons. Certainly if one experimentally reduces the size of the projection field, the magnitude of the naturally occurring cell death is accentuated to a proportional degree. In the case of the spinal motor neurons that innervate the hindlimb musculature it has been possible to reduce the amount of cell death in chick embryos by experimentally adding a supernumerary limb. Recent experiments suggest, however, that it may not be the formation of connections that is critical but rather the amount of trophic material available to the cells.

At a somewhat later stage in development there is a second adjustment, not in the size of the neuronal population as a whole but in the number of processes its cells maintain. The phenomenon of process (and synapse) elimination was first observed in the innervation of the limb muscles in young rats. Whereas in mature animals most muscle cells are innervated by a single axon, during the first postnatal week as many as five or six separate axons can be shown to form synapses with each muscle fiber. Over the course of the next two or three weeks the additional axons are successively eliminated, until only one axon survives. A comparable phase of process elimination has also been found in certain neuron-to-neuron connections both in the peripheral nervous system and in the brain. To cite just one example, in the cerebellum of adult animals each Purkinje cell receives only a single incoming nerve fiber of the class known as climbing fibers, but during the immediate postnatal period several such fibers may contact each Purkinje cell. Except in certain genetic mutations that affect the cerebellum all but one of these fibers are eliminated.

The finding that many early processes are later eliminated raises an interesting question: What determines which processes survive and which are eliminated? At present one can only surmise that during development fibers compete among themselves in some way. There is evidence to suggest that one factor that may give some fibers a competitive edge over the others is their functional activity. Certainly in many systems the final form of the relevant neuronal populations emerges only gradually from a rather amorphous structure, and it is often possible to alter markedly the final

appearance of the structure and its connections by interfering with its function during certain critical periods in its development. Two examples drawn from the sensory areas of the cerebral cortex will serve to make this point.

In the macaque monkey information from the retina reaches the fourth layer of the visual cortex by way of a structure called the lateral geniculate nucleus. At this level in the cortex the inputs from the two eyes are quite separate, a fact that has been directly demonstrated in experimental animals by injecting large amounts of a radioactively labeled amino acid into one eye. The retinal ganglion cells take up the labeled amino acid, incorporate it into protein and transport it to the lateral geniculate nucleus. Here some fraction of the label is released and becomes available for incorporation by the geniculate cells, which can then transport it along their axons to the visual cortex. In suitably prepared autoradiographs (in which the distribution of the labeled fibers reaching the cortex can be visualized) it is evident that the primary visual area is arranged into alternating eye-dominance bands, each band about 400 micrometers wide, that receive their input from either the right eye or the left eye. David H. Hubel, Torsten N. Wiesel and Simon LeVay of the Harvard Medical School have shown that if the eyelids of one eye of an experimental animal are sutured shut shortly after birth (so that the retina of the eye is never exposed to patterned illumination), the eye-dominance bands connected to the deprived eye are much narrower than normal bands. At the same time the bands connected with the open eye are correspondingly wider (the overall width of two adjoining bands remaining constant).

This result appears to be brought about partly by the shrinkage of the eye-dominance bands connected to the deprived eye, accompanied by a secondary expansion of those associated with the nondeprived, normal eye, and partly by the persistence of an earlier, more widespread distribution of the fibers from the nondeprived eye. If the inputs from the two eyes are examined at different stages in development, it can be shown that when the fibers from the lateral geniculate nucleus first reach the visual cortex, the inputs from one eye extensively overlap those from the other. It is not until about the end of the first postnatal month that the eye-dominance bands become clearly defined. In the light of this discovery (and the results of experiments in which the deprived eye is reopened and the other eye is sutured shut) it seems likely that the effect of visual deprivation is to place geniculocortical cells that connected with a deprived eye at some disadvantage, so that they become less effective in competing for synaptic sites on the target cells in the fourth layer of the cortex.

In the corresponding layer in the sensory cortex of the mouse the cells are arranged in a number of distinctive groupings called barrels. Physiological studies have shown that each barrel receives its input from a single whisker on the opposite side of the mouse's snout, the whiskers being among the most important sense organs in mice. Thomas A. Woolsey of the Washington University School of Medicine, who first recognized the importance of the barrels, has found that if a small group of whiskers is removed during the first few days after birth, the corresponding group of barrels in the cortex fails to develop. This is a particularly interesting finding because there are at least two intervening groups of neurons between the sensory neurons that innervate the whiskers and the neurons that constitute the cortical barrels.

These and many other observations make it clear that the developing brain is an extremely plastic structure. Although many regions may be "hardwired," others (such as the cerebral cortex) are open to a variety of influences, both intrinsic and environmental. The ability of the brain to reorganize itself in response to external influences or to localized injury is currently one of the most active areas in neurobiological research, not only because of its obvious relevance for such phenomena as learning and memory, and its bearing on the capacity of the brain to recover after injury, but also because of what it is likely to reveal about normal brain development.

Finally, it is worth pointing out that the development of the brain, like the development of most other biological structures, is not without error. I have already indicated that errors may appear during neuronal migration. There are also several known cases in which errors are made during the formation of connections. In the visual system it has been noted by a number of workers that some optic-nerve fibers that should cross the midline in the optic chiasm grow back aberrantly to the same side of the brain. In some of these situations if one eye is removed from an experimental animal early in development, the number of aberrantly directed fibers can be considerably increased. Since such aberrant fibers are often not seen in the mature brain, it looks as if the misdirected axons (and whatever inappropriate connections they form) are eliminated at later stages in development. How they are recognized as being erroneous and how they are subsequently removed remains a puzzle. Considering the complexity of the developmental mechanisms involved, it is hardly surprising that errors are found. What is surprising is that they appear infrequently and that they are often effectively eliminated.

VI

The Chemistry
of the Brain

The Chemistry of the Brain

BY LESLIE L. IVERSEN

Signals are sent from one neuron to another by diverse chemical transmitters. These chemical systems, overlaid on the neuronal circuits of the brain, add another dimension to brain function

Neurons share the biochemical machinery of all other living cells, including the ability to generate chemical energy from the oxidation of foodstuff and to repair and maintain themselves. Among the specialized features they possess and other cells do not are those that have to do with the special function of neurons as transmitters of nerve impulses, such as their need to maintain ionic gradients, involving a high rate of energy consumption, and those associated with the ability of neurons to manufacture and release a special array of chemical messengers known as neurotransmitters. At synapses, the microscopic regions of close proximity between the terminal of one neuron and the receiving surface of another, the arrival of an impulse causes a sudden release of molecules of transmitter from the terminal. The transmitter molecules then diffuse across the fluid-filled gap between the two cells and act on specific receptor sites in the postsynaptic membrane, thereby altering the electrical activity of the receiving neuron.

Some 30 different substances are known or suspected to be transmitters in the brain, and each has a characteristic excitatory or inhibitory effect on neurons. The transmitters are not randomly distributed throughout the brain but are localized in specific clusters of neurons whose axons project to other highly specific brain regions. The superimposition of these diverse chemically coded systems on the neuronal circuitry endows the brain with an extra dimension of modulation and specificity.

Considerable progress has been made in recent years in characterizing the various transmitter substances (although many more undoubtedly remain to be discovered), in mapping their distribution in the brain and in elucidating the molecular events of synaptic transmission. Such research has revealed that the behavioral effects of many drugs and neurotoxins arise from their ability to disrupt or modify chemical transmission between neurons. It has also hinted that the causes of mental illness may ultimately be traced to defects in the functioning of specific transmitter systems in the brain.

In terms of general energy metabolism the brain is the most active energy consumer of all body organs, a fact reflected in its large blood supply and oxygen uptake. Although the human brain represents only 2 percent of the total body weight, its rate of oxygen utilization (50 milliliters per minute) accounts for 20 percent of the total resting utilization of oxygen. This enormous expenditure of energy is thought to be due to the need to maintain the ionic gradients across the neuronal membrane on which the conduction of impulses in the billions of brain neurons depends. Moreover, there is no respite from this energy demand: the rate of brain metabolism is relatively constant day and night and may even increase somewhat during the dreaming phases of sleep. To put matters in perspective, however, the total energy equivalent of brain metabolism is only some 20 watts.

An important recent advance in studies of energy metabolism in the brain is the development by Louis Sokoloff and his colleagues at the National Institute of Mental Health of a method that makes it possible to visualize the rate of energy metabolism in brain cells. Neurons adjust the rate at which they take up glucose to fulfill their metabolic needs at the time. Hence active neurons take up glucose more rapidly than quiescent ones. The glucose taken up is normally metabolized rapidly, but a chemical analogue of glucose, 2-deoxyglucose, is taken up into the cells by the same uptake mechanism but is not metabolized there. If radioactively labeled deoxyglucose is injected into the bloodstream, it will accumulate in neurons, and the rate at which it accumulates can serve as an indicator of the cells' metabolic activity. The accumulation of radioactive deoxyglucose can be seen and measured by placing thin sections of frozen brain on radiation-sensitive film. Areas that are rich in labeled material show up when the film is developed. The technique has opened an entirely new realm in brain research, since it makes it possible to detect what cells in the brain were active during a given experimental procedure. For example, the precise areas of the brain receiving visual inputs from the left or right eye can be visualized by flashing a light into one eye or the other.

Whereas the other body organs are able to utilize a variety of alternative fuels (such as sugars, fats and amino acids), neurons can utilize only blood glucose. Moreover, whereas tissues such as muscle are able to function for short periods in the absence of oxygen, the brain is entirely dependent on oxidative metabolism. If the supply of oxygenated blood to the brain is interrupted, consciousness is lost within 10 seconds and permanent damage to the brain ensues. Similar effects result from any condition that lowers blood glucose, such as when a diabetic injects himself with an overdose of insulin. Although elaborate control mechanisms ensure that the blood pressure will remain stable and that

NEURONS CONTAINING NOREPINEPHRINE, a chemical transmitter in the brain, glow brilliantly in this section of rat brain viewed in the fluorescence microscope. The norepinephrine-containing cells, situated in a region of the brain stem called the locus coeruleus, were made visible by reacting them with glyoxylic acid, which converts norepinephrine into a fluorescent chemical derivative. Thousands of other neurons are also present in the field, but because they contain other transmitters they are not visible. The norepinephrine neurons in the locus coeruleus project their axons to many parts of the brain, including the cerebellum and the forebrain. They are thought to be involved in sleep, mood and brain reward. Micrograph was made by Floyd E. Bloom, Gary S. Jones and Jacqueline F. McGinty of the Salk Institute.

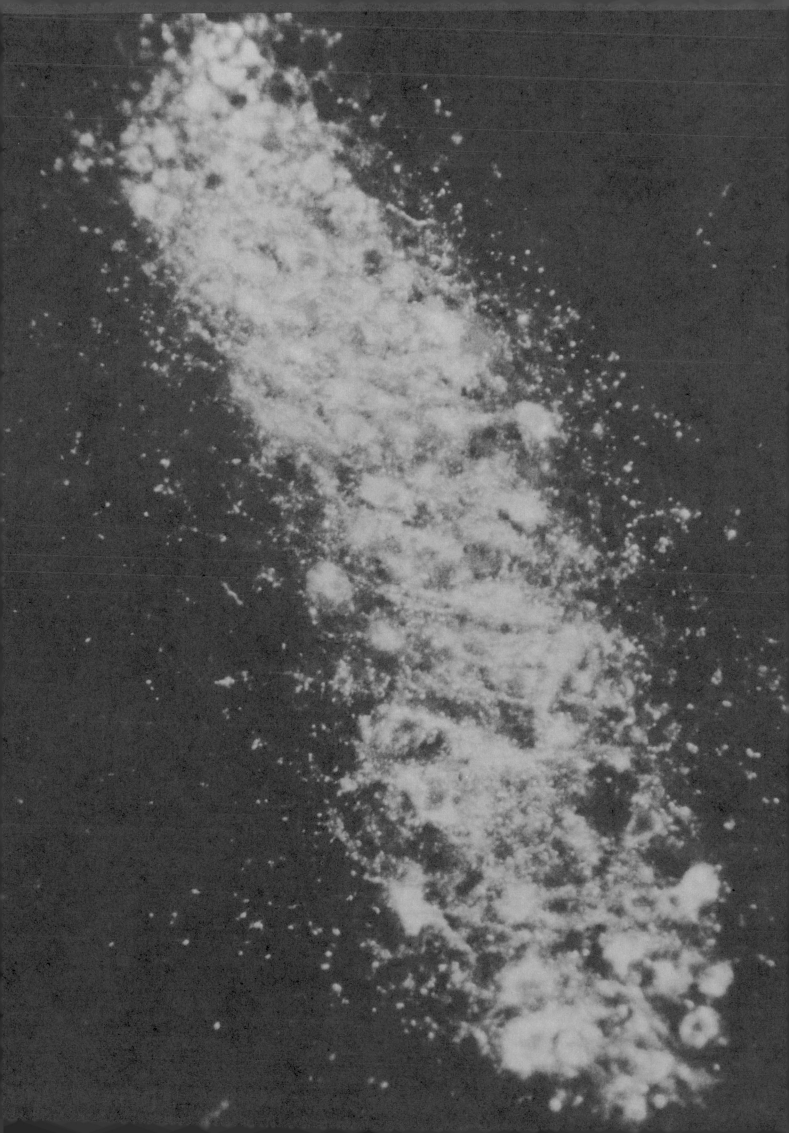

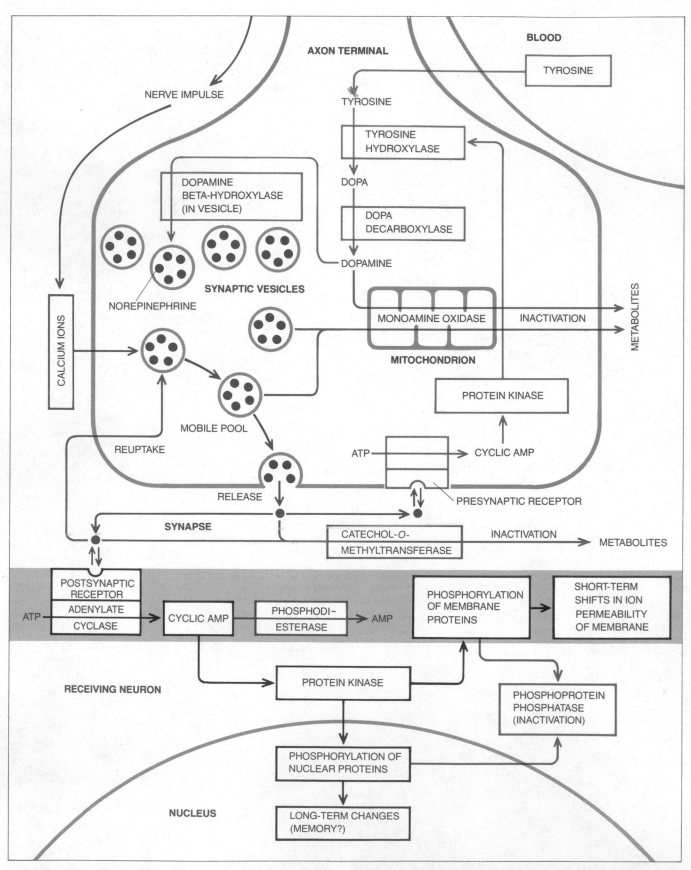

CHEMICAL TRANSMISSION across the synapse, the narrow gap between two neurons in the brain, involves an elaborate sequence of molecular events. Here the process of transmission at a norepinephrine synapse is diagrammed. First norepinephrine is manufactured from the amino acid tyrosine in three steps, each of which is catalyzed by an enzyme. The transmitter is then stored within membrane-bound vesicles in association with storage proteins (*indicated by green pathways*). The arrival in the axon terminal of a nerve impulse triggers an influx of calcium ions, which induces the release of norepinephrine from the vesicles into the synaptic space (*red pathways*).

The liberated transmitter molecules bind to specific receptor proteins embedded in the postsynaptic membrane, triggering a series of reactions that culminate in short-term (electrical) and long-term effects on the receiving neuron (*purple pathways*). The action of norepinephrine is then terminated by a variety of means, including rapid reuptake of the transmitter into the axon terminal and degradation by enzymes (*blue pathways*). The release of some norepinephrine into the synaptic space activates presynaptic receptors on the axon terminal, initiating production of cyclic AMP, which activates protein kinase, thus stimulating more norepinephrine production (*orange pathway*).

there will be constant levels of oxygen and glucose in the blood, it seems clear that the enormous behavioral flexibility made possible by the expanded size and capacity of the mammalian brain has been acquired during evolution at a high metabolic cost.

As cells go, neurons are exceedingly sensitive: their function can be disrupted by toxic substances that find their way into the bloodstream and also by small molecules that are normally present in the blood, such as amino acids. This sensitivity may explain why the brain is isolated from the general circulation by the selective filtration system known as the blood-brain barrier. The effectiveness of the barrier is due to the relative impermeability of the blood vessels in the brain and to the presence of tight sheaths of glial cells (the supporting cells of the brain) around the blood vessels. Although small molecules such as those of oxygen can pass readily through the barrier, most of the larger molecules required by brain cells, such as those of glucose, must be actively taken up by special transport mechanisms. The blood-brain barrier has important consequences for the design of drugs that act directly on the brain: if such substances are to cross the barrier, their molecules must be either very small or readily soluble in the fatty membranes of the glial cells. A few select regions of the brain are not shielded by the blood-brain barrier; they include structures that are specifically responsive to blood-borne hormones or whose job it is to monitor the chemical composition of the blood.

Within individual neurons other transport problems are presented by the fact that part of the cell is represented by extended thin fibers. The axon that carries the nerve impulse away from the cell body of a neuron can be millimeters or centimeters long. The neurons of the adult brain cannot be replaced and must last a lifetime, so that there must be mechanisms to renew all their components. This requirement calls for the synthesis by the cell of enzymes and other complex molecules, and such synthesis can proceed only in the region of the cell nucleus, that is, in the cell body of the neuron. Therefore replacing the components of the axon requires a means of transporting components substantial distances within the cell. Indeed, there is a constant movement of proteins and other components from the cell body down the entire length of the axon.

This phenomenon of axonal transport was discovered more than 30 years ago by Paul A. Weiss and his colleagues at the University of Chicago. Until that time it was generally assumed that the axoplasm—the jellylike fluid inside the axon—was merely an inert mechanical support for the excitable membrane that propagated the nerve impulse. When

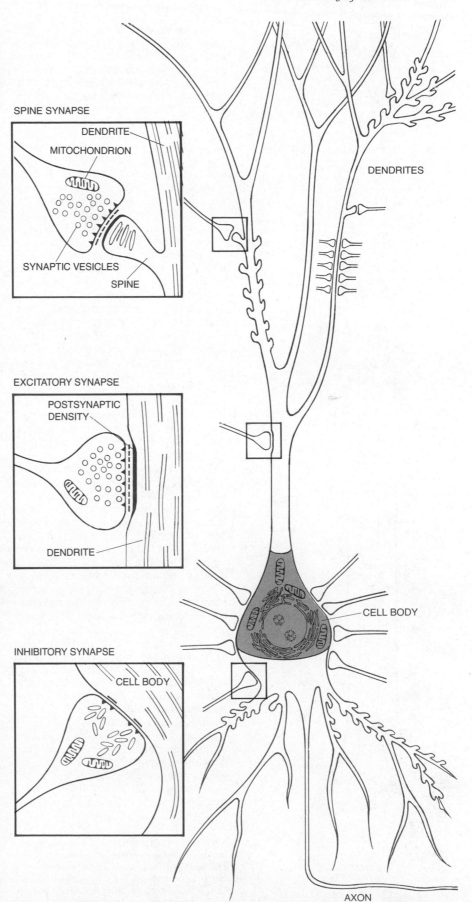

SPINE SYNAPSE

DENDRITE
MITOCHONDRION
SYNAPTIC VESICLES
SPINE

EXCITATORY SYNAPSE

POSTSYNAPTIC DENSITY
DENDRITE

INHIBITORY SYNAPSE

CELL BODY

DENDRITES

CELL BODY

AXON

SYNAPSES impinging on a typical neuron in the brain are either excitatory or inhibitory, depending on the type of transmitter that is released. Such synapses can be distinguished morphologically in the electron microscope: excitatory synapses tend to have round vesicles and a continuous dense thickening of the postsynaptic membrane, and inhibitory synapses tend to have flattened vesicles and a discontinuous postsynaptic density. Synapses can also be classified according to their position on the surface of the receiving neuron. They may be on the cell body, on the trunk of the dendrites, on "spines" projecting from the dendrites or on the axon.

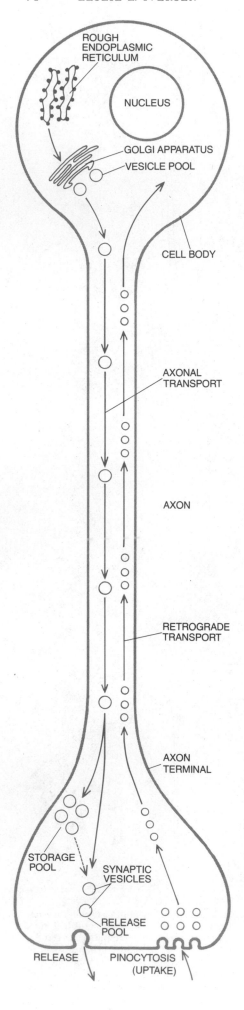

ROUGH
ENDOPLASMIC
RETICULUM

NUCLEUS

GOLGI APPARATUS

VESICLE POOL

CELL BODY

AXONAL
TRANSPORT

AXON

RETROGRADE
TRANSPORT

AXON
TERMINAL

STORAGE
POOL

SYNAPTIC
VESICLES

RELEASE
POOL

RELEASE   PINOCYTOSIS
                 (UPTAKE)

Weiss constricted the axon at a given point, however, he found that after several days the fiber bulged out on the side of the constriction toward the cell body and narrowed on the side away from the cell body. When he released the constriction, the dammed-up axoplasm resumed its flow.

It is now known that the axoplasm is an artery for a busy molecular traffic moving in both directions between the cell body of the neuron and its axon terminals. There are several different systems involved, including a slow-transport system in which material flows away from the cell body at a speed of about a millimeter a day, and a faster-transport system in which material flows in both directions at speeds of between 10 and 20 centimeters a day. The slow-transport system represents a bulk flow of axoplasm carrying components important for the growth and regeneration of the axon; the faster-transport system represents the flow of more specialized cellular components, including some of the enzymes involved in the manufacture of transmitters.

It is not yet understood how such differential rates of transport are achieved, but both the slow and the fast mechanisms seem to involve the numerous fibrous proteins in the axon that are visible in electron micrographs. By following the transport of radioactively labeled proteins outward along axons it has been possible to trace the precise anatomical connections between neurons in the brain. The connections between the terminals of a neuron in one region of the brain and the cell body in another region can also be mapped by means of the enzyme horseradish peroxidase, which has the special ability to travel rapidly up the axon in a retrograde fashion.

The functional chemistry of the brain is exceedingly difficult to study. Not only are the transmitter substances present in vanishingly small quantities but also the brain tissue is structurally and chemically so complex that it is not easy to isolate a given transmitter system for examination. New techniques have been developed, however, to overcome these formidable obstacles. One major advance came in the early 1960's with the

AXONAL TRANSPORT is responsible for moving cellular components such as vesicles and enzymes from their site of manufacture in the neuronal cell body to the axon terminals, which may be millimeters or centimeters away. Transport in the retrograde direction from the axon terminals to the cell body carries factors essential to health of the neuron. Axonal transport can be exploited to trace pathways by observing the movement along axons of radioactively labeled molecules or of enzymes such as horseradish peroxidase.

discovery by Victor P. Whittaker of the University of Cambridge and Eduardo De Robertis of the University of Buenos Aires that when brain tissue is gently disrupted by being homogenized in a sugar solution, many of the nerve terminals break away from their axons and form intact, closed particles named synaptosomes. The synaptosomes contain the mechanisms of synthesis, storage, release and transmitter inactivation associated with the nerve terminal, and they can be purified from the other neuronal components by spinning them in a centrifuge. This technique has enabled neurochemists to study the mechanisms of synaptic transmission in the test tube.

Perhaps the most far-reaching technical advance has been the development of methods that allow for the selective staining of neurons containing a particular transmitter. One approach is to convert the natural transmitter into a fluorescent derivative that will glow when it is exposed to ultraviolet radiation in the fluorescence microscope. A second approach is to inject radioactively labeled molecules of a transmitter into the brain of an experimental animal, where they are selectively taken up by the nerve terminals that release that transmitter; the radioactive terminals can then be detected by placing thin sections of the tissue on radiation-sensitive film. A third approach exploits the high specificity of antibodies. An enzyme involved in the synthesis of a particular transmitter is purified from brain tissue and injected into an experimental animal, where it induces the manufacture of antibodies that combine with it specifically. The antibodies are then purified, labeled with a fluorescent dye or some other marker and utilized to selectively stain neurons containing the relevant enzyme.

These selective-staining techniques have provided a flood of information about the detailed anatomical distribution of individual transmitters in the complex neuronal circuits of the brain. They have revealed that the transmitters are not distributed diffusely throughout the brain tissue but are highly localized in discrete centers and pathways. The best-mapped transmitters are the monoamines norepinephrine, dopamine and serotonin (so named because each contains a single amine group). As was first shown by Bengt Falck of the University of Lund and Nils-Åke Hillarp of the Karolinska Institute in Sweden, neurons containing monoamines will fluoresce green or yellow if the transmitters are converted into fluorescent derivatives by reacting them with formaldehyde or glyoxylic acid. Such studies have demonstrated that many of the norepinephrine-containing cells in the brain are concentrated in the small cluster of neurons in the brain stem known as the locus coeruleus. The axons of these neurons are highly branched and project to diverse regions, such as the hypothalamus, the cerebellum and the forebrain. The norepinephrine system has been implicated in the maintenance of arousal, in the brain system of reward, in dreaming sleep and in the regulation of mood.

The neurons containing the monoamine transmitter dopamine are concentrated in the regions of the midbrain known as the substantia nigra and ventral tegmentum. Many of the dopamine-containing neurons project their axons to the forebrain, where they are thought to be involved in regulating emotional responses. Other dopamine fibers terminate in the region near the center of the brain called the corpus striatum. In the corpus striatum dopamine appears to play a crucial role in the control of complex movements. The degeneration of the dopamine fibers projecting to this region gives rise to the muscular rigidity and tremors of Parkinson's disease.

The monoamine transmitter serotonin is concentrated in the cluster of neurons in the region of the brain stem known as the raphe nuclei. The neurons of this center project to the hypothalamus, the thalamus and many other brain regions. Serotonin is thought to be involved in temperature regulation, sensory perception and the onset of sleep.

Many other transmitters have been identified, some of which are designated "putative" because their involvement in synaptic transmission in the brain is still somewhat equivocal. For example, several amino acids—the building blocks of proteins—appear to act as transmitters. The common and abundant amino acids glutamic acid and aspartic acid exert powerful excitatory effects on most neurons and may well be the commonest excitatory transmitters at brain synapses. The simplest of all amino acids, glycine, is known to be an inhibitory transmitter in the spinal cord.

The commonest inhibitory transmitter in the brain is gamma-aminobutyric acid (GABA), an amino acid that is not incorporated into proteins. GABA is unique among amino acids in that it is manufactured almost exclusively in the brain and spinal cord. It has been estimated that as many as a third of the synapses in the brain employ GABA as a transmitter. Neurons that contain GABA can be identified in two ways: by labeling them with radioactive GABA or by staining them with antibodies against glutamic acid decarboxylase, the enzyme that catalyzes the manufacture of GABA. It is of interest to note that glutamic acid is a candidate excitatory transmitter in the brain, whereas GABA, which differs from it by a single chemical group, is an inhibitory transmitter. Clearly slight differences in the molecular structure of transmitters can give rise to completely different physiological effects.

The investigation of GABA mechanisms in the brain has been stimulated in recent years by the discovery by Thomas L. Perry of the University of British Columbia that a specific deficit in brain GABA occurs in Huntington's chorea, which is an inherited neurological syndrome. The uncontrolled movements of the disease are caused by progressive deterioration of the corpus striatum in middle life. Postmortem analysis has revealed that the brain damage involves a loss of inhibitory neurons that normally contain GABA, suggesting that a deficit

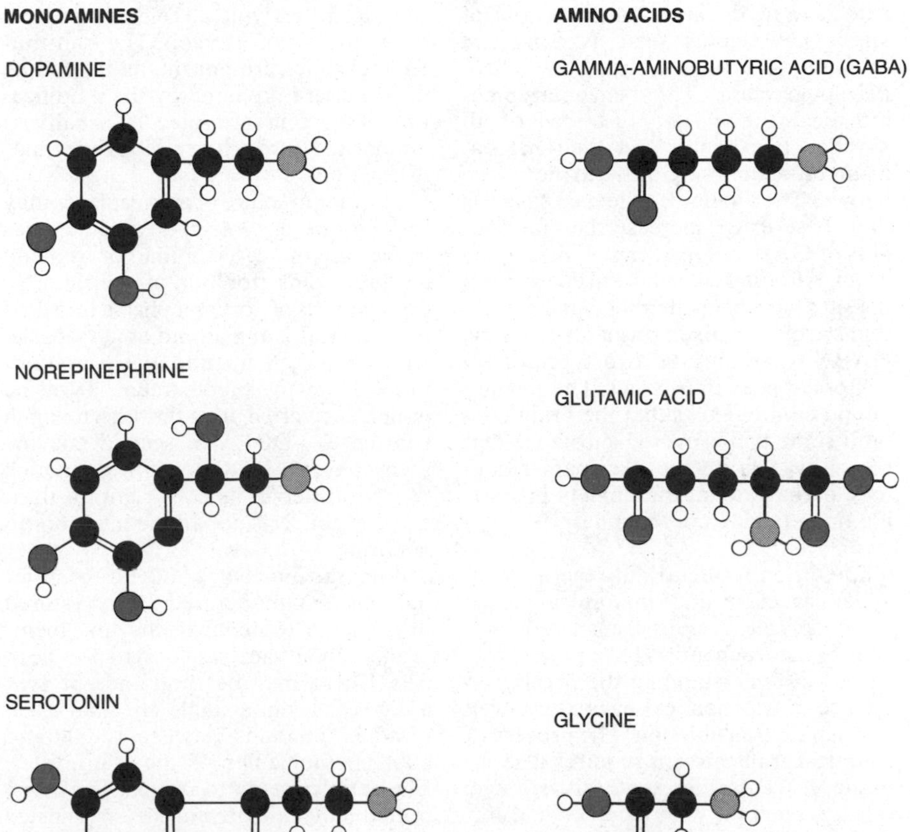

MONOAMINES

DOPAMINE

NOREPINEPHRINE

SEROTONIN

ACETYLCHOLINE

HISTAMINE

AMINO ACIDS

GAMMA-AMINOBUTYRIC ACID (GABA)

GLUTAMIC ACID

GLYCINE

TAURINE

● CARBON
● OXYGEN
● NITROGEN
Ⓢ SULFUR
○ HYDROGEN

TRANSMITTER CHEMICALS tend to be small molecules that incorporate a positively charged nitrogen atom. Each has a characteristic excitatory or inhibitory effect on neurons, although some transmitters are excitatory in one part of the brain and inhibitory in another. Histamine and taurine are considered putative transmitters because the experimental evidence for them is not yet complete. According to Dale's principle only one transmitter is released from all the terminals of an axon. Exceptions to this principle, however, have been found recently.

of the transmitter might be specifically responsible for the disease. Unfortunately attempts to treat patients by replacing the missing brain GABA is currently not possible, since GABA analogues that are capable of penetrating the blood-brain barrier have not yet been developed.

Recently GABA has also been implicated as a likely target for the actions of antianxiety agents such as diazepam (Valium) and other drugs of the benzodiazepine class. The benzodiazepines are the most widely prescribed of all psychoactive drugs, and their mechanism of action has hitherto not been known. The available evidence suggests that these drugs increase the effectiveness of GABA at its receptor sites in the brain. Although specific diazepam binding sites have been identified in the brain that are clearly distinguishable from the GABA receptors, the two types of receptors appear to interact. The intriguing possibility exists that the brain contains some undiscovered substance that normally acts on the diazepam receptors, perhaps a natural anxiety-producing or -relieving compound.

In addition to identifying the molecular structure and anatomical distribution of the various transmitter substances, neurochemists have made large strides in understanding the precise sequence of biochemical events involved in synaptic transmission. The process of chemical transmission requires a series of steps: transmitter synthesis, storage, release, reaction with receptor and termination of transmitter actions. Each of these steps has been characterized in detail, and drugs have been discovered that selectively enhance or block specific steps. This research has yielded insight into the mechanism of action of psychoactive drugs and also into how certain neurological and mental disorders might be related to specific defects in synaptic mechanisms.

The first step in chemical transmission is the synthesis of the transmitter molecules in the nerve terminals. Each neuron usually possesses only the biochemical machinery it needs to make one kind of transmitter, which it releases from all the terminals of its axon. The transmitter molecules are not manufactured de novo but are prepared by the modification of a precursor molecule, usually an amino acid, through a series of enzymatic reactions.

The manufacture of a transmitter may require one enzyme-catalyzed step (as in the case of acetylcholine) or as many as three steps (for norepinephrine). In the synthesis of norepinephrine the starting material is the amino acid tyrosine, which is taken up into the nerve terminal from the bloodstream. Tyrosine is first converted into the intermediate substance L-DOPA; a second enzyme then converts L-DOPA into dopamine (a transmitter in its own right); a third enzyme converts dopamine into norepinephrine.

After the molecules of the transmitter have been manufactured they are stored in the axon terminal in the tiny membrane-bound sacs called synaptic vesicles. There may be thousands of synaptic vesicles in a single terminal, each of which contains between 10,000 and 100,000 molecules of the transmitter. The vesicles serve to protect the transmitter molecules from enzymes inside the terminal that would otherwise destroy them.

The arrival of a nerve impulse at an axon terminal causes large numbers of transmitter molecules to be discharged from the terminal into the synaptic space. The mechanism of release is still controversial: some investigators believe the synaptic vesicles fuse directly with the presynaptic membrane and discharge their contents into the synaptic space; others contend that a mobile pool of transmitter molecules is liberated through special channels. In any case the nerve impulse is known to trigger release by increasing the permeability of the nerve terminal to calcium ions, which then rush into the terminal and activate the release mechanism.

The released transmitter molecules travel rapidly across the fluid-filled space between the axon terminal and the membrane of the receiving neuron. There they interact with specific receptor sites on the postsynaptic membrane. The receptors are actually large protein molecules embedded in the semifluid matrix of the cell membrane, with parts sticking out above and below the membrane like floating icebergs. A region on the surface of the receptor protein is precisely tailored to match the shape and configuration of the transmitter molecule, so that the latter fits into the former with the precision and specificity of a key entering a lock.

The interaction of the transmitter with its receptor alters the three-dimensional shape of the receptor protein, thereby initiating a sequence of events. The interaction may cause a neuron to become excited or inhibited, a muscle cell to contract or a gland cell to manufacture and secrete a hormone. In each case the receptor translates the message encoded by the molecular structure of the transmitter molecule into a specific physiological response. Some of the responses, such as the contraction of voluntary muscle, take place in a fraction of a second; others, such as the secretion

MESCALINE

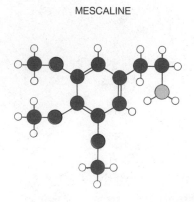

PSILOCYBIN

PHOSPHORUS

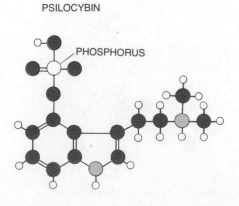

LYSERGIC ACID
DIETHYLAMIDE (LSD)

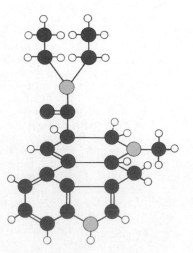

HALLUCINOGENIC DRUGS show a strong structural resemblance to the monoamine transmitters, suggesting that they may exert their potent effects on consciousness by mimicking these natural transmitters at synaptic receptors in the brain. Mescaline possesses the benzene-ring structure of dopamine and norepinephrine, and psilocybin and LSD incorporate the indole-ring structure of serotonin.

of a hormone, require a span of minutes and sometimes hours.

Many transmitter receptors have two functional components: a binding site for the transmitter molecule and a pore passing through the membrane that is selectively permeable to certain ions. The binding of the transmitter to the receptor changes its shape so that the pore is opened and ions inside and outside the cell membrane flow down their concentration gradients, resulting in either an excitatory or an inhibitory effect on the neuron's firing rate. Whether the electric potential generated by a transmitter is excitatory or inhibitory depends on the specific ions that move and the direction of their movement. Acetylcholine is excitatory at the synapse between nerve and muscle because it causes positively charged sodium ions to move into the cell and depolarize its negative resting voltage. GABA, on the other hand, has a receptor whose pore is selectively permeable to negatively charged chloride ions. When these ions flow through the open pores into the target cell, they increase the voltage across the membrane and temporarily inactivate the cell.

Other transmitters, such as dopamine and norepinephrine, appear to operate by a more elaborate mechanism. In the mid-1950's Earl W. Sutherland, Jr., and his colleagues at Case Western Reserve University demonstrated that these and other transmitters increase or decrease the concentration of a "second messenger" substance in the target cells. The second messenger then mediates the electrical or biochemical effects of the transmitter, or "first messenger." In a discovery that later brought him the 1971 Nobel prize in physiology and medicine, Sutherland identified the second-messenger substance as the small molecule cyclic adenosine monophosphate, or cyclic AMP.

According to Sutherland's hypothesis the receptor protein for norepinephrine (and many other transmitters) is coupled in the target-cell membrane to the enzyme adenylate cyclase, which catalyzes the conversion of the cellular energy-carrying molecule adenosine triphosphate (ATP) into cyclic AMP. Adenylate cyclase is usually inactive, but when norepinephrine binds to the postsynaptic receptor, the enzyme is automatically switched on and begins to rapidly convert ATP into cyclic AMP inside the cell. Cyclic AMP then acts on the biochemical machinery of the cell to initiate the physiological response characteristic of the transmitter.

The second-messenger system is therefore analogous to a relay race, in which the transmitter passes along its message to cyclic AMP at the cell membrane. Of course, the signal is passed not to one but to the many thousands of molecules of cyclic AMP that are gener-

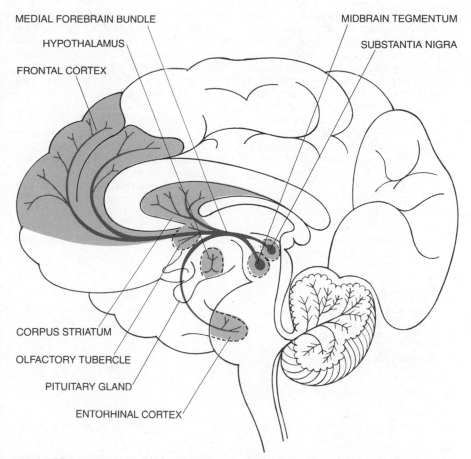

DOPAMINE PATHWAYS in the human brain are shown schematically. The neurons that contain dopamine have their cell bodies clustered in two small regions of the midbrain: the substantia nigra and the tegmentum. These neurons send out widely branching fibers that terminate in the corpus striatum, which regulates motor activity, and in the limbic forebrain, which is involved in emotion. A small set of dopamine neurons in the hypothalamus also regulates secretion of hormones from pituitary. Dopamine has been associated with two brain disorders: a deficiency of the transmitter in the corpus striatum causes the rigidity and tremor of Parkinson's disease, and an excess of dopamine in limbic forebrain may be involved in schizophrenia.

ated by the activated adenylate cyclase associated with each occupied receptor. As a result the very weak signal provided by the transmitter-receptor interaction is amplified several thousandfold inside the cell through the mass production of cyclic AMP.

The application of Sutherland's second-messenger theory to brain function is one of the most exciting areas in neurochemistry today. In 1971 Floyd E. Bloom and his co-workers at the National Institute of Mental Health demonstrated that cyclic AMP could affect signaling in neurons. Later Paul Greengard and his group at the Yale University School of Medicine implicated cyclic AMP in the synaptic actions of several brain transmitters, including norepinephrine, dopamine, serotonin and histamine. Greengard has proposed the unifying hypothesis that cyclic AMP activates specific enzymes in the target cell called protein kinases; these enzymes then act to catalyze the incorporation of phosphate groups into special proteins in the neuronal membrane, altering the permeability of the membrane to ions

and thereby changing the level of excitability of the target cell. Because the second-messenger system works relatively slowly on the time scale of neuronal events it is best suited for mediating the longer-lasting actions of transmitters in the brain such as slow shifts in membrane potential and perhaps the formation of long-term memories. Once cyclic AMP has relayed its message it is inactivated within the cell by the enzyme phosphodiesterase. Drugs that inhibit this enzyme therefore raise the level of cyclic AMP within the target cells and enhance the effect of the transmitter.

To sum up, there appear to be two basic types of transmitter receptor: rapidly acting receptors that mediate the transfer of information by controlling the permeability state of an ion pore, and longer-acting receptors that induce the formation of a second-messenger substance, which in turn mediates the effects of the transmitter inside the target neuron. Many transmitters possess two or more types of receptor. For example, the response to acetylcholine at the synapse between a motor neuron and a muscle cell is mediated by a simple flow of sodium ions across the membrane. In the brain, however, most of the effects of acetylcholine appear to be mediated by another second-messenger molecule: cyclic guanosine monophosphate, or cyclic GMP. Similarly, evidence recently acquired suggests that dopamine acts at two different types of receptor in the brain: the $D1$ receptor, which is coupled to a second-messenger cyclic-AMP system, and the $D2$ receptor, which is not.

Once a transmitter molecule has bound to its receptor it must be rapidly inactivated; otherwise it would act for too long and precise control of

transmission would be lost. Nerve fibers can conduct several hundred impulses per second only if the postsynaptic membrane recovers its resting voltage within a fraction of a millisecond. Some transmitters are inactivated by enzymes situated in the synaptic space. For example, acetylcholine is destroyed by the enzyme acetylcholinesterase, which can cleave 25,000 molecules of the transmitter per second. Norepinephrine is inactivated at the synapse by an entirely different mechanism.

Julius Axelrod and his colleagues at the National Institute of Mental Health found that after norepinephrine is released from the axon terminal it is rapidly pumped back inside. Then the recap-

tured molecules of norepinephrine either are destroyed by the enzymes catechol-O-methyltransferase (COMT) and monoamine oxidase (MAO) present in the nerve terminal or are recycled back into the synaptic vesicles. Similar reuptake mechanisms have since been identified for other transmitters, such as dopamine, serotonin and GABA. Reuptake has the obvious advantage over enzymatic degradation in that the transmitter molecules can be conserved through several cycles of release and recapture.

The working out of the steps of synaptic transmission has shed much light on the operation of psychoactive drugs. Some drugs exert their effects by either enhancing or inhibiting the release of a

Met-ENKEPHALIN
Tyr-Gly-Gly-Phe-Met

Leu-ENKEPHALIN
Tyr-Gly-Gly-Phe-Leu

SUBSTANCE P
Arg-Pro-Lys-Pro-Gln-Gln-Phe-Phe-Gly-Leu-Met-NH₂

NEUROTENSIN
p-Glu-Leu-Tyr-Glu-Asn-Lys-Pro-Arg-Arg-Pro-Tyr-Ile-Leu

β-ENDORPHIN
Tyr-Gly-Gly-Phe-Met-Thr-Ser-Glu-Lys-Ser-Gln-Thr-Pro-Leu-Val-Thr-Leu-Phe-Lys-Asn-Ala-Ile-Val-Lys-Asn-Ala-His-Lys-Lys-Gly-Gln

ACTH (CORTICOTROPIN)
Ser-Tyr-Ser-Met-Glu-His-Phe-Arg-Tyr-Gly-Lys-Pro-Val-Gly-Lys-Lys-Arg-Arg-Pro-Val-Lys-Val-Tyr-Pro-Asp-Gly-Ala-Glu-Asp-Glu-Leu-Ala-Glu-Ala-Phe-Pro-Leu-Glu-Phe-NH₂

ANGIOTENSIN II
Asp-Arg-Val-Tyr-Ile-His-Pro-Phe-NH₂

OXYTOCIN
Ile-Tyr-Cys / Gln-Asn-Cys-Pro-Leu-Gly-NH₂

VASOPRESSIN
Phe-Tyr-Cys / Gln-Asn-Cys-Pro-Arg-Gly-NH₂

VASOACTIVE INTESTINAL POLYPEPTIDE (VIP)
His-Ser-Asp-Ala-Val-Phe-Thr-Asp-Asn-Tyr-Thr-Arg-Leu-Arg-Lys-Gln-Met-Ala-Val-Lys-Lys-Tyr-Leu-Asn-Ser-Ile-Leu-Asn-NH₂

SOMATOSTATIN
Ala-Gly-Cys-Lys-Asn-Phe-Phe-Trp / Cys-Ser-Thr-Phe-Thr-Lys

THYROTROPIN RELEASING HORMONE (TRH)
p-Glu-His-Pro-NH₂

LUTEINIZING-HORMONE RELEASING HORMONE (LHRH)
p-Glu-His-Trp-Ser-Tyr-Gly-Leu-Arg-Pro-Gly-NH₂

BOMBESIN
p-Glu-Gln-Arg-Leu-Gly-Asn-Gln-Trp-Ala-Val-Gly-His-Leu-Met-NH₂

CARNOSINE
Ala-His

CHOLECYSTOKININ-LIKE PEPTIDE
Asp-Tyr-Met-Gly-Trp-Met-Asp-Phe-NH₂

Ala	ALANINE	Leu	LEUCINE
Arg	ARGININE	Lys	LYSINE
Asn	ASPARAGINE	Met	METHIONINE
Asp	ASPARTIC ACID	Phe	PHENYLALANINE
Cys	CYSTEINE	Pro	PROLINE
Gln	GLUTAMINE	Ser	SERINE
Glu	GLUTAMIC ACID	Thr	THREONINE
Gly	GLYCINE	Trp	TRYPTOPHAN
His	HISTIDINE	Tyr	TYROSINE
Ile	ISOLEUCINE	Val	VALINE

NEUROPEPTIDES are short chains of amino acids found in brain tissue. Many of them are localized in axon terminals and are released by a calcium-dependent process, suggesting that they are transmitters. Neuropeptides differ from previously identified transmitters, however, in that they appear to orchestrate complex phenomena such as thirst, memory and sexual behavior. Moreover, they play a multiplicity of roles in different parts of the body. For example, somatostatin inhibits the release of human growth hormone from the pituitary, regulates the secretion of insulin and glucagon by the pancreas and appears to function as a transmitter in the spinal cord and brain.

particular transmitter from axon terminals. For example, the potent stimulant amphetamine triggers the release from nerve terminals in the brain of dopamine, a transmitter associated with the arousal and pleasure systems in the brain. Excessive use of amphetamine by addicts can lead to disruption of thought processes, hallucinations and delusions of persecution, symptoms very similar to those found in some forms of schizophrenia. This and other evidence has led to the hypothesis that an overactivity in the brain dopamine systems may underlie the symptoms of schizophrenia.

Another intriguing finding is that the wide variety of antischizophrenic drugs that have been developed, such as chlorpromazine (Thorazine) and haloperidol (Haldol), share the property of binding tightly to dopamine receptors in the brain, thereby preventing the natural transmitter from activating them. This discovery has proved to be one of the most promising leads in modern schizophrenia research. The latest evidence suggests that schizophrenia is associated with an overproduction of dopamine or an overresponsiveness to the transmitter in certain regions of the brain. Work in my laboratory at the Neurochemical Pharmacology Unit of the British Medical Research Council and by T. J. Crow at the Medical Research Council's Clinical Research Centre in London and by Philip Seeman at the University of Toronto has revealed abnormally high concentrations of dopamine and dopamine receptors in the brains of deceased schizophrenics, particularly in the limbic system, a system of brain regions involved in emotional behavior. The dopamine pathways in these regions may therefore be a primary target for antipsychotic drugs.

Many psychoactive drugs may act by mimicking natural transmitters at their postsynaptic receptors. Many hallucinogenic drugs, for example, bear a structural resemblance to natural transmitters: mescaline is similar to norepinephrine and dopamine, and both LSD and psilocybin are related to serotonin. These drugs may therefore operate on monoamine mechanisms, although their precise modes of action are still not known. LSD is unusual because of its extraordinary potency: as little as 75 micrograms (a barely visible speck) is sufficient to induce hallucinations.

The methylxanthine drugs, such as caffeine and theophylline, are thought to exert their effects by acting through the second-messenger system. Specifically they inhibit the enzyme phosphodiesterase, which degrades cyclic AMP, so that they ultimately increase the amount of cyclic AMP that is generated in response to the transmitter. As a result these drugs exert a general mild stimulant action on the brain. Caffeine is the

HYPOTHETICAL GATING MECHANISM at the first synaptic relay in the spinal cord may regulate the transmission of pain information from the peripheral pain receptors to the brain. In the dorsal horn of the spinal cord, interneurons containing the peptide transmitter enkephalin make synapses onto the axon terminals of the pain neurons, which utilize substance P as their transmitter. Enkephalin released from the interneurons inhibits the release of substance P, so that the receiving neuron in the spinal cord receives less excitatory stimulation and hence sends fewer pain-related impulses to the brain. Opiate drugs such as morphine appear to bind to unoccupied enkephalin receptors, mimicking the pain-suppressing effects of enkephalin system.

principal active ingredient of coffee and tea; the weaker stimulant theophylline is found primarily in tea. Billions of pounds of coffee and tea are consumed each year, making the methylxanthines among the most widely used drugs.

Finally, certain drugs potentiate the effects of a transmitter by blocking its degradation in the synapse. One such group of drugs is represented by iproniazid (Marsilid) and other drugs that inhibit the enzyme monoamine oxidase, which degrades norepinephrine, dopamine and serotonin. As a result of the blockage of this enzyme the arousing effects of these monoamines are enhanced, accounting for the antidepressant actions of the drugs. A second group of antidepressant drugs, the tricyclics, also amplify the effects of norepinephrine and serotonin in the brain. These drugs, of which the best-known are imipramine (Tofranil) and amitriptyline (Elavil), block the reuptake of norepinephrine and serotonin from the synapse; the stimulant drug cocaine appears to work by the same mechanism. Such observations have suggested that depression may be associated with low levels of amine transmitters at brain synapses, whereas mania may be associated with excessively high levels of these transmitters.

The number of chemical-messenger systems known to exist in the brain has expanded dramatically in recent years with the discovery of a new family of brain chemicals: the neuropeptides. These molecules are chains of amino acids (ranging from two to 39 amino acids

long) that have been localized within neurons and are considered to be putative transmitter substances. Some of them were first identified as hormones secreted by the pituitary gland (ACTH, vasopressin), as local hormones in the gut (gastrin, cholecystokinin) or as hormones secreted by the hypothalamus to control the release of other hormones from the pituitary gland (luteinizing-hormone releasing hormone, somatostatin).

The newest and most exciting of the neuropeptides are the enkephalins and the endorphins: chemicals occurring naturally in the brain that bear a surprising similarity to morphine, the narcotic drug derived from the opium poppy. The discovery of these peptides followed the realization that certain regions of the brain bind opiate drugs with high affinity. The opiate receptors were detected by measuring the binding of radioactively labeled opiate compounds to fragments of neuronal membranes. Three research groups, led by Solomon H. Snyder and Candace B. Pert at the Johns Hopkins University School of Medicine, by Eric J. Simon at the New York University School of Medicine and by Lars Terenius at the University of Uppsala, developed such receptor-labeling techniques and found that opiate receptors were concentrated in those regions of the mammalian brain and spinal cord that are involved in the perception and integration of pain and emotional experience.

Then in 1975 John Hughes and Hans W. Kosterlitz of the University of Aberdeen isolated two naturally occurring

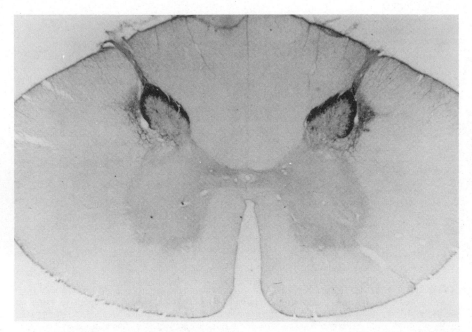

LOCALIZATION OF SUBSTANCE P in the spinal cord of the monkey was achieved by treating the tissue with specific antibodies that were labeled with a dark-staining chemical. The stain is present only in the dorsal horns of the spinal cord, which receive input from the peripheral pain fibers. The micrograph was made by Stephen Hunt of University of Cambridge.

peptides in the brain that bound tightly to the opiate receptors and named them enkephalins. Both enkephalins are chains of five amino acids; they are identical in sequence except for the terminal amino acid, which in one is methionine and in the other is leucine. Other morphinelike peptides, named endorphins, were subsequently isolated from the pituitary gland. Recent experiments have suggested that several procedures employed to treat chronic pain—acupuncture, direct electrical stimulation of the brain and even hypnosis—may act by eliciting the release of enkephalins or endorphins in the brain and spinal cord. This hypothesis is based on the finding that the effectiveness of all these procedures can be largely blocked by the administration of naloxone (Narcan), a drug that specifically blocks the binding of morphine to the opiate receptor.

Many of the neuropeptides found in the mammalian brain have been shown to be concentrated in the terminals of particular sets of neurons, and several are known to be released from axon terminals by a calcium-dependent process. Such findings, together with the observation that minute amounts of neuropeptides exert significant effects on neuronal activity or on the behavior of experimental animals, strongly suggest that these chemicals may well be a new family of transmitters. In most cases, however, the evidence is not yet strong enough to support a definite conclusion.

Perhaps the strongest candidate among the neuropeptides for transmitter status is substance P, a chain of 11 amino acids. It is present in a number of specific neuronal pathways in the brain and also in primary sensory fibers of peripheral nerves. Some of these sensory neurons, whose cell bodies lie in sensory ganglia on each side of the spinal cord, contain substance P and release it from their axon terminals at synapses with spinal-cord neurons. Because substance P excites those spinal neurons that respond most readily to painful stimuli the substance has been suggested to be a sensory transmitter that is specifically associated with the transmission of pain-related information from peripheral pain receptors into the central nervous system.

The morphinelike peptide enkephalin is also present in abundance in small neurons in the part of the spinal cord that receives the fiber input containing substance P. Thomas Jessel and I at the Neurochemical Pharmacology Unit of the Medical Research Council have shown that enkephalin and opiate drugs are able to suppress the release of substance P from sensory fibers. The enkephalin-containing neurons may therefore regulate the input of painful stimuli to the brain by modulating the release of substance P at the first relay in the central nervous system. Similar inhibitory interactions may also take place at higher levels of the brain. Substance P is not the only putative transmitter shown to be localized in sensory neurons; the others so far identified include angiotensin, cholecystokinin, somatostatin and glutamic acid. A bewildering chemical complexity is therefore beginning to emerge as more is learned about the sensory transmitters and their modulating mechanisms in the spinal cord.

A remarkable feature of the neuropeptides in the brain is the global nature of some of their effects. Administration of very small amounts of a neuropeptide (usually directly into the brain to circumvent the blood-brain barrier) can trigger a complex and highly specific pattern of behavior in experimental animals. For example, injection into the brain of nanogram amounts of the neuropeptide angiotensin II elicits intense and prolonged drinking behavior in animals that were not previously thirsty. Another peptide, luteinizing-hormone releasing hormone, induces characteristic female sexual behavior when it is injected into the brain of a female rat. Even more striking, as has been shown by David de Wied and his colleagues at the University of Utrecht, the administration of small amounts of the neuropeptide vasopressin markedly improves the memory of learned tasks in laboratory animals. Preliminary clinical trials of this agent are now in progress to ascertain whether it may have beneficial effects on human patients suffering from memory loss.

It therefore seems that the neuropeptides may be chemical messengers of a character different from that of the previously identified transmitters: they appear to represent a global means of chemical coding for patterns of brain activity associated with particular functions, such as body-fluid balance, sexual behavior and pain or pleasure. An unexpected observation is that biologically active peptides originally found in the gastrointestinal tract, such as gastrin, substance P, vasoactive intestinal polypeptide (VIP) and cholecystokinin, are also present in the central nervous system. Conversely some peptides originally found in the brain have later been found in the gut (somatostatin, neurotensin, enkephalins). It therefore appears that these peptides serve a multiplicity of roles, acting as local hormones or transmitters in the gastrointestinal tract and as global transmitters in the brain. Roger Guillemin of the Salk Institute has suggested that the multiple functions of neuropeptides may be due to the opportunism of the evolutionary process, in which a molecule that serves one function may be adapted to serve another function at a different time and place.

A number of other chemicals appear to play a modulatory role in neuronal communication. The prostaglandins, which consist of a five-carbon ring with two long carbon chains attached to it, are present at high levels in brain tissue and elicit a variety of excitatory and inhibitory effects on neurons, depending on the precise molecular structure of the prostaglandin and the identity of the target cell. Whereas the transmitters have rapid and transient effects, the prostaglandins elicit long-term shifts in the polarization of the neuronal membrane, suggesting that they play a modulatory role rather than a transmitter role. It is possible that they act in concert with transmitters to subtly alter their effects.

Still another set of chemicals plays a nutritive role rather than a messenger role. These "trophic" substances are thought to be secreted from nerve terminals and to maintain the viability of the target cell; other trophic substances are taken up by the nerve terminal and transported along the axon in a retrograde fashion to nourish the neuron itself. The well-known phenomenon of muscle atrophy after an innervating nerve has been severed may result from the inability of the muscle cells to obtain the trophic substances they require. A number of degenerative brain diseases may result from the failure of central neurons to exchange trophic substances. The best-characterized trophic substance to date is the nerve-growth factor (NGF), a protein that is essential for the differentiation and survival of peripheral sensory and sympathetic neurons and that may also be involved in maintaining central monoamine neurons.

Apart from the ever increasing list of chemical transmitters, the variety of different mechanisms by which transmitters can exert their effects is also becoming apparent. For example, instead of directly exciting or inhibiting a target neuron, a transmitter released from one nerve terminal can act presynaptically on an adjacent nerve terminal to increase or decrease the release of transmitter from that nerve terminal. It is also clear that there may be several different types of receptors for a given transmitter substance (some mediated by second-messenger systems and some not), accounting for the diverse excitatory or inhibitory effects of a given transmitter in different parts of the brain. Even the well-established concept (first suggested by Sir Henry Dale) that a neuron releases only one transmitter chemical from all its terminals may not be inviolable: a number of neuropeptides have been found to coexist in the same neurons with norepinephrine or serotonin. The functional significance of such dual-transmitter systems is not yet known. In addition the precise chemical disturbances that underlie such common disorders as epilepsy, senile dementia, alcoholism, schizophrenia and depression remain largely obscure. Although the study of transmitter systems in the brain has already provided major clues to the chemical mechanisms involved in learning, memory, sleep and mood, it seems clear that the most exciting discoveries lie ahead.

VII

Brain Mechanisms
of Vision

Brain Mechanisms of Vision

BY DAVID H. HUBEL AND TORSTEN N. WIESEL

A functional architecture that may underlie processing of sensory information in the cortex is revealed by studies of the activity and the organization in space of neurons in the primary visual cortex

Viewed as a kind of invention by evolution, the cerebral cortex must be one of the great success stories in the history of living things. In vertebrates lower than mammals the cerebral cortex is minuscule, if it can be said to exist at all. Suddenly impressive in the lowest mammals, it begins to dominate the brain in carnivores, and it increases explosively in primates; in man it almost completely envelops the rest of the brain, tending to obscure the other parts. The degree to which an animal depends on an organ is an index of the organ's importance that is even more convincing than size, and dependence on the cortex has increased rapidly as mammals have evolved. A mouse without a cortex appears fairly normal, at least to casual inspection; a man without a cortex is almost a vegetable, speechless, sightless, senseless.

Understanding of this large and indispensable organ is still woefully deficient. This is partly because it is very complex, not only structurally but also in its functions, and partly because neurobiologists' intuitions about the functions have so often been wrong. The outlook is changing, however, as techniques improve and as investigators learn how to deal with the huge numbers of intricately connected neurons that are the basic elements of the cortex, with the impulses they carry and with the synapses that connect them. In this article we hope to sketch the present state of knowledge of one subdivision of the cortex: the primary visual cortex (also known as the striate cortex or area 17), the most elementary of the cortical regions concerned with vision. That will necessarily lead us into the related subject of visual perception, since the workings of an organ cannot easily be separated from its biological purpose.

The cerebral cortex, a highly folded plate of neural tissue about two millimeters thick, is an outermost crust wrapped over the top of, and to some extent tucked under, the cerebral hemispheres. In man its total area, if it were spread out, would be about 1.5 square feet. (In a 1963 article in *Scientific American* one of us gave the area as 20 square feet and was quickly corrected by a neuroanatomist friend in Toronto, who said he thought it was 1.5 square feet—"at least that is what Canadians have.") The folding is presumably mainly the result of such an unlikely structure's having to be packed into a box the size of the skull.

A casual glance at cortical tissue under a microscope shows vast numbers of neurons: about 10^5 (100,000) for each square millimeter of surface, suggesting that the cortex as a whole has some 10^{10} (10 billion) neurons. The cell bodies are arranged in half a dozen layers that are alternately cell-sparse and cell-rich. In contrast to these marked changes in cell density in successive layers at different depths in the cortex there is marked uniformity from place to place in the plane of any given layer and in any direction within that plane. The cortex is morphologically rather uniform in two of its dimensions.

One of the first great insights about cortical organization came late in the 19th century, when it was gradually realized that this rather uniform plate of tissue is subdivided into a number of different regions that have very different functions. The evidence came from clinical, physiological and anatomical sources. It was noted that a brain injury, depending on its location, could cause paralysis or blindness or numbness or speech loss; the blindness could be total or limited to half or less of the visual world, and the numbness could involve one limb or a few fingers. The consistency of the relation between a given defect and the location of the lesion gradually led to a charting of the most obvious of these specialized regions, the visual, auditory, somatic sensory (body sensation), speech and motor regions.

In many cases a close look with a microscope at cortex stained for cell bodies showed that in spite of the relative uniformity there were structural variations, particularly in the layering pattern, that correlated well with the clinically defined subdivisions. Additional confirmation came from observations of the location (at the surface of the brain) of the electrical brain waves produced when an animal was stimulated by touching the body, sounding clicks or tones in the ear or flashing light in the eye. Similarly, motor areas could be mapped by stimulating the cortex electrically and noting what part of the animal's body moved.

This systematic mapping of the cortex soon led to a fundamental realization: most of the sensory and motor areas contained systematic two-dimensional maps of the world they represented. Destroying a particular small region of cortex could lead to paralysis of one arm; a similar lesion in another small region led to numbness of one hand or of the upper lip, or blindness in one small part of the visual world; if electrodes were placed on an animal's cortex, touching one limb produced a correspondingly localized series of electric potentials. Clearly the body was systematically mapped onto the somatic sensory and motor areas; the visual world was mapped onto the primary visual cortex, an area on the occipital lobe that in man and in the macaque monkey (the animal in which our investigations have mainly been conducted) covers about 15 square centimeters.

In the primary visual cortex the map is uncomplicated by breaks and discontinuities except for the remarkable split of the visual world down the exact middle, with the left half projected to the right cerebral cortex and the right half projected to the left cortex. The map of the body is more complicated and is still perhaps not completely understood. It is nonetheless systematic, and it is similarly crossed, with the right side of the body projecting to the left hemisphere and the left side projecting to the right hemisphere. (It is worth remarking that no one has the remotest idea why there should be this amazing tendency for nervous-system pathways to cross.)

An important feature of cortical maps is their distortion. The scale of the maps varies as it does in a Mercator projection, the rule for the cortex being that

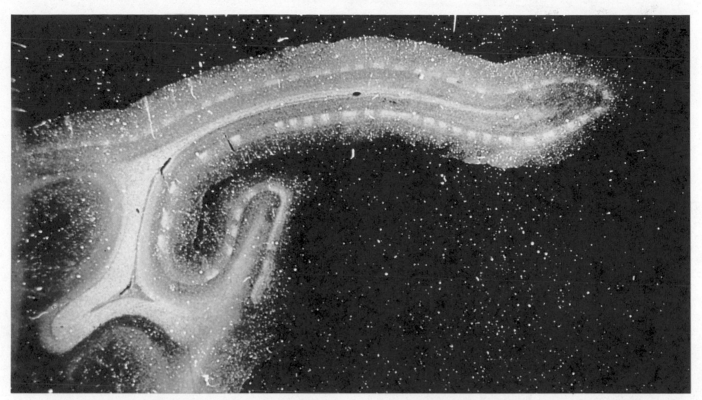

OCULAR-DOMINANCE COLUMNS, one of the two major systems that characterize the functional architecture of the primary visual cortex, are revealed as periodic bright patches in this dark-field autoradiograph of a section of macaque monkey cortex. The columns (actually curving slabs of cortex, seen here in cross section in a brain slice cut perpendicularly to the surface) are regions in which all neurons respond more actively to the right eye than to the left one; dark regions separating the bright patches are columns of left-eye prefer- ence. The autoradiograph was made by injecting a radioactively labeled amino acid into the right eye of an anesthetized animal. The amino acid was taken up by cell bodies in the retina and transported via the lateral geniculate nucleus, a way station in the brain, to cells in the cortex. A brain slice was coated with a photographic emulsion, which was exposed for several months and then developed. Exposed silver grains overlying the regions of radioactivity form the light-scattering patches that represent ocular-dominance columns.

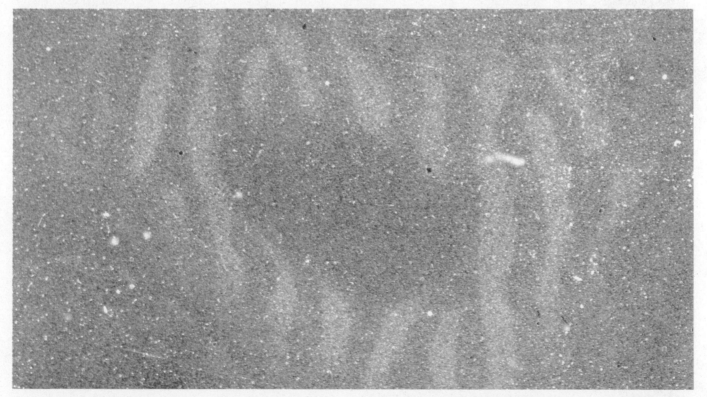

DOMINANCE PATTERN is seen face on in an axonal-transport autoradiograph of a brain section parallel, rather than perpendicular, to the surface of the primary visual cortex. As can be seen in the autoradiograph at the top of the page, the label is brightest in one layer of the folded cortex, layer IV. This is the level at which the axons bringing visual information to the cortex terminate and where the label therefore accumulates. This section was cut in a plane tangential to the dome-shaped surface of the cortex and just below layer IV, which therefore appears as a ring of roughly parallel bright bands. These are the radioactively labeled ocular-dominance regions, which are now seen from above instead of edge on. The actual width of the ocular-dominance regions is typically about .4 millimeter.

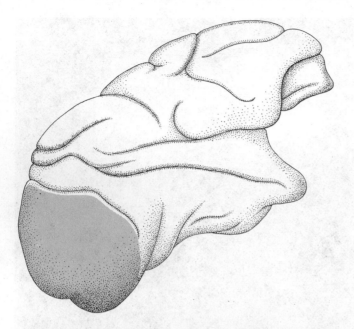 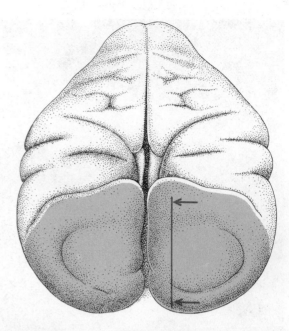

PRIMARY VISUAL CORTEX, also known as the striate cortex or area 17, is a region of the cerebral cortex: a layered plate of neurons that envelops the primate brain. In the macaque brain, seen here from the side (*left*) and from above and behind (*right*), the primary visual cortex (*colored areas*) occupies most of the exposed surface of the two occipital lobes. It also curves around the medial surface between the two cerebral hemispheres. It continues in a complex fold underneath the convex outer surface, as is shown in a parasagittal section (*see top illustration on opposite page*) that was cut along the colored line and is viewed in the direction indicated by the arrows.

the regions of highest discrimination or delicacy of function occupy relatively more cortical area. For the body surface, a millimeter of surface on the fingers, the lips or the tongue projects to more cortex than a millimeter of trunk, buttocks or back; in vision the central part of the retina has a representation some 35 times more detailed than the far peripheral part.

Important as the advances in mapping cortical projections were, they tended for some time to divert thought from the real problem of just how the brain analyzes information. It was as though the representation could be an end in itself instead of serving a more subtle purpose—as though what the cortex did was to cater to some little green man who sat inside the head and surveyed images playing across the cortex. In the course of this article we shall show that, for vision at least, the world is represented in a far more distorted way; any little green man trying to glean information from the cortical projection would be puzzled indeed.

The first major insight into cortical organization was nonetheless the recognition of this subdivision into areas having widely different functions, with a tendency to ordered mapping. Just how many such areas there are has been a subject of wide speculation. Anatomists' estimates have on the whole been rather high—up to several hundred areas, depending on the individual worker's sensitivity to fine differences in microscopic patterns and sometimes also on his ability to fool himself. Physiologists began with lower estimates, but lately, with more powerful mapping methods, they

have been revising their estimates upward. The important basic notion is that information on any given modality such as sight or sound is transmitted first to a primary cortical area and from there, either directly or via the thalamus, to successions of higher areas. A modern guess as to the number of cortical areas might be between 50 and 100.

The second major insight into cortical organization came from the work of the anatomist Santiago Ramón y Cajal and his pupil Rafael Lorente de Nó. This was the realization that the operations the cortex performs on the information it receives are local. What that means can best be understood by considering the wiring diagram that emerged from the Golgi method used by Cajal and Lorente de Nó. In essence the wiring is simple. Sets of fibers bring information to the cortex; by the time several synapses have been traversed the influence of the input has spread vertically to all cell layers; finally several other sets of fibers carry modified messages out of the area. The detailed connections between inputs and outputs differ from one area to the next, but within a given area they seem to be rather stereotyped. What is common to all regions is the local nature of the wiring. The information carried into the cortex by a single fiber can in principle make itself felt through the entire thickness in about three or four synapses, whereas the lateral spread, produced by branching trees of axons and dendrites, is limited for all practical purposes to a few millimeters, a small proportion of the vast extent of the cortex.

The implications of this are far-reaching. Whatever any given region of the cortex does, it does locally. At stages where there is any kind of detailed, systematic topographical mapping the analysis must be piecemeal. For example, in the somatic sensory cortex the messages concerning one finger can be combined and compared with an input from elsewhere on that same finger or with input from a neighboring finger, but they can hardly be combined with the influence from the trunk or from a foot. The same applies to the visual world. Given the detailed order of the input to the primary visual cortex, there is no likelihood that the region will do anything to correlate information coming in from both far above and far below the horizon, or from both the left and the right part of the visual scene. It follows that this cannot by any stretch of the imagination be the place where actual perception is enshrined. Whatever these cortical areas are doing, it must be some kind of local analysis of the sensory world. One can only assume that as the information on vision or touch or sound is relayed from one cortical area to the next the map becomes progressively more blurred and the information carried more abstract.

Even though the Golgi-method studies of the early 1900's made it clear that the cortex must perform local analyses, it was half a century before physiologists had the least inkling of just what the analysis was in any area of the cortex. The first understanding came in the primary visual area, which is now the best-understood of any cortical region and is still the only one where the analysis and consequent transformations of information are known in any detail. After describing the main transformations that take place in the primary visual cortex we shall go on to show how increasing understanding of these cortical functions has revealed an entire world of architectural order that is otherwise inaccessible to observation.

We can best begin by tracing the visual path in a primate from the retina to the cortex. The output from each eye is conveyed to the brain by about a million nerve fibers bundled together in the optic nerve. These fibers are the axons of the ganglion cells of the retina. The messages from the light-sensitive elements, the rods and cones, have already traversed from two to four synapses and have involved four other types of retinal cells before they arrive at the ganglion cells, and a certain amount of sophisticated analysis of the information has already taken place.

A large fraction of the optic-nerve fibers pass uninterrupted to two nests of cells deep in the brain called the lateral geniculate nuclei, where they make synapses. The lateral geniculate cells in turn send their axons directly to the primary visual cortex. From there, after several synapses, the messages are sent to a number of further destinations: neighboring cortical areas and also several targets deep in the brain. One contingent even projects back to the lateral geniculate bodies; the function of this feedback path is not known. The main point for the moment is that the primary visual cortex is in no sense the end of the visual path. It is just one stage, probably an early one in terms of the degree of abstraction of the information it handles.

As a result of the partial crossing of the optic nerves in the optic chiasm, the geniculate and the cortex on the left side are connected to the two left half retinas and are therefore concerned with the right half of the visual scene, and the converse is the case for the right geniculate and the right cortex. Each geniculate and each cortex receives input from both eyes, and each is concerned with the opposite half of the visual world.

To examine the workings of this visual pathway our strategy since the late 1950's has been (in principle) simple. Beginning, say, with the fibers of the optic nerve, we record with microelectrodes from a single nerve fiber and try to find out how we can most effectively influence the firing by stimulating the retina with light. For this one can use patterns of light of every conceivable size, shape and color, bright on a dark background or the reverse, and stationary or moving. It may take a long time, but sooner or later we satisfy ourselves that we have found the best stimulus for the cell being tested, in this case a ganglion cell of the retina. (Sometimes we are

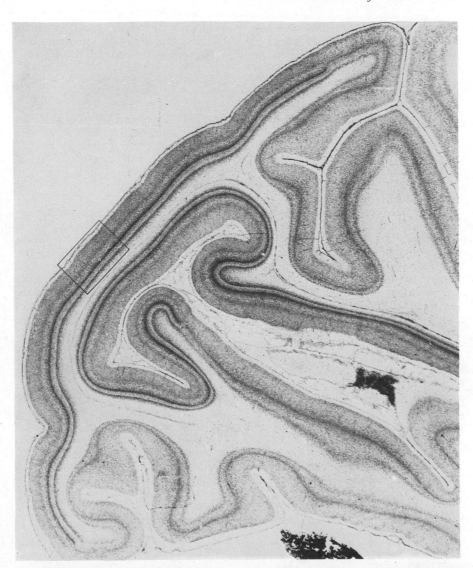

SECTION OF VISUAL CORTEX along the colored line in the illustration on the opposite page was stained by the Nissl method, which makes cell bodies but not fibers visible. The visual cortex is seen to be a continuous layered sheet of neurons about two millimeters thick. The black rectangle outlines a section like the one that is further enlarged in the illustration below.

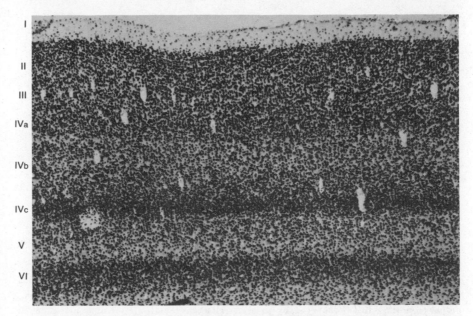

CROSS SECTION OF PRIMARY VISUAL CORTEX in the macaque, stained here by the Nissl method and enlarged about 35 diameters, shows the layered structure and gives the conventional designations of the six layers (*left*). The white gaps are sectioned blood vessels.

wrong!) We note the results and then go on to another fiber. After studying a few hundred cells we may find that new types become rare. Satisfied that we know roughly how the neurons at this stage work, we proceed to the next stage (in this case the geniculate) and repeat the process. Comparison of the two sets of results can tell us something about what the geniculate does. We then go on to the next stage, the primary cortex, and repeat the procedure.

Working in this way, one finds that both a retinal ganglion cell and a geniculate cell respond best to a roughly circular spot of light of a particular size in a particular part of the visual field. The size is critical because each cell's receptive field (the patch of retinal receptor cells supplying the cell) is divided, with an excitatory center and an inhibitory surround (an "on center" cell) or exactly the reverse configuration (an "off center" cell). This is the center-surround configuration first described by Stephen W. Kuffler at the Johns Hopkins University School of Medicine in 1953. A spot exactly filling the center of an on-center cell is therefore a more effective stimulus than a larger spot that invades the inhibitory area, or than diffuse light. A line stimulus (a bar of light) is effective if it covers a large part of the center region and only a small part of the surround. Because these cells have circular symmetry they respond well to such a line stimulus whatever its orientation. To sum up, the retinal ganglion cells and the cells of the lateral geniculate—the cells supplying the input to the visual cortex—are cells with concentric, center-surround receptive fields. They are primarily concerned not with assessing levels of illumination but rather with making a comparison between the light level in one small area of the visual scene and the average illumination of the immediate surround.

The first of the two major transformations accomplished by the visual cortex is the rearrangement of incoming information so that most of its cells respond not to spots of light but to specifically oriented line segments. There is a wide variety of cell types in the cortex, some simpler and some more complex in their response properties, and one soon gains an impression of a kind of hierarchy, with simpler cells feeding more complex ones. In the monkey there is first of all a large group of cells that behave (as far as is known) just like geniculate cells: they have circularly symmetrical fields. These cells are all in the lower part of one layer, called layer IV, which is precisely the layer that receives the lion's share of the geniculate input. It makes sense that these least sophisticated cortical cells should be the ones most immediately connected to the input.

Cells outside layer IV all respond best to specifically oriented line segments. A typical cell responds only when light falls in a particular part of the visual world, but illuminating that area diffusely has little effect or none, and small spots of light are not much better. The best response is obtained when a line that has just the right tilt is flashed in the region or, in some cells, is swept across the region. The most effective orientation varies from cell to cell and is usually defined sharply enough so that a change of 10 or 20 degrees clockwise or counterclockwise reduces the response markedly or abolishes it. (It is hard to convey the precision of this discrimination. If 10 to 20 degrees sounds like a wide range, one should remember that the angle between 12 o'clock and one o'clock is 30 degrees.) A line at 90 degrees to the best orientation almost never evokes any response.

Depending on the particular cell, the stimulus may be a bright line on a dark background or the reverse, or it may be a boundary between light and dark regions. If it is a line, the thickness is likely to be important; increasing it beyond some optimal width reduces the response, just as increasing the diameter of a spot does in the case of ganglion and geniculate cells. Indeed, for a particular part of the visual field the geniculate receptive-field centers and the optimal cortical line widths are comparable.

Neurons with orientation specificity vary in their complexity. The simplest, which we call "simple" cells, behave as though they received their input directly from several cells with center-surround, circularly symmetrical fields—the type of cells found in layer IV. The response properties of these simple cells, which respond to an optimally oriented line in a narrowly defined location, can most easily be accounted for by requiring that the centers of the incoming center-surround fields all be excitatory or all be inhibitory, and that they lie along a straight line. At present we have no direct evidence for this scheme, but it is attractive because of its simplicity and because certain kinds of indirect evidence support it. According to the work of Jennifer S. Lund of the University of Washington School of Medicine, who in the past few years has done more than anyone else to advance the Golgi-stain anatomy of this cortical area, the cells in layer IV project to the layers just above, which is roughly where the simple cells are found.

The second major group of orientation-specific neurons are the far more numerous "complex" cells. They come in a number of subcategories, but their main feature is that they are less particular about the exact position of a line.

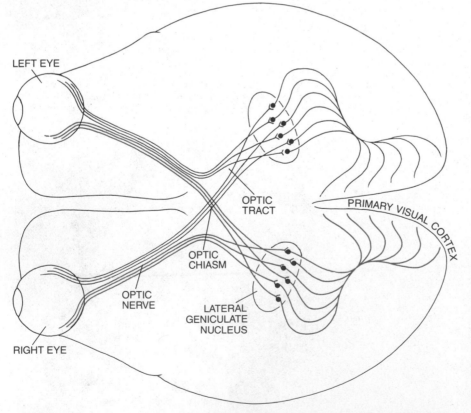

LEFT EYE

OPTIC TRACT

PRIMARY VISUAL CORTEX

OPTIC CHIASM

OPTIC NERVE

LATERAL GENICULATE NUCLEUS

RIGHT EYE

VISUAL PATHWAY is traced schematically in the human brain, seen here from below. The output from the retina is conveyed, by ganglion-cell axons bundled in the optic nerves, to the lateral geniculate nuclei; about half of the axons cross over to the opposite side of the brain, so that a representation of each half of the visual scene is projected on the geniculate of the opposite hemisphere. Neurons in the geniculates send their axons to the primary visual cortex.

RIGHT EYE

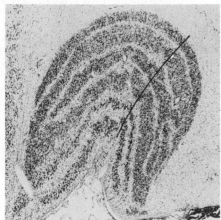

LEFT EYE

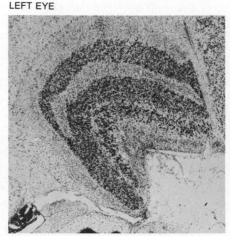

RIGHT EYE

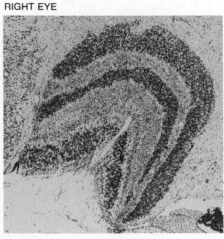

LATERAL GENICULATE NUCLEUS of a normal monkey (*left*) is a layered structure in which cells in layers 1, 4 and 6 (numbered from bottom to top) receive their input from the eye on the opposite side and those in layers 2, 3 and 5 receive information from the eye on the same side. The maps are in register, so that the neurons along any radius (*black line*) receive signals from the same part of the visual scene. The layered nature of the input is demonstrated in the two geniculates of an animal that had vision in the left eye only (*two micrographs at right*): in each geniculate cells in the three layers with input from right eye have atrophied. Geniculates are enlarged 10 diameters.

Complex cells behave as though they received their input from a number of simple cells, all with the same receptive-field orientation but differing slightly in the exact location of their fields. This scheme readily explains the strong steady firing evoked in a complex cell as a line is kept in the optimal orientation and is swept across the receptive field. With the line optimally oriented many cells prefer one direction of movement to the opposite direction. Several possible circuits have been proposed to explain this behavior, but the exact mechanism is still not known.

Although there is no direct evidence that orientation-sensitive cells have anything to do with visual perception, it is certainly tempting to think they represent some early stage in the brain's analysis of visual forms. It is worth asking which cells at this early stage would be expected to be turned on by some very simple visual form, say a dark blob on a light background. Any cell whose receptive field is entirely inside or outside the boundaries of such an image will be completely unaffected by the figure's presence because cortical cells effectively ignore diffuse changes in the illumination of their entire receptive fields.

The only cells to be affected will be those whose field is cut by the borders. For the circularly symmetrical cells the ones most strongly influenced will be those whose center is grazed by a boundary (because for them the excitatory and inhibitory subdivisions are most unequally illuminated). For the orientation-specific cells the only ones to be activated will be those whose optimal orientation happens to coincide with the prevailing direction of the border. And among these the simple cells will be much more exacting than the complex ones, responding optimally only when the border falls along a line separating an excitatory and an inhibitory region. It is important to realize that this part of the cortex is operating only locally, on bits of the form; how the entire form is analyzed or handled by the brain—how this information is worked on and synthesized at later stages, if indeed it is—is still not known.

The second major function of the monkey visual cortex is to combine the inputs from the two eyes. In the lateral geniculate nuclei a neuron may re-

a

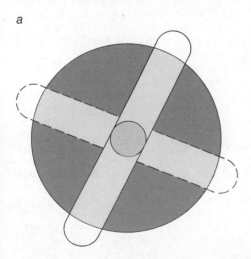

b

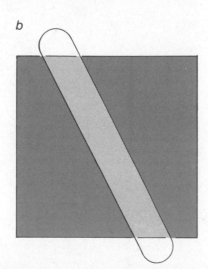

c

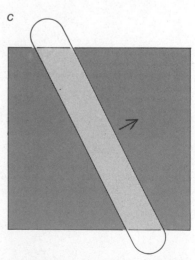

RECEPTIVE FIELDS of various cells in the visual pathway are compared. Retinal ganglion cells and neurons in the lateral geniculate nucleus have circular fields with either an excitatory center and an inhibitory surround (*a*) or the opposite arrangement. A spot of light falling on the center stimulates a response from such a cell; so does a bar of light falling on the field in any orientation, provided it falls on the center. In the visual cortex there is a hierarchy of neurons with increasingly complex response properties. The cortical cells that receive signals directly from the geniculate have circularly symmetrical fields. Cortical cells farther along the pathway, however, respond only to a line stimulus in a particular orientation. A "simple" cell (*b*) responds to such a line stimulus only in a particular part of its field. A "complex" cell (*c*) responds to a precisely oriented line regardless of where it is in its field and also to one moving in a particular direction (*arrow*).

spond to stimulation of the left eye or of the right one, but no cell responds to stimulation of both eyes. This may seem surprising, since each geniculate receives inputs from both eyes, but the fact is that the geniculates are constructed in a way that keeps inputs from the two eyes segregated. Each geniculate body is divided into six layers, three left-eye layers interdigitated with three right-eye ones. The opposite-side half of the visual world is mapped onto each layer (with the six maps in precise register, so that in a radial pathway traversing the six layers the receptive fields of all the cells encountered have virtually identical positions in the visual field). Since any one layer has input from only one eye, the individual cells of that layer must be monocular.

Even in the visual cortex the neurons to which the geniculate cells project directly, the circularly symmetrical cells in layer IV, are all (as far as we can tell) strictly monocular; so are all the simple cells. Only at the level of the complex cells do the paths from the two eyes converge, and even there the blending of information is incomplete and takes a special form. About half of the complex cells are monocular, in the sense that any one cell can be activated only by stimulating one eye. The rest of the cells can be influenced independently by both eyes.

If one maps the right-eye and left-eye receptive fields of a binocular cell (by stimulating first through one eye and then through the other) and compares the two fields, the fields turn out to have identical positions, levels of complexity, orientation and directional preference; everything one learns about the cell by stimulating one eye is confirmed through the other eye. There is only one exception: if first one eye and then the other are tested with identical stimuli, the two responses are usually not quantitatively identical; in many cases one eye is dominant, consistently producing a higher frequency of firing than the other eye.

From cell to cell all degrees of ocular dominance can be found, from complete monopoly by one eye through equality to exclusive control by the other eye. In the monkey the cells with a marked eye preference are somewhat commoner than the cells in which the two eyes make about equal contributions. Apparently a binocular cell in the primary visual cortex has connections to the two eyes that are qualitatively virtually identical, but the density of the two sets of connections is not necessarily the same.

It is remarkable enough that the elaborate sets of wiring that produce specificity of orientation and of direction of movement and other special properties

should be present in two duplicate copies. It is perhaps even more surprising that all of this can be observed in a newborn animal. The wiring is mostly innate, and it presumably is genetically determined. (In one particular respect, however, some maturation of binocular wiring does take place mostly after birth.)

We now turn to a consideration of the way these cells are grouped in the cortex. Are cells with similar characteristics—complexity, receptive-field position, orientation and ocular dominance—grouped together or scattered at random? From the description so far it will be obvious that cells of like complexity tend to be grouped in layers, with the circularly symmetrical cells low in layer IV, the simple cells just above them and the complex cells in layers II, III, V and VI. Complex cells can be further subcategorized, and the ones found in each layer are in a number of ways very different.

These differences from layer to layer take on added interest in view of the important discovery, confirmed by several physiologists and anatomists during the past few decades, that fibers projecting from particular layers of the cortex have particular destinations. For example, in the visual cortex the deepest layer, layer VI, projects mainly (perhaps only) back to the lateral geniculate body; layer V projects to the superior colliculus, a visual station in the midbrain; layers II and III send their projections to other parts of the cortex. This relation between layer and projection site probably deserves to be ranked as a third major insight into cortical organization.

The next stimulus variable to be considered is the position of the receptive field in the visual field. In describing the lateral geniculate nucleus we pointed out that in each layer the opposite-half visual field forms an ordered topographical map. In the projection from lateral geniculate to primary visual cortex this order is preserved, producing a cortical map of the visual field. Given this ordered map it is no surprise that neighboring cells in this part of the cortex always have receptive fields that are close together; usually, in fact, they overlap. If one plunges a microelectrode into the cortex at a right angle to the surface and records from cell after cell (as many as 100 or 200 of them) in successively deeper layers, again the receptive fields mostly overlap, with each new field heaped on all the others. The extent of the entire pile of fields is usually several times the size of any one typical field.

There is some variation in the size of these receptive fields. Some of the variation is tied to the layering: the largest fields in any penetration tend to be in

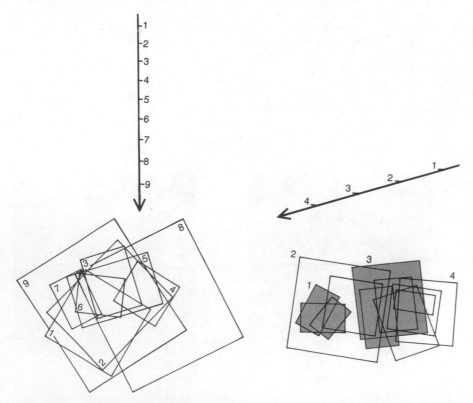

POSITIONS OF RECEPTIVE FIELDS (*numbered from 1 to 9*) **of cortical neurons mapped by an electrode penetrating at roughly a right angle to the surface are essentially the same** (*left*), **although the fields are different sizes and there is some scatter. In an oblique penetration** (*right*) **from two to four cells were recorded, at .1-millimeter intervals, at each of four sites** (*numbered from 1 to 4*) **one millimeter apart. Each group includes various sizes and some scatter, but now there is also a systematic drift: fields of each successive group of cells are somewhat displaced.**

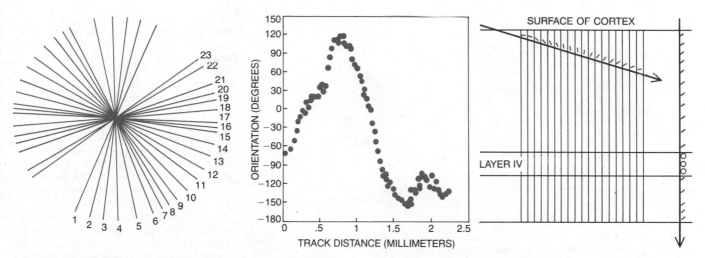

ORIENTATION PREFERENCES of 23 neurons encountered as a microelectrode penetrated the cortex obliquely are charted (*left*); the most effective tilt of the stimulus changed steadily in a counterclockwise direction. The results of a similar experiment are plotted (*center*); in this case, however, there were several reversals in direction of rotation. The results of a large number of such experiments, together with the observation that a microelectrode penetrating the cortex perpendicularly encounters only cells that prefer the same orientation (apart from the circularly symmetrical cells in layer IV, which have no preferred orientation), suggested that the cortex is subdivided into roughly parallel slabs of tissue, with each slab, called an orientation column, containing neurons with like orientation specificity (*right*).

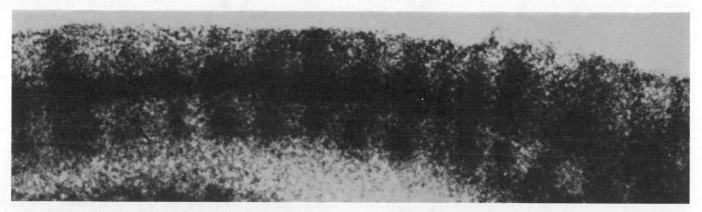

ORIENTATION COLUMNS are visualized as anatomical structures in a deoxyglucose autoradiograph made by the authors and Michael P. Stryker. Radioactively labeled deoxyglucose was injected into a monkey; it was taken up primarily by active neurons, and an early metabolite accumulated in the cells. Immediately after the injection the animal was stimulated with a pattern of vertical stripes, so that cells responding to vertical lines were most active and became most radioactive. In this section perpendicular to surface active-cell regions are narrow bands about .5 millimeter apart. Layer IV (with no orientation preference) is, as expected, uniformly radioactive.

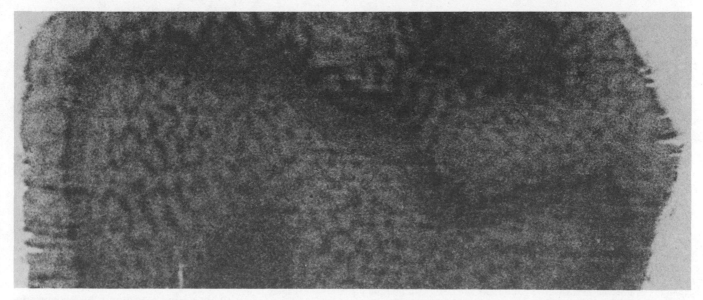

ORIENTATION PATTERN, seen face on, is unexpectedly complex. This deoxyglucose autoradiograph is of a section tangential to the somewhat curved layers of the cortex. The darker regions represent continuously labeled layer IV. In the other layers the orientation regions are intricately curved bands, something like the walls of a maze seen from above, but distance from one band to next is uniform.

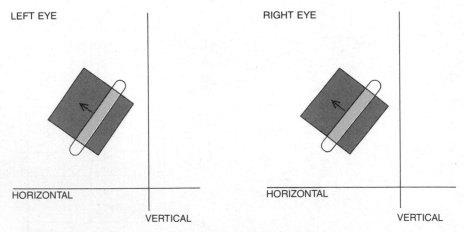

LEFT EYE RIGHT EYE

HORIZONTAL HORIZONTAL

VERTICAL VERTICAL

BINOCULAR CELL in the cortex can be influenced independently by both eyes or more strongly by both eyes together. Here the left-eye and right-eye fields are mapped for a complex cell whose receptive field is in the upper left quadrant of the visual field. (The lines represent the horizontal and vertical meridians of the field, intersecting at the point of fixation.) The two receptive fields are identical, but the amount of response may differ depending on whether the left eye or the right eye is stimulated. Preference for one eye is called ocular dominance.

layers III, V and VI. The most important variation, however, is linked to eccentricity, or the distance of a cell's receptive field from the center of gaze. The size of the fields and the extent of the associated scatter in the part of the cortex that maps the center of gaze are tiny compared to the size and amount of scatter in the part that maps the far periphery. We call the pile of superimposed fields that are mapped in a penetration beginning at any point on the cortex the "aggregate field" of that point. The size of the aggregate field is obviously a function of eccentricity.

If the electrode penetrates in an oblique direction, almost parallel to the surface, the scatter in field position from cell to cell is again evident, but now there is superimposed on the scatter

a consistent drift in field position, its direction dictated by the topographical map of the visual fields. And an interesting regularity is revealed: it turns out that moving the electrode about one or two millimeters always produces a displacement in visual field that is roughly enough to take one into an entirely new region. The movement in the visual field, in short, is about the same as the size of the aggregate receptive field. For the primary visual cortex this holds wherever the recording is made. At the center of gaze the fields and their associated scatter are tiny, but so is the displacement corresponding to a one-millimeter movement along the cortex. With increasing eccentricity (farther out in the visual field) both the field and scatter and the displacement become larger, in parallel fashion. It seems that every-

where a block of cortex about one or two millimeters in size is what is needed to take care of a region of the visual world equivalent to the size of an aggregate field.

These observations suggest the way the visual cortex solves a basic problem: how to analyze the visual scene in detail in the central part and much more crudely in the periphery. In the retina, which has the same problem, for obvious optical reasons the number of millimeters corresponding to a degree of visual field is constant. The retina handles the central areas in great detail by having huge numbers of ganglion cells, each subserving a tiny area of central visual field; the layer of ganglion cells in the central part of the retina is thick, whereas in the outlying parts of the retina it is very thin. The cortex, in contrast, seems to want to be uniform in thickness everywhere. Here there are none of the optical constraints imposed on the retina, and so area is simply allotted in amounts corresponding to the problem at hand.

The machinery in any square millimeter of cortex is presumably about the same as in any other. A few thousand geniculate fibers enter such a region, the cortex does its thing and perhaps 50,000 fibers leave—whether a small part of the visual world is represented in great detail or a larger part in correspondingly less detail. The uniformity of the cortex is suggested, as we indicated at the outset, by the appearance of stained sections. It is compellingly confirmed when we examine the architecture further, looking specifically at orientation and at ocular dominance.

For orientation we inquire about groupings of cells just as we did with field position, looking first at two cells sitting side by side. Two such cells almost invariably have the same optimal stimulus orientation. If the electrode is inserted in a direction perpendicular to the surface, all the cells along the path of penetration have identical or almost identical orientations (except for the cells deep in layer IV, which have no optimal orientation at all). In two perpendicular penetrations a millimeter or so apart, however, the two orientations observed are usually different. The cortex must therefore be subdivided by some kind of vertical partitioning into regions of constant receptive-field orientation. When we came on this system almost 20 years ago, it intrigued us because it fitted so well with the hierarchical schemes we had proposed to explain how complex cells are supplied by inputs from simple cells: the circuit diagrams involve connections between cells whose fields cover the same part of the visual world and that respond to the same line orientation. It seemed eminently reasonable that strongly inter-

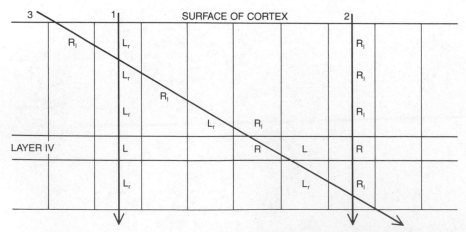

3 1 SURFACE OF CORTEX 2

LAYER IV

GROUPING OF CELLS according to ocular dominance was revealed by physiological studies. In one typical vertical penetration of the cortex (*1*) a microelectrode encounters only cells that respond preferentially to the left eye (*L$_r$*) and, in layer IV, cells that respond only to the left eye (*L*); in another vertical penetration (*2*) the cells all have right-eye dominance (*R$_l$*) or, in layer IV, are driven exclusively by the right eye (*R*). In an oblique penetration (*3*) there is a regular alternation of dominance by one eye or the other eye. Repeated penetrations suggest that the cortex is subdivided into regions with a cross-sectional width of about .4 millimeter and with walls perpendicular to the cortical surface and layers: the ocular-dominance columns.

connected cells should be grouped together.

If the cortex is diced up into small regions of constant receptive-field orientation, can one say anything more about the three-dimensional shape of the regions than that their walls are perpendicular to the surface? Are neighboring regions related in any systematic way or are regions subserving all the possible orientations scattered over the cortex at random? We began to study these questions simply by penetrating the cortex obliquely or parallel to the surface. When we first did this experiment in about 1961, the result was so surprising that we could hardly believe it. Instead of a random assortment of successive orientations there was an amazing orderliness. Each time the electrode moved forward as little as 25 or 50 micrometers (thousandths of a millimeter) the optimal orientation changed by a small step, about 10 degrees on the average; the steps continued in the same direction, clockwise or counterclockwise, through a total angle of anywhere from 90 to 270 degrees. Occasionally such a sequence would reverse direction suddenly, from a clockwise progression to a counterclockwise one or vice versa. These reversals were unpredictable, usually coming after steady progressions of from 90 to 270 degrees.

Since making this first observation we have seen similar order in almost every monkey. Either there is a steady progression in orientation or, less frequently, there are stretches in which orientation stays constant. The successive changes in orientation are small enough so that it is hard to be sure that the regions of constant orientation are finite in size; it could be that the optimal orientation changes in some sense continuously as the electrode moves along the cortex.

We became increasingly interested in the three-dimensional shape of these regional subdivisions. From considerations of geometry alone the existence of small or zero changes in every direction during a horizontal or tangential penetration points to parallel slabs of tissue containing cells with like orientation specificity, with each slab perpendicular to the surface. The slabs would not necessarily be planar, like slices of bread; seen from above they might well have the form of swirls, which could easily explain the reversals in the direction of orientation changes. Recording large numbers of cells in several parallel electrode penetrations seemed to confirm this prediction, but it was hard to examine more than a tiny region of brain with the microelectrode.

Fortunately an ideal anatomical method was invented at just the right time for us. This was the 2-deoxyglucose technique for assessing brain activity, devised by Louis Sokoloff and his group at the National Institute of Mental Health and described elsewhere in this issue [see "The Chemistry of the Brain," by Leslie L. Iversen, page 70]. The method capitalizes on the fact that brain cells depend mainly on glucose as a source of metabolic energy and that the closely similar compound 2-deoxyglucose can to some extent masquerade as glucose. If deoxyglucose is injected into an animal, it is taken up actively by neurons as though it were glucose; the more active the neuron, the greater the uptake. The compound begins to be metabolized, but for reasons best known to biochemists the sequence stops with a metabolite that cannot cross the cell wall and therefore accumulates within the cell.

The Sokoloff procedure is to inject an animal with deoxyglucose that has been labeled with the radioactive isotope carbon 14, stimulate the animal in a way calculated to activate certain neurons

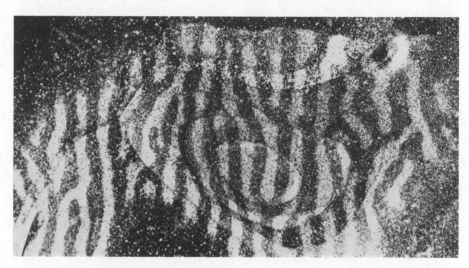

ANATOMICAL CONFIRMATION of ocular-dominance columns came from various staining methods and from axonal-transport autoradiographs such as those shown in color on page 85. This composite autoradiograph visualizing the pattern over an area some 10 millimeters wide was made by cutting out and pasting together the regions representing layer IV in a number of parallel sections; the one in bottom illustration on page 85 and others at different depths.

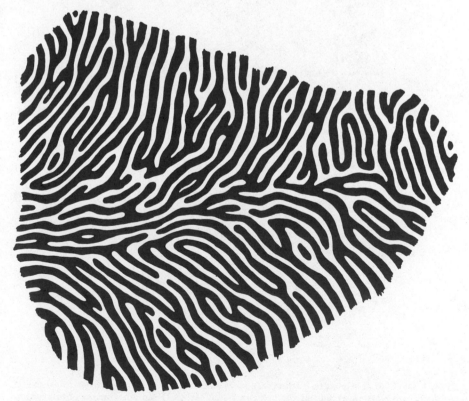

RECONSTRUCTION of the ocular-dominance pattern over the entire exposed part of the right primary visual cortex was made by the authors and Simon LeVay from a series of sections stained by a reduced-silver method he developed. The left-hand margin is at the medial edge of occipital lobe, where cortex folds downward; pattern is enlarged about six diameters.

and then immediately examine the brain for radioactivity, which reveals active areas where cells will have taken up more deoxyglucose than those in quiescent areas. The usual way of examining the brain for this purpose is to cut very thin slices of it (as one would for microscopic examination) and press them against a photographic plate sensitive to the radioactive particles. When the film is developed, any areas that were in contact with radioactive material are seen as dark masses of developed silver grains. Together with Michael P. Stryker we adapted the Sokoloff method to our problem, injecting an anesthetized animal with deoxyglucose and then moving a pattern of black and white vertical stripes back and forth 1.5 meters in front of the animal for 45 minutes. We then cut the brain into slices, either perpendicular to the surface of the cortex or parallel to it.

The autoradiographs quickly confirmed the physiological results. Sections cut perpendicular to the surface showed narrow bands of radioactivity about every 570 micrometers (roughly half a millimeter), extending through the full thickness of the cortex. Evidently these were the regions containing cells responsive to vertical lines. The deep

part of layer IV was uniformly radioactive, as was expected from the fact that the cells in the layer have circularly symmetrical receptive fields and show no orientation selectivity.

Sections cut parallel to the surface showed an unexpectedly complex set of periodically spaced bands, often swirling, frequently branching and rejoining, only here and there forming regular parallel slabs. What was particularly striking was the uniformity of the distance from one band to the next over the entire cortex. This fitted perfectly with the idea of a uniform cortex. Moreover, the distance between stripes fitted well with the idea that the cortical machinery must repeat itself at least every millimeter. If the distance were, for example, 10 millimeters from vertical through 180 degrees and back to vertical, sizable parts of the visual field would lack cells sensitive to any given orientation, making for a sketchy and extremely bizarre representation of the visual scene.

The final variable whose associated architecture needs to be considered is eye preference. In microelectrode studies neighboring cells proved almost invariably to prefer the same eye. If in vertical penetrations the first cell we en-

countered preferred the right eye, then so did all the cells, right down to the bottom of layer VI; if the first cell preferred the left eye, so did all the rest. Any penetration favored one eye or the other with equal probability. (Since the cells of layer IV are monocular, there it was a matter not of eye preference but of eye monopoly.) If the penetration was oblique or horizontal, there was an alternation of left and right preferences, with a rather abrupt switchover about every half millimeter. The cortex thus proved to be diced up into a second set of regions separated by vertical walls that extend through the full cortical thickness. The ocular-dominance system was apparently quite independent of the orientation system, because in oblique or tangential penetrations the two sequences had no apparent relation to each other.

The basis of these ocular-dominance columns, as they have come to be called, seems to be quite simple. The terminals of geniculate fibers, some subserving the left eye and others the right, group themselves as they enter the cortex so that in layer IV there is no mixing. This produces left-eye and right-eye patches at roughly half-millimeter intervals. A neuron above or below layer IV receives connections from that layer from up to about a millimeter away in every direction. Probably the strongest connections are from the region of layer IV closest to the neuron, so that it is presumably dominated by whichever eye feeds that region.

Again we were most curious to learn what these left-eye and right-eye regions might look like in three dimensions; any of several geometries could lead to the cross-sectional appearance the physiology had suggested. The answer first came from studies with the silver-degeneration method for mapping connections, devised by Walle J. H. Nauta of the Massachusetts Institute of Technology. Since then we have found three other independent anatomical methods for demonstrating these columns.

A particularly effective method (because it enables one to observe in a single animal the arrangement of columns over the entire primary visual cortex) is based on the phenomenon of axonal transport. The procedure is to inject a radioactively labeled amino acid into an area of nervous tissue. A cell body takes up the amino acid, presumably incorporates it into a protein and then transports it along the axon to its terminals. When we injected the material into one eye of a monkey, the retinal ganglion cells took it up and transported it along their axons, the optic-nerve fibers. We could then examine the destinations of these fibers in the lateral geniculate nuclei by coating tissue slices with a silver emulsion and developing the emulsion; the radioactive label showed up clearly in

BLOCK OF CORTEX about a millimeter square and two millimeters deep (*light color*) can be considered an elementary unit of the primary visual cortex. It contains one set of orientation slabs subserving all orientations and one set of ocular-dominance slabs subserving both eyes. The pattern is reiterated throughout the primary visual area. The placing of the boundaries (at the right or the left eye, at a vertical, horizontal or oblique orientation) is arbitrary; representation of the slabs as flat planes intersecting at right angles is an oversimplification.

the three complementary layers of the geniculate on each side.

This method does not ordinarily trace a path from one axon terminal across a synapse to the next neuron and its terminals, however, and we wanted to follow the path all the way to the cortex. In 1971 Bernice Grafstein of the Cornell University Medical College discovered that after a large enough injection in the eye of a mouse some of the radioactive material escaped from the optic-nerve terminals and was taken up by the cells in the geniculate and transported along their axons to the cortex. We had the thought that a similarly large injection in a monkey, combined with autoradiography, might demonstrate the geniculate terminals from one eye in layer IV of the visual cortex.

Our first attempt yielded dismayingly negative results, with only faint hints of a few silver grains visible in layer IV. It was only after several weeks that we realized that by resorting to dark-field microscopy we could take advantage of the light-scattering properties of silver grains and so increase the sensitivity of the method. We borrowed a dark-field condenser, and when we looked at our first slide under the microscope, there shining in all their glory were the periodic patches of label in layer IV [*see top illustration on page 85*].

The next step was to try to see the pattern face on by sectioning the cortex parallel to its surface. The monkey cortex is dome-shaped, and so a section parallel to the surface and tangent to layer IV shows that layer as a circle or an oval, while a section below layer IV shows it as a ring. By assembling a series of such ovals and rings from a set of sections one can reconstruct the pattern over a wide expanse of cortex.

From the reconstructions it was immediately obvious that the main overall pattern is one of parallel stripes representing terminals belonging to the injected eye, separated by gaps representing the other eye. The striping pattern is not regular like wallpaper. (We remind ourselves occasionally that this is, after all, biology!) Here and there a stripe representing one eye branches into two stripes, or else it ends blindly at a point where a stripe from the other eye branches. The irregularities are commonest near the center of gaze and along the line that maps the horizon. The stripes always seem to be perpendicular to the border between the primary visual cortex and its neighbor, area 18, and here the regularity is greatest. Such general rules seem to apply to all macaque brains, although the details of the pattern vary from one individual to the next and even from one hemisphere to the other in the same monkey.

The width of a set of two stripes is constant, about .8 millimeter, over the

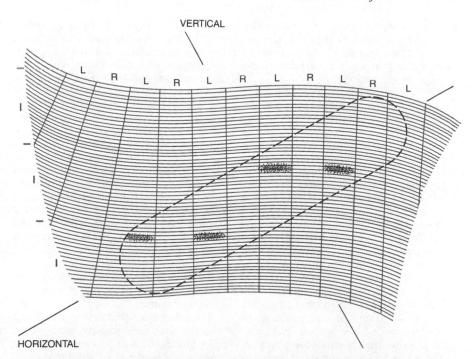

HYPOTHETICAL PATTERN OF CORTICAL ACTIVITY that might result from stimulation of the left eye with a single short horizontal line, placed in the upper left quadrant of the visual field, is shown by the colored patches on a diagram of an area of the right cortex, seen face on. The area receiving input from the object in the visual field is indicated by the broken black line. If ocular-dominance and orientation columns are arrayed as shown, activated cells will be those that respond optimally to approximately horizontal stimuli from the left eye.

entire primary visual cortex, once more emphasizing the uniformity of the cortex. Again the widths fit perfectly with the idea that all of the apparatus needed to look after an area the size of an aggregate field must be contained within any square millimeter of cortex. The two techniques, deoxyglucose labeling and amino acid transport, have the great advantage of being mutually compatible, so that we have been able to apply both together, one to mark orientation lines and the other to see the ocular-dominance columns. The number of brains examined so far is too small to justify any final conclusions, but the two systems appear to be quite independent, neither parallel nor at right angles but intersecting at random.

The function served by ocular-dominance columns is still a mystery. We know there are neurons with all grades of eye preference throughout the entire binocular part of the visual fields, and it may be that a regular, patterned system of converging inputs guarantees that the distribution will be uniform, with neither eye favored by accident in any one place. Why there should be all these grades of eye preference everywhere is itself not clear, but our guess is that it has something to do with stereoscopic depth perception.

Given what has been learned about the primary visual cortex, it is clear that one can consider an elementary piece of cortex to be a block about a millimeter square and two millimeters deep. To know the organization of this chunk of tissue is to know the organization for all of area 17; the whole must be mainly an iterated version of this elementary unit. Of course the elementary unit should not be thought of as a discrete, separable block. Whether the set of orientation slabs begins with a slab representing a vertical orientation, an oblique one or a horizontal one is completely arbitrary; so too is whether an ocular-dominance sequence begins with a left-plus-right pair of dominance slabs or a right-plus-left pair. The same thing is true for a unit crystal of sodium chloride or for any complex repetitive pattern such as is found in wallpaper.

What, then, does the visual scene really look like as it is projected onto the visual cortex? Suppose an animal fixes its gaze on some point and the only object in the visual field is a straight line above and a bit to the left of the point where the gaze is riveted. If each active cell were to light up, and if one could stand above the cortex and look down at it, what would the pattern be? To make the problem more interesting, suppose the pattern is seen by one eye only. In view of the architecture just described the pattern turns out to be not a line but merely a set of regularly spaced patches [*see illustration above*]. The reasoning can be checked directly by exposing a monkey with one eye closed to a set of vertical stripes and making a deoxyglucose autoradiograph. The resulting pattern should not be a great surprise: it is a set of regularly spaced patches, which simply represents the intersection of the two sets of column systems. Imagine the surprise and bewilderment of a little green man looking at such a version of the outside world!

Why evolution has gone to the trouble of designing such an elaborate architecture is a question that continues to fascinate us. Perhaps the most plausible notion is that the column systems are a solution to the problem of portraying more than two dimensions on a two-dimensional surface. The cortex is dealing with at least four sets of values: two for the x and y position variables in the visual field, one for orientation and one for the different degrees of eye preference. The two surface coordinates are used up in designating field position; the other two variables are accommodated by dicing up the cortex with subdivisions so fine that one can run through a complete set of orientations or eye preferences and meanwhile have a shift in visual-field position that is small with respect to the resolution in that part of the visual world.

The strategy of subdividing the cortex with small vertical partitions is certainly not limited to the primary visual area. Such subdivisions were first seen in the somatic sensory area by Vernon B. Mountcastle of the Johns Hopkins University School of Medicine about 10 years before our work in the visual area. In the somatic sensory area, as we pointed out above, the basic topography is a map of the opposite half of the body, but superimposed on that there is a twofold system of subdivisions, with some areas where neurons respond to the movement of the joints or pressure on the skin and other areas where they respond to touch or the bending of hairs. As in the case of the visual columns, a complete set here (one area for each kind of neuron) occupies a distance of about a millimeter. These subdivisions are analogous to ocular-dominance columns in that they are determined in the first instance by inputs to the cortex (from either the left or the right eye and from either deep receptors or receptors in the upper skin layers) rather than by connections within the cortex, such as those that determine orientation selectivity and the associated system of orientation regions.

The columnar subdivisions associated with the visual and somatic sensory systems are the best-understood ones, but there are indications of similar vertical subdivisions in some other areas: several higher visual areas, sensory parietal regions recently studied by Mountcastle and the auditory region, where Thomas J. Imig, H. O. Adrián and John F. Brugge of the University of Wisconsin Medical School and their colleagues have found subdivisions in which the two ears seem alternately to add their information or to compete.

For most of these physiologically defined systems (except the visual ones) there are so far no anatomical correlates. On the other hand, in the past few years several anatomists, notably Edward G. Jones of the Washington University School of Medicine and Nauta and Patricia Goldman at M.I.T., have shown that connections from one region of the cortex to another (for example from the somatic sensory area on one side to the corresponding area on the other side) terminate in patches that have a regular periodicity of about a millimeter. Here the columns are evident morphologically, but one has no idea of the physiological interpretation. It is clear, however, that fine periodic subdivisions are a very general feature of the cerebral cortex. Indeed, Mountcastle's original observation of that feature may be said to supply a fourth profound insight into cortical organization.

It would surely be wrong to assume that this account of the visual cortex in any way exhausts the subject. Color, movement and stereoscopic depth are probably all dealt with in the cortex, but to what extent or how is still not clear. There are indications from work we and others have done on depth and from work on color by Semir Zeki of University College London that higher cortical visual areas to which the primary area projects directly or indirectly may be specialized to handle these variables, but we are a long way from knowing what the handling involves.

What happens beyond the primary visual area, and how is the information on orientation exploited at later stages? Is one to imagine ultimately finding a cell that responds specifically to some very particular item? (Usually one's grandmother is selected as the particular item, for reasons that escape us.) Our answer is that we doubt there is such a cell, but we have no good alternative to offer. To speculate broadly on how the brain may work is fortunately not the only course open to investigators. To explore the brain is more fun and seems to be more profitable.

There was a time, not so long ago, when one looked at the millions of neurons in the various layers of the cortex and wondered if anyone would ever have any idea of their function. Did they all work in parallel, like the cells of the liver or the kidney, achieving their objectives by pure bulk, or were they each doing something special? For the visual cortex the answer seems now to be known in broad outline: Particular stimuli turn neurons on or off; groups of neurons do indeed perform particular transformations. It seems reasonable to think that if the secrets of a few regions such as this one can be unlocked, other regions will also in time give up their secrets.

ACTUAL PATTERN of cortical activity was elicited by exposing only the left eye to a set of vertical stripes. The deoxyglucose autoradiograph is of a tangential section in the outer layers of the cortex. The pattern of regularly spaced dark patches of radioactivity represents intersection of ocular-dominance and orientation systems. Magnification is about eight diameters.

VIII

Brain Mechanisms
of Movement

Brain Mechanisms of Movement

BY EDWARD V. EVARTS

How do the brain and the spinal cord bring about the movements of the body? They not only issue commands to muscles but also receive feedback signals that help to orchestrate the commands

One of the first facts to be established about the control of movement by the brain more than a century ago was that body movements can be caused by signals to the spinal cord from a specific region of the brain: the motor area of the cerebral cortex. The movements can range in scale from the gross muscular adjustments required for manual labor or rapid locomotion to the tiny adjustments of the finger muscles that make it possible to do surgery under the microscope.

These motor-cortex outputs are themselves the result of inputs from elsewhere; they come not only from other cortical areas, such as the area for touch, but also from subcortical structures, the cerebellum and the basal ganglia, which send signals to the motor cortex by way of still another subcortical area, the thalamus. A major part of current research on the brain's mechanisms of movement is aimed at a better understanding of how the inputs from these various cortical and subcortical structures work together to control the final outputs from the motor cortex to the spinal cord and thence to the muscles. Here I shall review the present state of this understanding, which is significant on two counts. First, it relates to fundamental questions about the overall organization of the brain. Second, it bears on the treatment and possible prevention of such neurological disorders as Parkinson's disease and Huntington's chorea (two of several disorders involving the basal ganglia) and the many manifestations of stroke, of multiple sclerosis and of numerous other disorders that result from damage to the cerebellum.

What are the elementary requirements for movement? The first is muscle; the second is a signaling system that makes muscle contract in an orderly manner. To begin with muscle, not all muscles work the same way. Consider the muscles of the human eye and arm. Eye muscles must operate with great speed and precision in quickly orienting the eyeball to within a few minutes of

arc. At the same time eye muscle does not have to cope with such external demands as weight lifting. The fine control needed in eye movement calls for a high innervation ratio: the ratio of the number of neurons with axons terminating on the outer membrane of muscle cells to the number of cells in the muscle.

For eye muscle the innervation ratio is about one to three, which means that the axon terminals of a single motor neuron release their chemical transmitter to no more than three individual muscle cells. (A motor neuron is a neuron whose cell body is in the spinal cord and whose axon terminates on muscle-cell membrane.) In contrast to this high innervation ratio the axon terminals of a single motor neuron that innervates a limb muscle such as a biceps muscle may deliver transmitter to hundreds of muscle fibers; the muscle may therefore have the low ratio of one to many hundreds. As a result the output of the motor unit in limb muscle—the single twitch caused by a single impulse that releases transmitter from the terminals of a single motor neuron—is correspondingly coarse.

Muscle motor units also differ in their susceptibility to fatigue. At one extreme are slow-twitch motor units with great resistance to fatigue. Such units can remain active for long periods, but they generate relatively little muscle tension. At the opposite extreme are fast-twitch motor units; they can generate a large peak muscle tension but fatigue rapidly.

These fast-twitch units tend to be innervated by motor neurons with axons of above-average diameter and velocity of nerve-impulse conduction.

Within a single muscle the fibers of slow and fast motor units are intermixed. In 1968 the Swedish investigators E. Kugelberg and L. Edstrom discovered a way of telling which individual motor fibers belonged to which motor unit. By prolonged stimulation of a single motor-neuron axon they induced prolonged contraction in the muscle fibers of a single motor unit. The contraction depleted the supply of the energy-storing compound glycogen in the individual muscle fibers. When the tissue was stained for glycogen, the fibers of the depleted motor unit appeared as white "ghosts" mixed with pink-staining fibers that still contained a normal supply of glycogen.

This is known as a histochemical effect, that is, a demonstration of the biochemical reaction of a living microanatomical structure. For example, taking Kugelberg and Edstrom's approach, Robert E. Burke and his colleagues at the National Institutes of Health have found that fast-twitch muscle units stain histochemically as if their contractile fibers use up the energy source adenosine triphosphate, or ATP, by enzymatically breaking it down faster than slow-twitch motor units do. This enzymatic breakdown is thought to be one of the important factors that determine the intrinsic

THREE WHITE "GHOSTS" in the micrograph on the opposite page are markers deliberately created to assist the study of a major aspect of the relation between the brain and movement: the chemistry of muscle contraction following the firing of a motor neuron. The micrograph shows a cat leg muscle that has been sectioned perpendicular to its long axis. The ghosts are individual muscle fibers in a single motor unit of the leg muscle. Earlier study of the unit indicated that it was "slow twitch" muscle, the kind that generates small forces but is extremely resistant to fatigue. The three fibers have been made markers by prolonged stimulation of the motor neuron that controls their contraction, thus depleting their supply of glycogen, the stored form of glucose, a muscle energy source. Staining has colored pink all the muscle fibers in the section with a normal supply of glycogen. Micrographs of other sections of the same muscle, including the same three markers, appear on page 100. They have been stained to determine the relation between the chemical and mechanical properties of the muscle fibers. The micrographs were made by Robert E. Burke and Peter Tsairis at the National Institutes of Health.

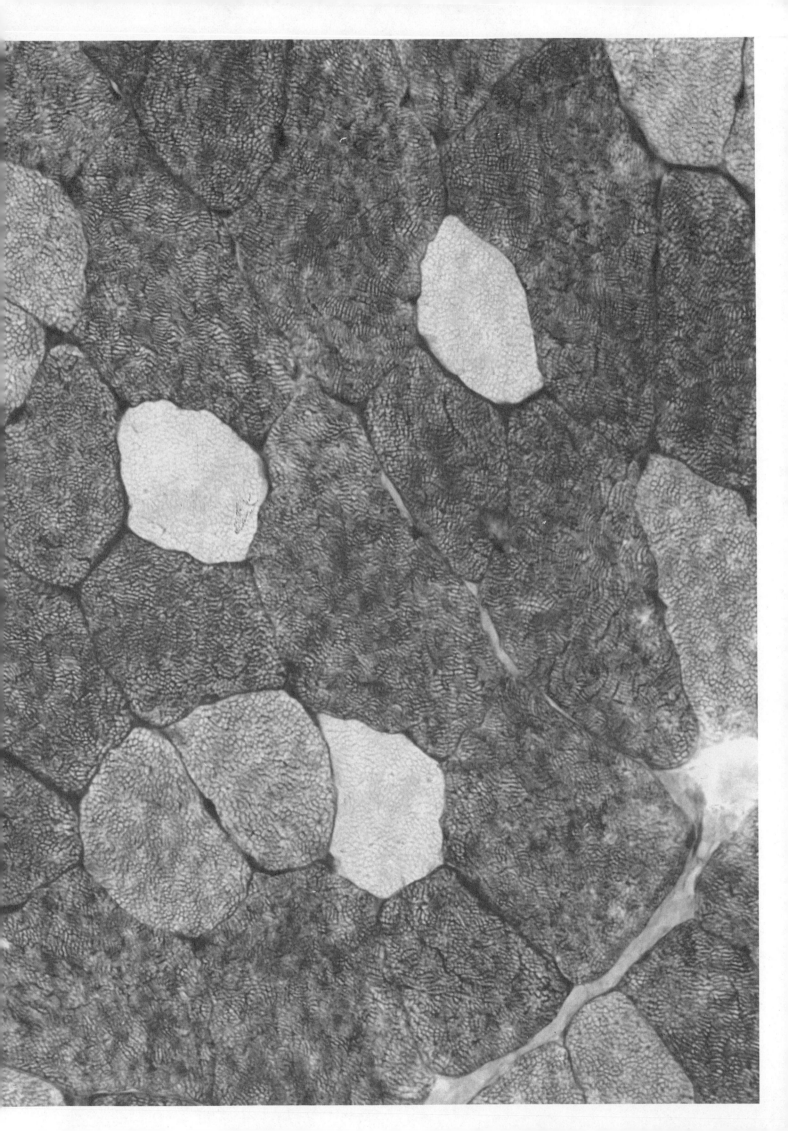

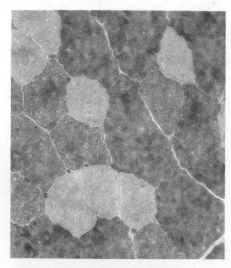
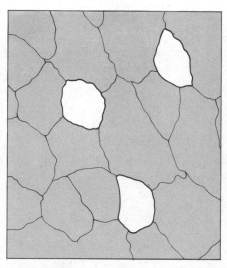

SECOND SECTION of leg muscle was stained to determine the relative ability of muscle-fiber proteins to metabolize the energy-supplying compound adenosine triphosphate (ATP). Dark staining implies a greater metabolic ability. The three marker fibers are only lightly stained (*see map at right*). This lesser ability is characteristic of the slow-twitch fibers in cat muscle.

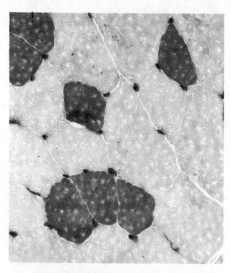
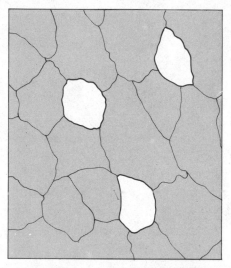

THIRD SECTION is stained to indicate the ability of muscle proteins to metabolize ATP after modification by an acidic pretreatment. The approximate reversal of staining intensities from those seen in the second section provides further information about muscle-fiber chemistry.

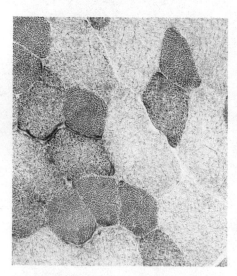
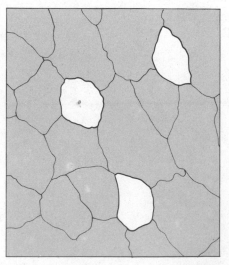

FOURTH SECTION has been stained to indicate the relative capacity of the muscle fibers for oxidative metabolism as measured by the presence of a key enzyme in the cell's mitochondria. The three fibers of the slow-twitch unit (*see map*) are among the heavily stained fibers; this is consistent with the great resistance to fatigue that characterizes slow-twitch motor units.

speed of muscle contraction. Thus the histochemical finding helps to explain the difference in the speeds of twitch contraction. Histochemical studies of other enzymes involved in the breakdown of sugars and fats similarly help to explain the very large differences in the resistance to fatigue among the two kinds of motor units.

What is the importance of these contrasting motor-unit properties to the organization of movement? Consider how the motor units of a muscle are sequentially "recruited" in the course of a movement. In general muscle tension is regulated in two ways. One way is through the control of the number of motor units recruited to act. The other is through the control of the firing frequency of the motor units that have been recruited. Slow-twitch units, resistant to fatigue and generating relatively little tension, are the first to be recruited. The last motor units to be recruited are the fast-twitch units, those that generate large peak tensions but are quickly fatigued.

Elwood Henneman of the Harvard Medical School has made major contributions to a general understanding of the significance of the order in which the motor units are recruited. He notes that small muscle tensions are generated and precisely controlled by the selective mobilization of varying numbers of small motor units. The difference between smaller and larger motor units is not trivial. For example, the largest motor unit in the human calf muscle develops 200 times more tension than the smallest. When the total muscle output must be increased, Henneman learned, the larger motor units are activated, so that larger individual increments of tension are provided. This means that as the total tension rises fewer additional motor units are needed to furnish it. Of course, when circumstances require that the overall tension output of the muscle rise abruptly, little recruitment order is evident and virtually all motor units in the muscle are activated simultaneously.

So much for the different kinds of muscle and their motor units. Let us now consider what makes the units twitch. The muscular contractions depend on the ability of the transmitter acetylcholine, which is released at the neuromuscular junction with each motor-neuron impulse, to excite a muscle-cell impulse. Blocking the transmission at the junction, for example with the alkaloid curare, eliminates muscular contraction. Experiments that illustrate such blockage have been done with human subjects. They were given curare while their respiration was maintained artificially. During the period of curare paralysis acetylcholine continued to be released by the motor-neuron axons, but the curare prevented the interaction of the transmitter and its receptors on the muscle-cell membrane. As a result the subjects' muscles ceased to respond to the commands of their cerebral cortex. The subjects continued to have thoughts and feelings, but there were no external signs of these cerebral activities. Speech, facial expression, the ability to direct the gaze—all these forms of behavior depend on muscular contraction.

Many current concepts of the brain mechanisms of movement have evolved from the work of the British physiologist Charles Scott Sherrington early in this century on the function of the motor neuron in certain reflexive forms of motor activity such as scratching and walking. Signals from many different areas of the brain often impinge on the same few spinal-cord motor neurons. Recognizing this fact, Sherrington characterized motor neurons as the "final common pathway" linking the brain with muscle action. He studied muscle movement in animals whose spinal cord was severed, effectively separating the motor neurons from the brain.

Sherrington found that within a few months after a dog's spinal cord was severed a scratch reflex could be elicited by such mechanical stimuli as tickling the animal's skin or lightly pulling on its hair anywhere within a large saddle-shaped region of the upper body. In describing these responses he stated that the movements were "executed without obvious impairment of direction or rhythm." Sherrington's work on the scratch reflex led to today's concept of the "triggered movement" based on a "central program" involving a spinal rhythm generator. Not long afterward another British physiologist, Graham Brown, showed that rhythmical limb movements similar to those involved in walking were also possible in dogs deprived of connections between the brain and the spinal cord. Evidently spinal rhythm generators existed for walking as well as for scratching.

Many current investigations of the neurophysiology of locomotion are aimed at clarifying the interaction between what may be termed central programs from the brain and sensory feedback from outside the nervous system. Indeed, Sherrington's work was particularly concerned with the ways motorneuron activity could be regulated by sensory feedback. He introduced the term "proprioception" to describe sensory inputs arising in the course of centrally driven movements when "the stimuli to the receptors were delivered by the organism itself." Sherrington chose the prefix "proprio-" (from the Latin *proprius,* "one's own") because he believed the major function of the proprioceptors was to provide feedback information on the organism's own movements.

Muscle proprioceptors are of two kinds. One kind senses elongation and the other senses tension. The length re-

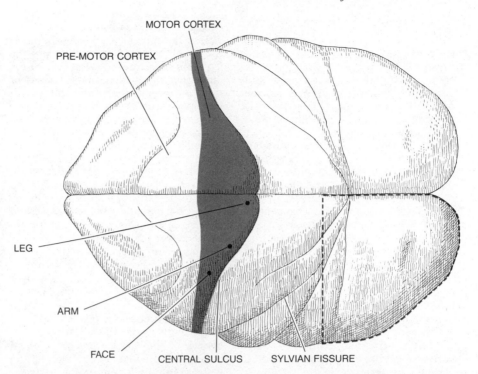

BRAIN OF THE MACAQUE MONKEY is seen from the top. Labeling indicates various subdivisions of the motor area of this brain's cerebral cortex. Pie-slice lines (*color*) indicate the section of brain that has been removed in the illustration below to reveal subcortical structures.

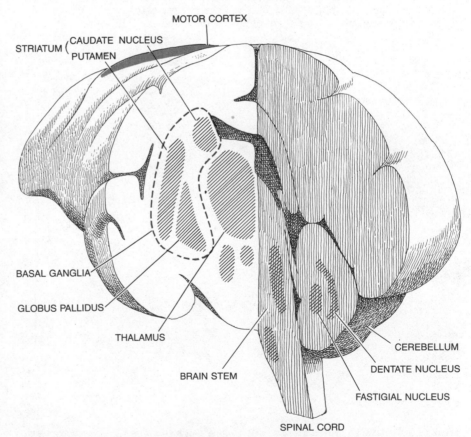

MACAQUE'S BRAIN is seen from the rear with one 90-degree pie slice removed to expose some details of its subcortical structures. Broken line in color surrounds the basal ganglia of the left hemisphere: the caudate and putamen segments of the striatum and the adjacent globus pallidus. Nearer the center line is the left thalamus, and astride the center line is the sectioned right half of the cerebellum, with its interior components, the dentate and fastigial nuclei, exposed to view. The motor section of the cerebral cortex (*color*) is a phylogenetically recent brain structure compared with the basal ganglia and the cerebellum. Research now in progress indicates that the firing of motor-cortex neurons is mediated by signals sent to the motor cortex by way of the thalamus from these phylogenetically older subcortical structures.

ceptors of muscles send fibers into the spinal cord to form synapses on motor neurons that terminate on the same muscles. Hence any increased length-receptor activity that results from muscle elongation activates the motor neurons of the elongated muscle. That gives rise to a muscular contraction that opposes the elongation.

The tension receptors, the second kind of proprioceptor, sense force rather than elongation; their activation leads to the inhibition of the associated motor neurons. Thus when an increase in muscle tension activates these receptors, their response acts on the associated motor neurons and gives rise to a reduction in force. Both the length receptors and the tension receptors may therefore be viewed as components of what an engineer would call a negative-feedback control system. This particular system maintains its stability by resisting changes in muscle length and tension.

It will clarify the operation of such a negative-feedback servomechanism to consider an example of the system in action. Imagine a man who is trying, in the absence of any external disturbance, to hold his arm steady while it is extended straight out to the side of his body. Slight unintended fluctuations in position will of course take place, particularly as the arm gets tired. For example,

occasional involuntary decreases of tension in the muscles opposing the force of gravity will lead to increases in the length of those muscles. Because of the increase in muscle length the activity of the proprioceptive length receptors will increase, while at the same time (because of the decrease in muscle tension) the activity of the proprioceptive tension receptors will decrease.

Although these are opposite directions of change, their central effect is not subtractive but additive: the increased firing of the length receptors excites the motor neurons affecting the muscle, and the decreased firing of the force receptors removes the inhibition of the same neurons. This synergistic action of the two kinds of proprioceptive receptors takes effect when muscle-length changes are a consequence of involuntary changes of muscle tension due to internal causes, but it does not take effect if the length and tension changes are a consequence of the application or removal of an external force. For example, an increase in muscle length due to an increased external load gives rise to an increase in length-receptor activity associated with an increase, rather than a decrease in the activity of the tension receptors. In coining the word proprioceptor Sherrington was calling attention to the important differences in neural

organization that underlie active movement as opposed to passive. In this context "active" refers to a subject's own movements and "passive" to displacements produced by external forces.

Sherrington's concept of the relation between the length receptors in muscle and movement in general was dramatically demonstrated when the Swedish physiologist L. Leksell discovered the role played by special neurons known as gamma motor neurons. Unlike the ordinary, or alpha, motor neurons, which act on the muscle fibers that contract powerfully, the gamma motor neurons act on specialized small muscle fibers that regulate the sensitivity of length receptors. Hence motor neurons also are of two kinds. One kind acts on the muscles that generate bodily movements (alphas) and the other serves to optimize the performance of the proprioceptive muscle-length receptors (gammas).

Thus different kinds of muscles, different kinds of motor neurons and their associated control systems provide the elementary components of voluntary and reflex body movements. The relations between these components can be studied in the laboratory with a wide range of animal subjects. For example, much current work on the control of movement relies on mollusks and on arthropods such as insects and crustaceans. In these invertebrate animals the simplicity of the nervous system offers distinct advantages to the investigator. Invertebrates, however, lack a cerebral cortex and its related structures. To learn how the brain signals to the motor neurons and so controls human movements requires information obtained from animals that have not only a cerebral cortex but also that specialized cerebral subdivision—the motor cortex—where the control of movement is engineered.

The motor cortex was first recognized in 1870, when it was discovered that electrical stimulation of the cerebral cortex could elicit body movements. The stimulus experiments confirmed a conclusion that had already been reached by the British neurologist John Hughlings Jackson on the basis of clinical observations. Hughlings Jackson had noted that an irritative lesion of the cerebral cortex on one side of the brain could cause epileptic movements of the opposite side of the body. The first stimulus experiments, performed with dogs as subjects, were confirmed for monkeys in 1873 by the British neurologist David Ferrier.

These motor-cortex studies had a remarkable impact on neurological thinking. To appreciate that impact fully one must realize that before 1870 the cerebral cortex was widely believed to be the repository only of thoughts. Hughlings

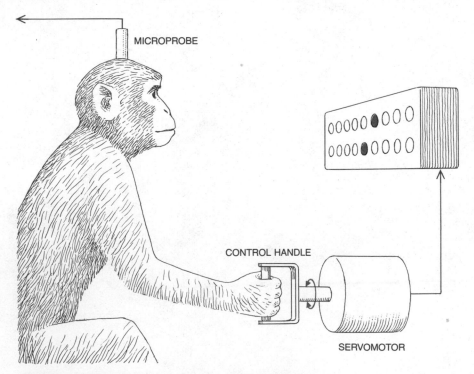

MONKEY SUBJECTS proved amenable to training that involved precise muscular response to stimuli. In this experiment one of nine lamps in the top row of a two-row display was illuminated by the experimenter. By twisting a handle the monkey was able to "follow" the upper lamp to the left or the right and was rewarded when the two lighted lamps were aligned. A microprobe, inserted among the motor-cortex cells associated with precise manipulation, recorded the activity of the cells involved in the muscular response. Even a small voluntary movement was accompanied by a striking increase in motor-cortex activity; the proportion of brain cells that fired was far greater than the proportion of spinal-cord motor neurons involved.

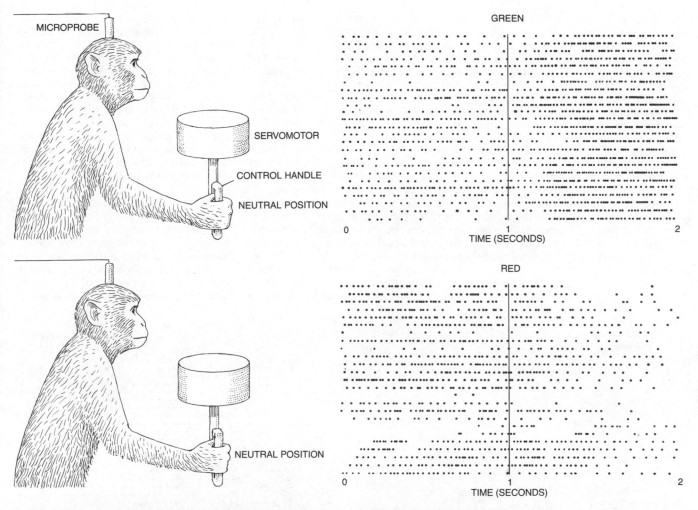

GREEN

0   1   2
TIME (SECONDS)

RED

0   1   2
TIME (SECONDS)

MICROPROBE

SERVOMOTOR

CONTROL HANDLE

NEUTRAL POSITION

NEUTRAL POSITION

"GETTING SET" EXPERIMENT involved additional training of monkey subjects. They were taught to keep a handle fixed in a "neutral" position and to prepare to push it forward at some indefinite time after a signal light flashed green (*top*) or to pull it back sometime after the light flashed red (*bottom*). The activity of one motor-cortex neuron was recorded for one second before and one second after the signal lights flashed; its impulses are depicted by the horizontal rows of dots, and each row records a single presentation of the stimulus. As these raster displays show, getting set to push caused an increase in neuron activity and getting set to pull caused a decrease.

Jackson stated the consensus of the time as follows: "There seems to be an insuperable objection to the notion that the cerebral hemispheres are for movements.... The reason, I suppose, is that the convolutions [of the cortex] are considered to be *not* for *movements* but for *ideas*."

The next step was in 1874. It was the discovery of a special set of giant neurons that provided a pathway between the motor cortex and the spinal cord. In that year the Russian anatomist Vladimir Betz detected some extraordinarily large neurons in the motor cortex of monkeys and human beings. These neurons are now known as Betz cells. It was found that the axons of Betz cells descend through the brain and make direct connections with spinal-cord motor neurons, particularly those controlling the muscles that serve human beings for the precise movements of manipulation and speech. Further investigation proved that a seemingly disproportionate part of the motor cortex is devoted to the control of a very small percentage

of the total musculature of the human body, as the famous motor-cortex "homunculus" maps made by Wilder Penfield and his colleagues at the Montreal Neurological Institute so graphically demonstrate. It has now been shown that there are some direct connections from motor-cortex neurons to spinal-cord motor neurons in the thoracic region, an area where many of the motor neurons drive the intercostal respiratory muscles.

At first it seems odd that motor-cortex neurons, devoted in the main to the control of precise movements, should terminate on motor neurons controlling an action as automatic and primitive as breathing. As the British physiologist Charles Phillips points out, however, these brain-to-spinal-cord connections are probably related not to respiration but to the use of respiratory muscles in such skilled activities as speech and song. Thus the motor-cortex projection provides new controls for muscles conditioned to old reflex patterns. As Hughlings Jackson recognized a century

ago, the loss of corticospinal connections does not in itself paralyze muscles. Rather it prevents the use of the muscles in connection with certain movements. Specifically, destruction of the corticospinal projection to thoracic motor neurons does not affect the use of the respiratory muscles for respiration even though the muscles have been rendered useless for speech.

Within the past decade much has been learned about the control the motor cortex exercises over voluntary movement. The new information is largely the product of ingenious techniques that allow the placement of microelectrodes in the brain of an animal subject, usually a monkey, that is capable of executing skilled movements. Employing these techniques, Christoph Fromm of the University of Düsseldorf has worked with me at the National Institute of Mental Health in examining motor-cortex features that underlie the critical role played by this part of the cerebral cortex in the precise control of hand movements. It is the same kind of precise control that enables a surgeon looking through the dissecting microscope to move a surgical instrument with an accuracy of within a small fraction of a millimeter.

It seemed to Fromm and me that if motor-cortex output was what controlled precise small movements, then the motor-cortex neurons would have to be strongly modulated by even the most minute fluctuations in the activity of the muscles. Furthermore, precise manual control depends strongly on sensory feedback from the hand, and so we favored the view that motor-cortex activity during precisely controlled manual movements should be under continuous closed-loop control by negative feedback.

To see if our conjectures were correct we began by training monkeys to move a handle with precision. Rotating the handle controlled a visual display; the monkeys were rewarded for precision of manual performance. During each test we recorded the impulses from Betz cells of the subjects' motor cortex. We found that the smallest movement of the handle was accompanied by a striking intensification of Betz-cell activity. For example, the fraction of motor-cortex neurons that fired during the control of these fine movements was far larger than the fraction of spinal-cord motor neurons involved in the movement.

We noted a second feature underlying the role of the motor cortex in the control of precise movements. It is a negative-feedback system that automatically regulates the output of the motor cortex. The system is preferentially focused on the motor-cortex neurons controlling the most precise small movements. The anatomical pathways that return the negative feedback to the motor cortex have yet to be traced in detail. One source of the signals, however, is the sensory area of the cerebral cortex, which is directly behind the motor cortex and is connected to it through a number of linkages. Areas of the sensory cortex that receive inputs from the subject's hand evidently relay signals to the motor cortex, completing one loop in this feedback system, although probably not the only loop.

The motor-cortex controls we have considered so far are of critical importance in generating and stabilizing the most precise human movements. What happens when a subject wants to carry out a movement that runs counter to a normal reflex reaction? To investigate this question Jun Tanji of Hokkai-

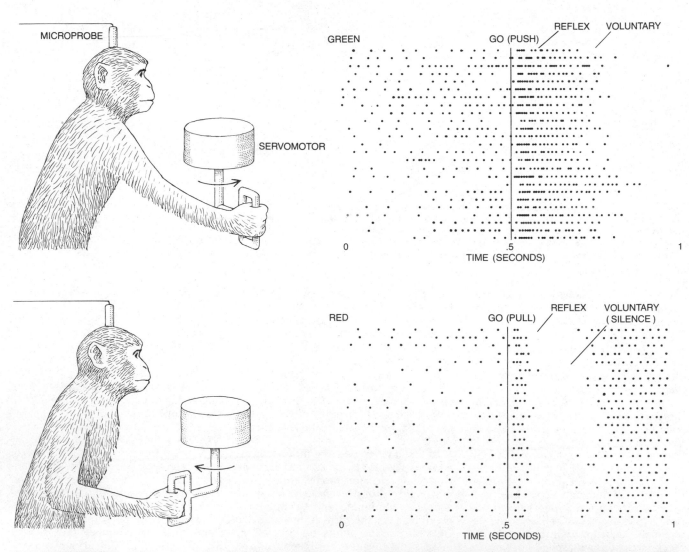

"GO" EXPERIMENT, an extension of the getting-set experiment, was designed to examine the relation between voluntary and reflex responses. The "go" signal, a motor-driven displacement of the handle from its neutral position, came from one second to five seconds after the getting-set light was turned on. Motor-cortex neuron activity was recorded before and after the "go" signal for a total duration of one second. Whether the handle motion elicited a push reaction (top) or a pull reaction (bottom), the immediate response of the monkey was purely reflex, as is shown by the increased neuron activity immediately after stimulus (at .5 second) in the raster displays. Within 40 milliseconds this reflex response was replaced by the voluntary neuron "silence" associated with the getting-set cue for pull (white area in bottom raster). Following both the brief reflex response and the more extended voluntary response (push) seen in the top raster the subject returned the handle to the neutral position before the next trial; this required a pull and produced the silence area visible in the top raster (far right). The similar push return to neutral accounts for the resumption of neural activity seen in the bottom raster.

do University and I studied the activity of motor-cortex neurons of monkeys that had been trained to react to the involuntary movement of their arm. Training sometimes called for a muscular response that was exactly opposite to a normal reflex response. To use a human analogy, imagine a man standing upright. He has been instructed that when the experimenter pushes him, he is to lean forward without moving his feet. The subject will first get set to move forward and then wait for the experimenter's push. If the push comes from behind, the subject's reflex response to preserve his equilibrium will make him lean backward. For the subject to generate a centrally programmed movement forward, as he has been instructed, he must

now shift out of the closed-loop mode of response that preserves equilibrium into an open-loop mode of response that will result in his pitching forward (in this case into a net or the arms of someone waiting to catch him).

Tanji and I trained monkeys to respond to a similar sequence of events. The subjects began by precisely positioning a handle and holding it immobile for a few seconds. During this brief period the subjects' motor-cortex output to the arm muscles was regulated by negative feedback in the closed-loop mode. Then a colored lamp was switched on; its color was a cue that told the monkey how to react to an impending external displacement of the handle. If the light was red, the subject

was to pull the handle back; if it was green, the subject was to push the handle forward. The monkeys were rewarded for correct responses to movements of the handles after the two cues had been received. It took them about 200 milliseconds to get set in response to the cues.

We recorded the firing of motor-cortex neurons and found that after getting set the monkeys needed only 40 milliseconds to respond correctly to the handle movements. In the brief interval following the movement the motor-cortex control abruptly shifted from the closed-loop mode of feedback (which reflexively provides for postural stability) to the open-loop mode that was necessary to generate the preprogrammed movement.

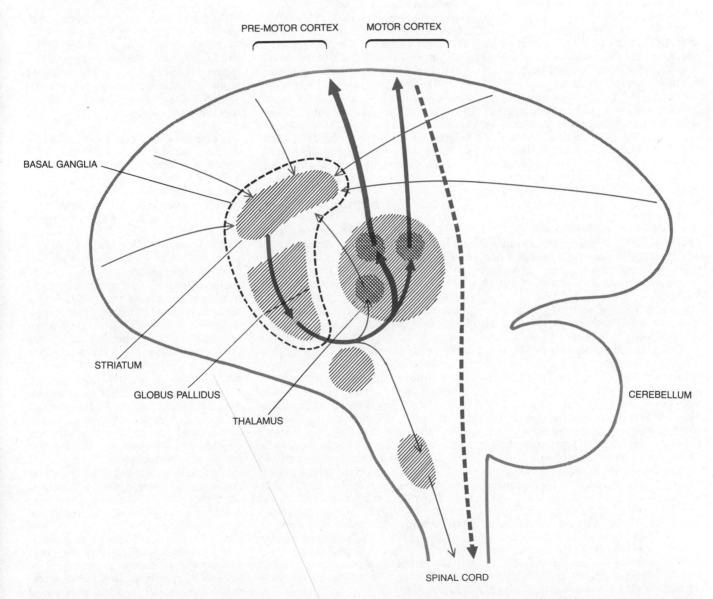

PATHWAYS between various areas of the cerebral cortex and certain subcortical structures are traced in this schematic profile of a monkey brain. Thin arrows indicate inputs to the basal ganglia (*structures within black boundary*) that convey many forms of information from the cerebral cortex. One component, the striatum, is a major link between association areas of the cortex and the motor area. The output of the striatum is passed to the two-part globus pallidus (*thick arrow*); this component in turn provides inputs to another subcortical structure, the thalamus, particularly to two of its nuclei: the ventralis lateralis and ventralis anterior (*thick and less thick arrows*). Thalamic output goes particularly to the pre-motor areas of the cortex (*thick arrow*); additional outputs (*less thick arrow*) go to the motor cortex for relay to the motor neurons of the spinal cord (*broken arrow*). Subcortical inputs play an important part in central motor programming.

The sensory area of the cerebral cortex therefore plays a role in relaying signals that control motor-cortex output in the closed-loop mode. The sensory area does not, however, provide the signals that underlie open-loop preprogrammed movements occurring in spite of (rather than because of) the reflex consequences of sensory input. The signals related to preprogrammed movements reach the motor cortex from subcortical structures, specifically from the cerebellum by way of the thalamus. Peter L. Strick did experiments at the National Institute of Mental Health showing that the pathway running from cerebellum to thalamus to cortex is involved in centrally programmed open-loop control. Following much the same experimental design that Tanji and I had, Strick recorded the activity of single neurons in certain structures of the cerebellum.

Strick trained his monkeys to make arm movements on cue, the cue being the actual displacement of the subject's arm by an externally arranged movement of the handle it grasped. When the monkeys were additionally preprogrammed to move the handle in a particular direction, by means of the system of red and green lights, Strick found that the preprogramming had profound effects on the responses of certain neurons in the cerebellum called dentate neurons: the neurons fired within 30 milliseconds after the arm-displacement cue was given. The dentate-neuron signal thus had an interval of 10 milliseconds available for traversing the thalamus and initiating the centrally programmed activity of the motor cortex (apparent after a 40-millisecond interval following the cue).

Strick's findings are consistent with those of W. Thomas Thatch, Jr., of Washington University. While at the National Institute of Mental Health, Thatch was the first to demonstrate that neurons in the cerebellum fired well in advance of the muscular action of a subject trained to respond to a visual cue. The role of signals from the cerebellum in generating motor-cortex activity has also been demonstrated experimentally by Vernon B. Brooks and his colleagues at the University of Western Ontario. They artificially reduced the temperature of the cerebellum in monkeys and then allowed the temperature to return to normal. The activity of motor-cortex neurons was measured before, during and after the cooling of the cerebellum. Brooks and his colleagues found that when the cerebellum was cooled, the firing of motor-cortex neurons (and the related preprogrammed movement) in response to cues was delayed.

In addition to transmitting outputs from the cerebellum to the motor cortex the thalamus relays signals from another subcortical structure. This is the large set of cell groups collectively known as the basal ganglia. While at the National Institute of Mental Health, Mahlon R. DeLong of Johns Hopkins University demonstrated that cells of the basal ganglia fire well in advance of volitional movements by subjects responding to cues. The finding is consistent with evidence from human neurological disorders that the basal ganglia are critically important to the earliest stages of initiating movement: the stages when, by processes not yet understood, an abstract thought is translated into a concrete motor action.

Reflexes and voluntary movements are not opposites. This was recognized by Hughlings Jackson a century ago when he wrote that volitional movements are subject to the laws of reflex action. Nevertheless, if voluntary movement cannot be defined by exclusion, that is, as something that does not involve a reflex, how can it be defined? The most succinct statement I know is one put forward by the Swedish neurophysiologist Ragnar Granit in his recent book *The Purposive Brain:* "What is volitional in voluntary movement is its purpose." From this viewpoint the volitional features of a motor act should be considered in terms of the goal of the action. Meanwhile the actual events that underlie the achievement of the goal are built up from a variety of reflex processes.

I recently discussed this point with a Russian cyberneticist, Victor Gurfinkel. He too defines volitional movement in relation to its goal. In describing the kinds of process that underlie voluntary movement he told me of some kinesiological studies aimed at assessing the motor-control characteristics of the "best pistol shots in the Red Army." Gurfinkel noted that an essential characteristic of a marksman is his ability to stabilize his gun. Studies of the electromyographic and kinematic characteristics of the army marksmen showed that although many parts of their body moved, the pistol was virtually immobile. All kinds of reflex mechanisms stabilized the position of the marksman's hand in space: the vestibulo-ocular system, the vestibulospinal system and so on. Gurfinkel's example of the marksman recalls a view of William James's regarding the essence of volitional movement. Writing almost a century ago, he said: "The marksman ends by thinking only of the exact position of the goal, the singer only of the perfect sound, the balancer only of the point of the pole whose oscillations he must counteract."

Here one finds remarkable agreement among scholars of widely different backgrounds, disciplines and eras. Granit shares the opinions of James and Gurfinkel. Granit and Gurfinkel accept the Sherringtonian notion that purpos-ive movements are built on a base of reflex processes. This was also the view of the British neurologist Kinnier Wilson. Writing in 1928, he pointed out that a "large part of every voluntary movement is both involuntary and outside consciousness."

What, then, are the features that differentiate goal-directed movements from purposeless ones? Surely there are many kinds of involuntary movement, for example those associated with certain neurological disorders. This has been noted in several forms of basal-ganglia disease. Marked impairment of voluntary movement is characteristic: either movements fail to occur when they are wanted or occur when they are not wanted. In patients with Huntington's chorea, as Wilson pointed out, unwanted movements occur that resemble the movements "executed at the bidding of volition. Each fresh movement appears to be directed to an end—which is never attained." The muscular events associated with the unwanted movements resemble the events associated with volitional movement in a healthy subject. The movements of chorea, however, are aimless.

In essence it is clear that the laws of reflex action, which have long been known to operate at the level of the spinal-cord motor neuron, also operate at the level of the motor cortex during volitional movements. Motor-cortex neurons in turn are impinged on by transcortical inputs. Thus the mammalian motor cortex, phylogenetically a new part of the brain, is subject to the same laws of reflex action that characterize the brain's older components. In addition the motor cortex can be driven by a second major set of inputs. These inputs underlie the internally generated motor programs that are a product of activity in the basal ganglia and the cerebellum and reach the motor cortex by way of the thalamus.

Hence of the two major classes of inputs that impinge on the motor cortex of the brain and generate the stream of impulses passed along to the spinal cord, the class of inputs that operate automatically—the transcortical loop—seems the simplest to understand: it operates according to Sherringtonian principles of reflex action. The second class of inputs, originating in the basal ganglia and the cerebellum and passing to the motor cortex by way of the thalamus, presents a more complicated picture. In order to understand voluntary movement we need to comprehend the kinds of information processed by these subcortical structures and to discover how the outputs of the cerebellum and the basal ganglia interact in the thalamus. To students of the brain mechanisms of movement these are the problems that are now uppermost.

IX

Specializations of the Human Brain

Specializations of the Human Brain

BY NORMAN GESCHWIND

Certain higher faculties, such as language, depend on specialized regions in the human brain. On a larger scale the two cerebral hemispheres are specialized for different kinds of mental activity

The nervous systems of all animals have a number of basic functions in common, most notably the control of movement and the analysis of sensation. What distinguishes the human brain is the variety of more specialized activities it is capable of learning. The preeminent example is language: no one is born knowing a language, but virtually everyone learns to speak and to understand the spoken word, and people of all cultures can be taught to write and to read. Music is also universal in man: people with no formal training are able to recognize and to reproduce dozens of melodies. Similarly, almost everyone can draw simple figures, and the ability to make accurate renderings is not rare.

At least some of these higher functions of the human brain are governed by dedicated networks of neurons. It has been known for more than 100 years, for example, that at least two delimited regions of the cerebral cortex are essential to linguistic competence; they seem to be organized explicitly for the processing of verbal information. Certain structures on the inner surface of the underside of the temporal lobe, including the hippocampus, are apparently necessary for the long-term retention of memories. In some cases the functional specialization of a neural system seems to be quite narrowly defined: hence one area on both sides of the human cerebral cortex is concerned primarily with the recognition of faces. It is likely that other mental activities are also associated with particular neural networks. Musical and artistic abilities, for example, appear to depend on specialized systems in the brain, although the circuitry has not yet been worked out.

Another distinctive characteristic of the human brain is the allocation of functions to the two cerebral hemispheres. That the human brain is not fully symmetrical in its functioning could be guessed from at least one observation of daily experience: most of the human population favors the right hand, which is controlled by the left side of the brain. Linguistic abilities also reside mainly on the left side. For these reasons the left cerebral hemisphere was once said to be the dominant one and the right side of the brain was thought to be subservient. In recent years this concept has been revised as it has become apparent that each hemisphere has its own specialized talents. Those for which the right cortex is dominant include some features of aptitudes for music and for the recognition of complex visual patterns. The right hemisphere is also the more important one for the expression and recognition of emotion. In the past few years these functional asymmetries have been matched with anatomical ones, and a start has been made on exploring their prevalence in species other than man.

In man as in other mammalian species large areas of the cerebral cortex are given over to comparatively elementary sensory and motor functions. An arch that extends roughly from ear to ear across the roof of the brain is the primary motor cortex, which exercises voluntary control over the muscles. Parallel to this arch and just behind it is the primary somatic sensory area, where signals are received from the skin, the bones, the joints and the muscles. Almost every region of the body is represented by a corresponding region in both the primary motor cortex and the somatic sensory cortex. At the back of the brain, and particularly on the inner surface of the occipital lobes, is the primary visual cortex. The primary auditory areas are in the temporal lobes; olfaction is focused in a region on the underside of the frontal lobes.

The primary motor and sensory areas are specialized in the sense that each one is dedicated to a specified function, but the functions themselves are of general utility, and the areas are called on in a great variety of activities. Moreover, homologous areas are found in all species that have a well-developed cerebral cortex. My main concern in this article is with certain regions of the cortex that govern a narrower range of behavior. Some of these highly specialized areas may be common to many species but others may be uniquely human.

A series of experiments dealing with learning in monkeys illustrates how fine the functional distinction can be between two networks of neurons. A monkey can be taught to choose consistently one object or pattern from a pair. The task is made somewhat more difficult if the objects are presented and then withdrawn and the monkey is allowed to indicate its choice only after a delay during which the objects are hidden behind a screen. It has been found that performance on this test is impaired markedly if a small region of the frontal lobes is destroyed on both sides of the brain. Difficulty can also be introduced into the experiment by making the patterns complex but allowing a choice to be made while the patterns are still in sight. Damage to a quite different area of the cortex reduces ability to carry out this task, but it has no effect on the delay test.

These experiments also illustrate one of the principal means for acquiring information about the functions of the brain. When a particular site is damaged by disease or injury, a well-defined deficiency in behavior sometimes ensues. In many cases one may conclude that some aspects of the behavior affected are normally dependent on the part of the brain that has been destroyed. In man the commonest cause of brain damage is cerebral thrombosis, or stroke: the occlusion of arteries in the brain, which results in the death of the tissues the blocked arteries supply. By 1920 the study of patients who had sustained such damage had led to the identification of several functional regions of the brain, including the language areas.

The study of the effects of damage to the brain is still an important method of investigating brain function, but other techniques have since been developed. One of the most important was brought to a high level of development by the German neurosurgeon Otfrid Foerster and by Wilder Penfield of the Montreal Neurological Institute. They studied the responses in the conscious patient un-

REPRODUCED BY LEFT HAND
(RIGHT HEMISPHERE)

MODEL PATTERN

REPRODUCED BY RIGHT HAND
(LEFT HEMISPHERE)

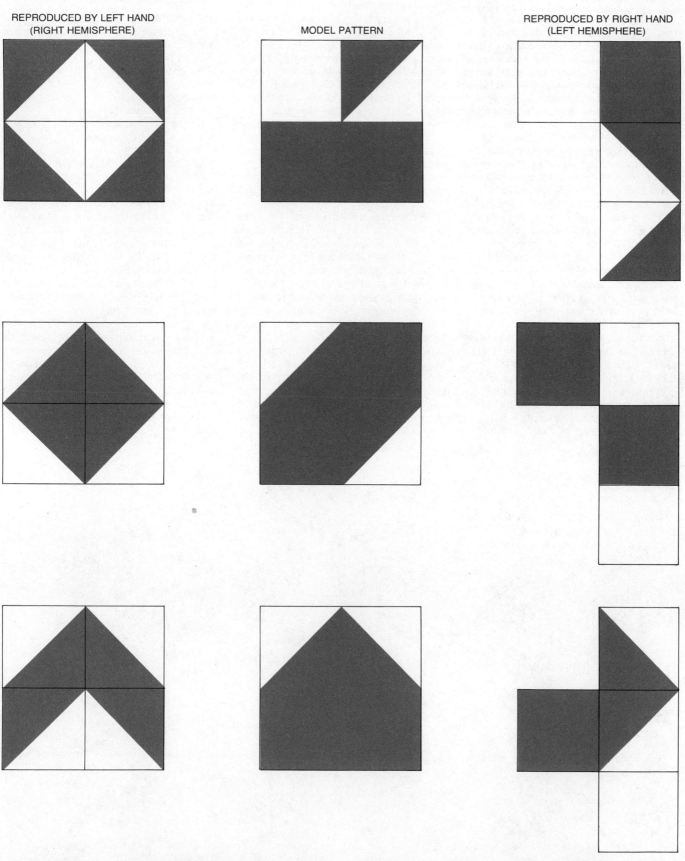

CAPABILITIES OF THE TWO HEMISPHERES of the human cerebral cortex were tested in a subject whose hemispheres had been surgically isolated from each other. The surgical procedure consisted in cutting the two main bundles of nerve fibers that connect the hemispheres: the corpus callosum and the anterior commissure. In the test each of the patterns in the middle column was presented to the subject, who was asked to reproduce it by assembling colored blocks. The assembly was carried out either with the right hand alone (which communicates mainly with the left hemisphere) or with the left hand alone (which is controlled primarily by the right hemisphere). Errors were equally frequent with either hand, but the kinds of error typical of each hand were quite different. The results suggest that each side of the brain may bring a separate set of skills to bear on such a task, a finding consistent with other evidence that the hemispheres are specialized for different functions. What is equally apparent, however, is that neither hemisphere alone is competent in the analysis of such patterns; the two hemispheres must cooperate. The test was conducted by Edith Kaplan of the Boston Veterans Administration Hospital.

dergoing brain surgery that follow electrical stimulation of various sites in the brain. In this way they were able to map the regions responsible for a number of functions. Apart from the importance of this technique for the study of the brain, it is of clinical benefit since it enables the surgeon to avoid areas where damage might be crippling.

Surgical procedures developed for the control of severe epilepsy have also contributed much information. One method of treating persistent epileptic seizures (adopted only when other therapies have failed) is to remove the region of the cortex from which the seizures arise. The functional deficits that sometimes result from this procedure have been studied in detail by Brenda Milner of the Montreal Neurological Institute.

The specializations of the hemispheres can be studied in people who have sustained damage to the commissures that connect the two sides of the brain, the most important of these being the corpus callosum. In the first such cases, studied at the end of the 19th century by Jules Déjerine in France and by Hugo Liepmann in Germany, the damage had been caused by strokes. More recently isolation of the hemispheres by surgical sectioning of the commissures

has been employed for the relief of epilepsy. Studies of such "split brain" patients by Roger W. Sperry of the California Institute of Technology and by Michael S. Gazzaniga of the Cornell University Medical College have provided increasingly detailed knowledge of the functions of the separated hemispheres. Doreen Kimura, who is now at the University of Western Ontario, pioneered in the development of a technique, called dichotic listening, that provides information about hemispheric specialization in the intact human brain.

The specialized regions of the brain that have been investigated in the greatest detail are those involved in language. In the 1860's the French investigator Paul Broca pointed out that damage to a particular region of the cortex consistently gives rise to an aphasia, or speech disorder. The region is on the side of the frontal lobes, and it is now called the anterior language area, or simply Broca's area. Broca went on to make a second major discovery. He showed that whereas damage to this area on the left side of the brain leads to aphasia, similar damage to the corresponding area on the right side leaves the faculty of speech intact. This finding

has since been amply confirmed: well over 95 percent of the aphasias caused by brain damage result from damage to the left hemisphere.

Broca's area is adjacent to the face area of the motor cortex, which controls the muscles of the face, the tongue, the jaw and the throat. When Broca's area is destroyed by a stroke, there is almost always severe damage to the face area in the left hemisphere as well, and so it might be thought that the disruption of speech is caused by partial paralysis of the muscles required for articulation. That some other explanation is required is easily demonstrated. First, damage to the corresponding area on the right side of the brain does not cause aphasia, although a similar weakness of the facial muscles results. Furthermore, in Broca's aphasia it is known that the muscles that function poorly in speech operate normally in other tasks. The evidence is quite simple: the patient with Broca's aphasia can speak only with great difficulty, but he can sing with ease and often with elegance. The speech of a patient with Broca's aphasia also has features, such as faulty grammar, that cannot be explained by a muscular failure.

Another kind of aphasia was identified in 1874 by the German investiga-

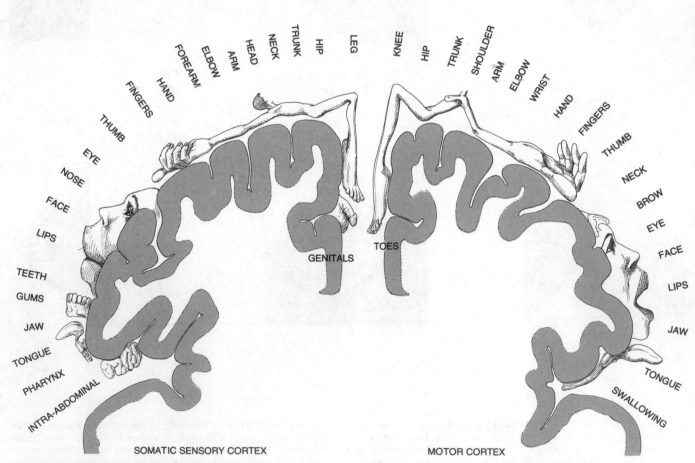

SOMATIC SENSORY CORTEX   MOTOR CORTEX

SOMATIC SENSORY AND MOTOR REGIONS of the cerebral cortex are specialized in the sense that every site in these regions can be associated with some part of the body. In other words, most of the body can be mapped onto the cortex, yielding two distorted homunculi. The distortions come about because the area of the cortex dedicated to a part of the body is proportional not to that part's actual size but to the precision with which it must be controlled. In man the motor and somatic sensory regions given over to the face and to the hands are greatly exaggerated. Only half of each cortical region is shown: the left somatic sensory area (which receives sensations primarily from the right side of the body) and the right motor cortex (which exercises control over movement in the left half of the body).

tor Carl Wernicke. It is associated with damage to another site in the cortex, also in the left hemisphere, but in the temporal lobe rather than the frontal lobe. This region, which is now called Wernicke's area, lies between the primary auditory cortex and a structure called the angular gyrus, which probably mediates between visual and auditory centers of the brain. It has since been learned that Wernicke's area and Broca's area are connected by a bundle of nerve fibers, the arcuate fasciculus.

A lesion in either Broca's area or Wernicke's area leads to a disruption of speech, but the nature of the two disorders is quite different. In Broca's aphasia speech is labored and slow and articulation is impaired. The response to a question will often make sense, but it generally cannot be expressed as a fully formed or grammatical sentence. There is particular difficulty with the inflection of verbs, with pronouns and connective words and with complex grammatical constructions. As a result the speech has a telegraphic style. For example, a patient asked about a dental appointment said, hesitantly and indistinctly: "Yes... Monday... Dad and Dick... Wednesday nine o'clock... 10 o'clock... doctors... and... teeth." The same kinds of errors are made in writing.

In Wernicke's aphasia speech is phonetically and even grammatically normal, but it is semantically deviant. Words are often strung together with considerable facility and with the proper inflections, so that the utterance has the recognizable structure of a sentence. The words chosen, however, are often inappropriate, and they sometimes include nonsensical syllables or words. Even when the individual words are correct, the utterance as a whole may express its meaning in a remarkably roundabout way. A patient who was asked to describe a picture that showed two boys stealing cookies behind a woman's back reported: "Mother is away here working her work to get her better, but when she's looking the two boys looking in the other part. She's working another time."

From an analysis of these defects Wernicke formulated a model of language production in the brain. Much new information has been added in the past 100 years, but the general principles Wernicke elaborated still seem valid. In this model the underlying structure of an utterance arises in Wernicke's area. It is then transferred through the arcuate fasciculus to Broca's area, where it evokes a detailed and coordinated program for vocalization. The program is passed on to the adjacent face area of the motor cortex, which activates the appropriate muscles of the mouth, the lips, the tongue, the larynx and so on.

Wernicke's area not only has a part

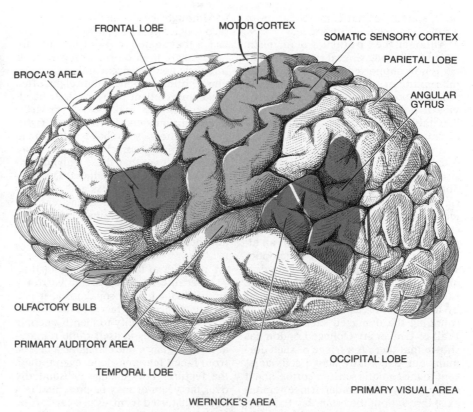

MAP OF THE HUMAN CORTEX shows regions whose functional specializations have been identified. Much of the cortex is given over to comparatively elementary functions: the generation of movement and the primary analysis of sensations. These areas, which include the motor and somatic sensory regions and the primary visual, auditory and olfactory areas, are present in all species that have a well-developed cortex and are called on in the course of many activities. Several other regions (*dark color*) are more narrowly specialized. Broca's area and Wernicke's area are involved in the production and comprehension of language. The angular gyrus is thought to mediate between visual and auditory forms of information. These functional specializations have been detected only on the left side of the brain; the corresponding areas of the right hemisphere do not have the same linguistic competence. The right hemisphere, which is not shown, has its own specialized abilities, including the analysis of some aspects of music and of complex visual patterns. The anatomical regions associated with these faculties, however, are not as well defined as the language areas. Even in the left hemisphere the assignment of functions to sites in the cortex is only approximate; some areas may have functions in addition to those indicated, and some functions may be carried out in more than one place.

in speaking but also has a major role in the comprehension of the spoken word and in reading and writing. When a word is heard, the sound is initially received in the primary auditory cortex, but the signal must pass through the adjacent Wernicke's area if it is to be understood as a verbal message. When a word is read, the visual pattern (from the primary visual cortex) is transmitted to the angular gyrus, which applies a transformation that elicits the auditory form of the word in Wernicke's area. Writing a word in response to an oral instruction requires information to be passed along the same pathways in the opposite direction: from the auditory cortex to Wernicke's area to the angular gyrus.

This model explains many of the symptoms that characterize the aphasias. A lesion in Broca's area disturbs the production of speech but has a much smaller effect on comprehension. Damage to Wernicke's area, on the other hand, disrupts all aspects of the use of language. The effects of certain rarer lesions are also in accord with the model. For example, destruction of the arcuate fasciculus, disconnecting Wernicke's area from Broca's area, leaves speech fluent and well articulated but semantically aberrant; Broca's area is operating but it is not receiving information from Wernicke's area. Because the latter center is also functional, however, comprehension of spoken and written words is almost normal. Writing is disrupted in all aphasias where speech is abnormal, but the neural circuits employed in writing are not known in detail.

Lesions in the angular gyrus have the effect of disconnecting the systems involved in auditory language and written language. Patients with injuries in certain areas of the angular gyrus may speak and understand speech normally, but they have difficulty with written language. The comprehension of a written word seems to require that the auditory form of the word be evoked in Wernicke's area. Damage to the angular gyrus seems to interrupt communication between the visual cortex and Wernicke's area, so that comprehension of written language is impaired.

Although the partitioning of linguistic functions among several sites in the cortex is now supported by much evidence, the rigidity of these assignments should not be overemphasized. The pessimistic view that damage to tissue in these areas inevitably leads to a permanent linguistic impairment is unwarranted. Actually a considerable degree of recovery is often observed. The neural tissue destroyed by an arterial thrombosis cannot be regenerated, but it seems the functions of the damaged areas can often be assumed, at least in part, by other regions. In some cases the recovery probably reflects the existence of an alternative store of learning on the opposite side of the brain, which remains dormant until the dominant side is injured. In other cases the function is taken over by neurons in areas adjacent to or surrounding the damaged site. Patrick D. Wall of University College London has shown that there is a fringe of such dormant but potentially active cells adjacent to the somatic sensory cortex, and it seems likely that similar fringe regions exist throughout the brain. Jay P. Mohr, who is now at the University of Southern Alabama, and his co-workers have shown that the prospects for recovery from Broca's aphasia are quite good provided the region destroyed is not too large. One interpretation of these findings suggests that regions bordering on Broca's area share its specialization in latent form.

Although the detailed mechanism of recovery is not known, it has been established that some groups of patients are more likely than others to regain their linguistic competence. Children, particularly children younger than eight, often make an excellent recovery. Left-handed people also make better progress than right-handers. Even among right-handers those who have left-handed parents, siblings or children are more likely to recover than those with no family history of left-handedness. The relation between handedness and recovery from damage to the language areas suggests that cerebral dominance for handedness and dominance for language are not totally independent.

A disorder of the brain that is startling because its effects are so narrowly circumscribed is prosopagnosia; it is a failure to recognize faces. In the normal individual the ability to identify people from their faces is itself quite remarkable. At a glance one can name a person from facial features alone, even though the features may change substantially over the years or may be presented in a highly distorted form, as in a caricature. In a patient with prosopagnosia this talent for association is abolished.

What is most remarkable about the disorder is its specificity. In general it is accompanied by few other neurological symptoms except for the loss of some part of the visual field, sometimes on both sides and sometimes only in the left half of space. Most mental tasks, in-

cluding those that require the processing of visual information, are done without particular difficulty; for example, the patient can usually read and correctly name seen objects. What he cannot do is look at a person or at a photograph of a face and name the person. He may even fail to recognize his wife or his children. It is not the identity of familiar people that has been lost to him, however, but only the connection between the face and the identity. When a familiar person speaks, the patient knows the voice and can say the name immediately. The perception of facial features is also unimpaired, since the patient can often describe a face in detail and can usually match a photograph made from the front with a profile of the same person. The deficiency seems to be confined to forming associations between faces and identities.

The lesions that cause prosopagnosia are as stereotyped as the disorder itself. Damage is found on the underside of both occipital lobes, extending forward to the inner surface of the temporal lobes. The implication is that some neural network within this region is specialized for the rapid and reliable recognition of human faces. It may seem that a disproportionate share of the brain's resources is being devoted to a rather limited task. It should be kept in mind, however, that the recognition of people as individuals is a valuable talent in a highly social animal, and there has probably been strong selectional pressure to improve its efficiency.

Similar capacities probably exist in other social species. Gary W. Van Hoesen, formerly in my department at the Harvard Medical School and now at the University of Iowa College of Medicine, has begun to investigate the neurological basis of face recognition in the rhesus monkey. So far he has demonstrated that the monkeys can readily discriminate between other monkeys on the basis of facial photographs. The neural structures called into play by this task have not, however, been identified.

Until recently little was known about the physiological basis of memory, one of the most important functions of the human brain. Through the study of some highly specific disorders, however, it has been possible to identify areas or structures in the brain that are involved in certain memory processes. For example, the examination of different forms of anterograde amnesia—an inability to learn new information—has revealed the role of the temporal lobes in memory. In particular, the striking disability of a patient whom Milner has studied for more than 25 years demonstrates the importance in memory of structures on the inner surface of the temporal lobes, such as the hippocampus.

In 1953 the patient had submitted to a radical surgical procedure in which

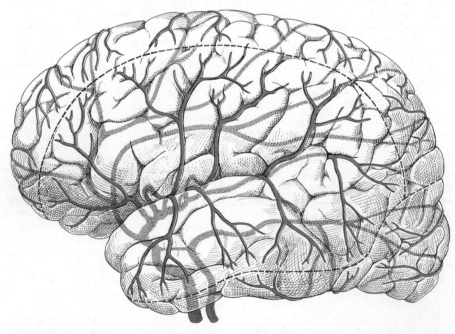

VASCULAR SYSTEM OF THE BRAIN has had an important part in the mapping of functional regions in the cerebral cortex. The normal functions of an area can often be inferred from the disturbance or impairment of behavior that results when the area is damaged. The commonest cause of such damage is the occlusion of an artery supplying the cortex, which leads to the death of the tissue nourished by that artery. Broca's area and Wernicke's area were identified in this way about 100 years ago, when patients with distinctive aphasias, or speech defects, were found by postmortem examination to have damage in those areas of the left hemisphere.

much of the hippocampus and several associated structures in both temporal lobes were destroyed. After the operation the skills and knowledge the patient had acquired up to that time remained largely intact, and he was and still is able to attend normally to ongoing events. In fact, he seems to be able to register limited amounts of new information in the usual manner. Within a short time, however, most of the newly learned information ceases to be available to him.

Milner has interviewed and tested the patient at intervals since the operation, and she has found that his severe anterograde amnesia has changed very little during that time. He has also exhibited an extensive although patchy retrograde amnesia (about the years before the operation), but that has improved appreciably. In the absence of distraction he can retain, say, a three-digit number for many minutes by means of verbal rehearsal or with the aid of an elaborate mnemonic device. Once his attention has been momentarily diverted, however, he cannot remember the number or the mnemonic device to which he devoted so much effort. He cannot even remember the task itself. Living from moment to moment, he has not been able to learn his address or to remember where the objects he uses every day are kept in his home. He fails to recognize people who have visited him regularly for many years.

The bilateral surgery that resulted in this memory impairment is, for obvious reasons, no longer done, but similar lesions on the inner surface of the temporal lobes have occasionally resulted from operations on one side of the brain in a patient with unsuspected damage to the opposite lobe. Comparable memory deficits result, and so the role of the inner surface of the temporal lobes in memory function is now widely accepted. Moreover, the fact that these patients generally retain their faculties of perception supports the distinction made by many workers between a short-term memory process and a long-term process by which more stable storage of information is achieved. It is clearly the second process that is impaired in the patients described above, but the nature of the impairment is a matter of controversy. Some think the problem is a failure of consolidation, that is, transferring information from short-term to long-term storage. Others hold that the information is transferred and stored but cannot be retrieved. The ultimate resolution of these conflicting theories will require a clearer specification of the neural circuitry of memory.

At a glance the brain appears to have perfect bilateral symmetry, like most other organs of the body. It might therefore be expected that the two halves of the brain would also be functionally equivalent, just as the two kid-

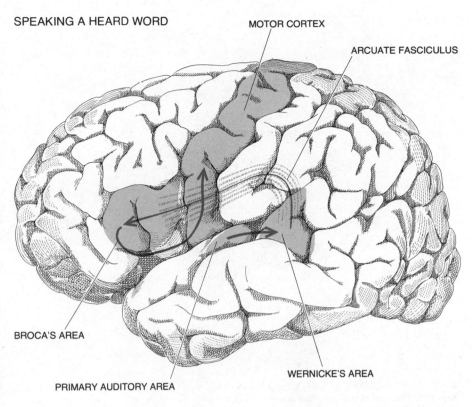

SPEAKING A HEARD WORD

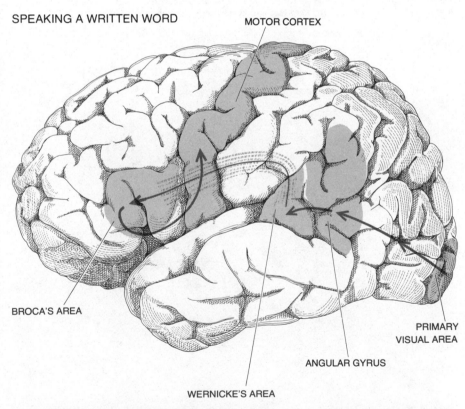

SPEAKING A WRITTEN WORD

LINGUISTIC COMPETENCE requires the cooperation of several areas of the cortex. When a word is heard (*upper diagram*), the sensation from the ears is received by the primary auditory cortex, but the word cannot be understood until the signal has been processed in Wernicke's area nearby. If the word is to be spoken, some representation of it is thought to be transmitted from Wernicke's area to Broca's area, through a bundle of nerve fibers called the arcuate fasciculus. In Broca's area the word evokes a detailed program for articulation, which is supplied to the face area of the motor cortex. The motor cortex in turn drives the muscles of the lips, the tongue, the larynx and so on. When a written word is read (*lower diagram*), the sensation is first registered by the primary visual cortex. It is then thought to be relayed to the angular gyrus, which associates the visual form of the word with the corresponding auditory pattern in Wernicke's area. Speaking the word then draws on the same systems of neurons as before.

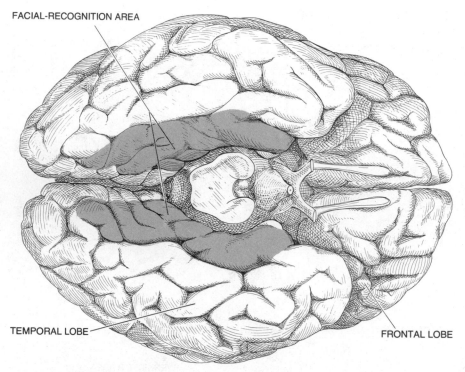

FACIAL-RECOGNITION AREA

TEMPORAL LOBE

FRONTAL LOBE

RECOGNITION OF FACES is a faculty that seems to be governed by regions on the underside of the temporal and occipital lobes on both sides of the cortex, which is seen here from below. A lesion that destroys this area impairs the ability to identify a person by facial features but has almost no other effects. There is often some loss of vision, but the patient can read, can name objects on sight and can even match a full-face portrait with a profile of the same person. People can also be recognized by their voices. The only ability that is lost is the ability to recognize people by their faces, and that loss can be so severe that close relatives are not recognized.

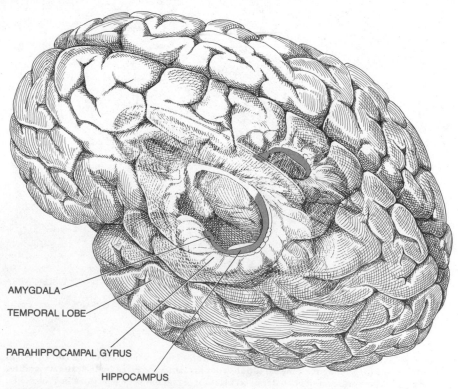

AMYGDALA

TEMPORAL LOBE

PARAHIPPOCAMPAL GYRUS

HIPPOCAMPUS

CERTAIN MEMORY PROCESSES appear to be associated with structures on the inner surface of the temporal lobes, such as the hippocampus (*color*). Bilateral lesions of these areas have been shown to cause a severe and lasting memory disorder characterized by the inability to learn new information. Patients with lesions of this type appear to have undiminished powers of perception, but they are largely incapable of incorporating new information into their long-term store. Acute lesions in this region of a single temporal lobe sometimes result in similar but less persistent memory disorders that reflect the contrasting specializations of the hemispheres: the type of information that cannot be learned varies according to the side the lesion is on.

neys or the two lungs are. Actually many of the more specialized functions are found in only one hemisphere or the other. Even the apparent anatomical symmetry turns out to be illusory.

In the primary motor and sensory areas of the cortex the assignment of duties to the two hemispheres follows a simple pattern: each side of the brain is concerned mainly with the opposite side of the body. Most of the nerve fibers in the pathways that radiate from the motor and somatic sensory areas cross to the opposite side of the nervous system at some point in their course. Hence the muscles of the right hand and foot are controlled primarily by the left motor cortex, and sensory impulses from the right side go mainly to the left somatic sensory cortex. Each ear has connections to the auditory cortex on both sides of the brain, but the connections to the contralateral side are stronger. The distribution of signals from the eyes is somewhat more complicated. The optic nerves are arranged so that images from the right half of space in both eyes are projected onto the left visual cortex; the left visual field from both eyes goes to the right hemisphere. As a result of this pattern of contralateral connections the sensory and motor functions of the two hemispheres are kept separate, but they are largely symmetrical. Each half of the brain is concerned with half of the body and half of the visual field.

The distribution of the more specialized functions is quite different, and it is profoundly asymmetrical. I have indicated above that linguistic ability is dependent primarily on the left hemisphere. There is reason to believe the right side of the brain is more important for the perception of melodies, one item of evidence being the ease with which aphasic patients with left-hemisphere damage can sing. The perception and analysis of nonverbal visual patterns, such as perspective drawings, is largely a function of the right hemisphere, although the left hemisphere also makes a distinctive contribution to such tasks. These asymmetries are also reflected in partial memory defects that can result from lesions in a single temporal lobe. A left temporal lobectomy can impair the ability to retain verbal material but can leave intact the ability to remember spatial locations, faces, melodies and abstract visual patterns.

In everyday life this lateralization of function can seldom be detected because information is readily passed between the hemispheres through several commissures, including the corpus callosum. Even when the interconnections are severed, the full effects of cerebral dominance can be observed only in laboratory situations, where it is possible to ensure that sensory information reaches only one hemisphere at a time and that a motor response comes from only one hemisphere. Under these conditions a

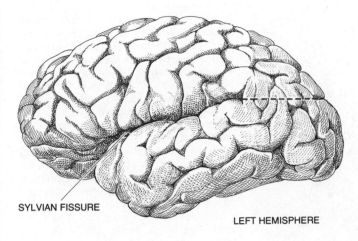
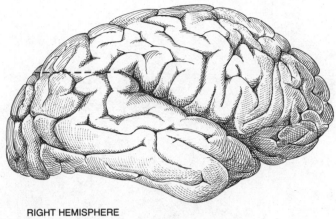
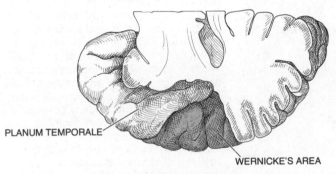
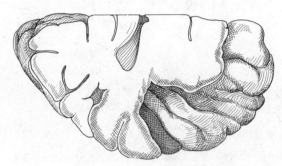

SYLVIAN FISSURE

LEFT HEMISPHERE   RIGHT HEMISPHERE

PLANUM TEMPORALE

WERNICKE'S AREA

ANATOMICAL ASYMMETRY of the cortex has been detected in the human brain and may be related to the distinctive functional specializations of the two hemispheres. One asymmetry is readily observed in the intact brain: the sylvian fissure, which defines the upper margin of the temporal lobe, rises more steeply on the right side of the brain. A more striking asymmetry is found on the planum temporale, which forms the upper surface of the temporal lobe, and which can be seen only when the sylvian fissure is opened. The posterior part of the planum temporale is usually much larger on the left side. The enlarged region is part of Wernicke's area, suggesting that the asymmetry may be related to the linguistic dominance of the left hemisphere. The distribution of the asymmetries varies with handedness.

remarkable pattern of behavior is observed. If an object is placed in a patient's left hand or if it is presented only to his left visual field, he cannot say its name. The failure is not one of recognition, since the patient is able to match related objects, but the perception received only in the right hemisphere cannot be associated with a name that is known only to the left hemisphere.

The specialization of the isolated hemispheres should not be overstated, however. The right half of the brain does have some rudimentary linguistic ability. Moreover, there are doubtless many tasks where the two hemispheres ordinarily act in concert. In one test administered after surgical isolation of the hemispheres the patient is asked to reproduce a simple pattern by assembling colored blocks. In some cases errors are frequent whether the task is completed with the left hand or the right, but they are characteristically different kinds of errors. It appears that neither hemisphere alone is competent in this task and that the two must cooperate.

One of the most surprising recent findings is that different emotional reactions follow damage to the right and left sides of the brain. Lesions in most areas on the left side are accompanied by the feelings of loss that might be expected as a result of any serious injury. The patient is disturbed by his disability and often is depressed. Damage in much of the right hemisphere sometimes leaves the patient unconcerned with his condition. Guido Gainotti of the Catholic University of Rome has made a detailed compilation of these differences in emotional response.

Emotion and "state of mind" are often associated with the structures of the limbic system, at the core of the brain, but in recent years it has been recognized that the cerebral cortex, particularly the right hemisphere of the cortex, also makes an important contribution. Lesions in the right hemisphere not only give rise to inappropriate emotional responses to the patient's own condition but also impair his recognition of emotion in others. A patient with damage on the left side may not be able to comprehend a statement, but in many cases he can still recognize the emotional tone with which it is spoken. A patient with a disorder of the right hemisphere usually understands the meaning of what is said, but he often fails to recognize that it is spoken in an angry or a humorous way.

Although cerebral dominance has been known in the human brain for more than a century, comparable asymmetries in other species have been recognized only in the past few years. A pioneer in this endeavor is Fernando Nottebohm of Rockefeller University, who has studied the neural basis of singing in songbirds. In most of the species he has studied so far, but not in all of them, the left side of the brain is more important for singing. Examples of dominance in mammals other than man have also been described, although in much less detail. Under certain conditions damage to the right side of the brain in rats alters emotional behavior, as Victor H. Denenberg of the University of Connecticut has shown. Dominance of the left cerebral cortex for some auditory tasks has been discovered in one species of monkey by James H. Dewson III, who is now at Stanford University. Michael Petersen and other investigators at the University of Michigan and at Rockefeller University have shown that the left hemisphere is dominant in the recognition of species-specific cries in Japanese macaques, which employ an unusual variety of such signals. So far, however, no definitive example of functional asymmetry has been described in the brains of the great apes, the closest relations of man.

For many years it was the prevailing view of neurologists that the func-

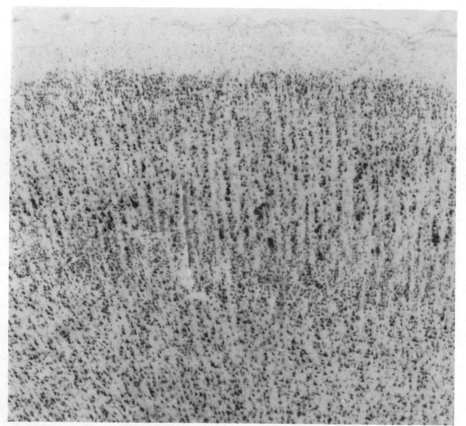

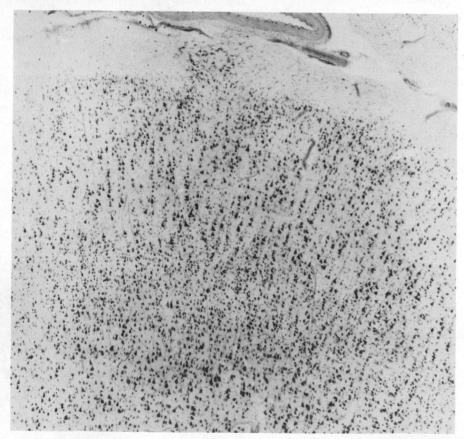

ABNORMAL CELLULAR ARCHITECTURE has been found in a language area of a patient with a developmental reading disorder. The top photomicrograph is a section of the normal cortex from the posterior portion of the planum temporale, the region that makes up part of Wernicke's area. Several layers can be perceived and the cells have a characteristic columnar organization. The bottom photograph is a section from the same region in a patient with dyslexia. One peculiarity is the presence of nerve-cell bodies in the most superficial layer (*near top of photograph*), where they are normally absent. Moreover, throughout the tissue the arrangement of cells is disrupted. The abnormality was found by Albert M. Galaburda of the Harvard Medical School and Thomas Kemper of the Boston University School of Medicine.

tional asymmetries of the brain could not be correlated with anatomical asymmetries. If there were any significant differences between the hemispheres, it was assumed, they would have been noted long ago by surgeons or pathologists. About 10 years ago my colleague Walter Levitsky and I decided to look into this matter again, following some earlier observations by the German neurologist Richard Arwed Pfeifer. We examined 100 human brains, paying particular attention to a region called the planum temporale, which lies on the upper surface of the temporal lobe and is hidden within the sylvian fissure that runs along each side of the brain. Our study was concerned only with gross anatomy, and we employed no instruments more elaborate than a camera and a ruler; nevertheless, we found unequivocal evidence of asymmetry. In general the length and orientation of the sylvian fissures is different on opposite sides of the head. What is more significant, the posterior area of the planum temporale, which forms part of Wernicke's area, is generally larger on the left side. The differences are not subtle and can easily be seen with the unaided eye.

Juhn A. Wada of the University of British Columbia subsequently showed that the asymmetry of the planum temporale can be detected in the human fetus. It therefore appears that the enlargement of the left planum cannot be a response to the development of linguistic competence in childhood. On the contrary, the superior linguistic talent of the left hemisphere may result from the anatomical bias.

More recently my colleague Albert M. Galaburda has discovered that the enlargement of the left planum can be explained in terms of the cellular organization of the tissue. On the planum is a region with a distinctive cellular architecture, designated *Tpt*. Galaburda found that the extent of the *Tpt* region is considerably greater in the left hemisphere; in the first brain he examined it was more than seven times as large on the left side as it was on the right.

Galaburda and Thomas Kemper of the Boston University School of Medicine also examined the brain of an accident victim who had suffered from persistent dyslexia. He found that the *Tpt* areas in the two hemispheres were of approximately equal size. Furthermore, the cellular structure of the *Tpt* area on the left side was abnormal. The neurons in the normal cortex are arranged in a sequence of layers, each of which has a distinctive population of cells. In the brain of the dyslexic the strata were disrupted, one conspicuous anomaly being the presence of cell bodies of neurons in the most superficial layer of the cortex, where they are normally absent. Islands of cortical tissue were also found in the white matter of the brain, where they do not belong. Although no firm conclusion can be drawn from a single case, it does seem striking that a structural abnormality would be found in the language area of a patient who was known to have a linguistic disability.

A new line of research on brain asymmetry has lately been opened by my colleague Marjorie J. LeMay. She has devised several methods for detecting anatomical asymmetry in the living person. One of these methods is cerebral arteriography, in which a substance opaque to X rays is injected into the bloodstream and the distribution of the substance is monitored as it flows through the cranial arteries. Arteriography is often employed in the diagnosis of brain tumors and other brain diseases, and the arteriograms LeMay examined had been made for diagnostic purposes. One of the cranial arteries (the middle cerebral artery) follows the groove of the sylvian fissure, and LeMay showed that the position of the artery in the arteriogram reveals the length and orientation of the fissure. She found that in most people the middle cerebral artery on the right side of the head is inclined more steeply and ultimately ascends higher than the corresponding artery on the left side.

LeMay has also detected brain asymmetries by computed axial tomography, the process whereby an image of the skull in cross section is reconstructed from a set of X-ray projections. In these images a peculiar, skewed departure from bilateral symmetry is observed. In right-handed people the right frontal lobe is usually wider than the left, but the left parietal and occipital lobes are wider than the right. The inner surface of the skull itself bulges at the right front and the left rear to accommodate the protuberances.

LeMay has even reported finding asymmetries in cranial endocasts made from the fossil skulls of Neanderthal man and other hominids. A ridge on the inner surface of the skull corresponds to the sylvian fissure; where the ridge is preserved well enough to make an impression in an endocast LeMay finds the same pattern of asymmetry that is observed in modern man, suggesting that hemispheric dominance had already emerged at least 30,000 years ago. LeMay and I have shown that asymmetries of the sylvian fissures exist in the great apes but not in monkeys. (Grace H. Yeni-Komshian and Dennis A. Benson of the Johns Hopkins University School of Medicine have reported similar findings.) If a functional correlative to this anatomical bias can be discovered, an animal model of cerebral dominance in the anthropoid apes would become available.

One of the most commonplace manifestations of cerebral dominance is also one of the most puzzling: the phenomenon of handedness. Many animals exhibit a form of handedness; for example, if a monkey is made to carry out a task with only one hand, it will consistently use the same one. In any large population of monkeys, however, left- and right-handed individuals are equally common. In the human population no more than 9 percent are left-handed. This considerable bias toward right-handedness may represent a unique specialization of the human brain.

The genetics and heritability of handedness is a controversial topic. In mice Robert V. Collins of the Jackson Laboratory in Bar Harbor, Me., has shown that continued inbreeding of right-handed animals does not increase the prevalence of right-handedness in their offspring. The pattern in man is quite different. Marian Annett of the Lanchester Polytechnic in England has proposed a theory in which one allele of a gene pair favors the development of right-handedness, but there is no complementary allele for left-handedness. In the absence of the right-favoring allele handedness is randomly determined.

Studies undertaken by LeMay and her co-workers have revealed that the distribution of brain asymmetries in left-handed people is different from that in right-handers. In right-handed individuals, and hence in most of the population, the right sylvian fissure is higher than the left in 67 percent of the brains examined. The left fissure is higher in 8 percent and the two fissures rise to approximately equal height in 25 percent. In the left-handed population a substantial majority (71 percent) have approximate symmetry of the sylvian fissures. Among the remainder the right fissure is still more likely to be the higher (21 percent v. 7 percent). The asymmetries observed by tomography also have a different distribution in right-handers and left-handers. Again in the left-handed segment of the population the asymmetries tend to be less pronounced. These findings are in qualitative agreement with the theory proposed by Annett.

If functions as narrowly defined as facial recognition are accorded specific neural networks in the brain, it seems likely that many other functions are represented in a similar way. For example, one of the major goals of child rearing is to teach a set of highly differentiated responses to emotional stimuli, such as anger and fear. The child must also be taught the appropriate responses to stimuli from its internal milieu, such as hunger or fullness of the bladder or bowel. Most children learn these patterns of behavior just as they learn a language, suggesting that here too special-purpose processors may be present. As yet little is known about such neural systems. Indeed, even as the mapping of specialized regions continues, the next major task must be confronted: that of describing their internal operation.

X

Disorders of
the Human Brain

Disorders of the Human Brain

BY SEYMOUR S. KETY

They can result from inherited metabolic defect, vascular disease, infection, tumor and trauma. The frontier in the study of mental illness is the relation between genetic and environmental factors

In a structure as complex as the human brain a multitude of things can go wrong. The wonder is that for most people the brain functions effectively and unceasingly for more than 60 years. It speaks for the resiliency, redundancy and self-restorative nature of the brain's mechanisms. The fact remains that disorders of the brain do sometimes arise in its structural architecture or in its electrical and chemical processes. More than a century ago pathologists were able to recognize disorders that involve damage to the gross anatomical structure of the brain, damage resulting from hemorrhage, pressure, displacement, inflammation, degeneration and atrophy. The microscope and selective chemical stains made it possible to see how morphological damage contributes to the starvation, degeneration and death of neurons and to the interruption of the pathways connecting them.

Investigations of brain disorders were hampered for many years by the absence of techniques for studying the living brain. What little was known about such disorders came from studies at autopsy. The discovery of X rays at the end of the 19th century enabled investigators to look inside the living brain. Gross structural defects in the ventricles, or cavities, of the brain can now be detected by pneumoencephalography: the X-ray technique in which the fluid that normally surrounds the brain and fills the ventricles is replaced with air to reveal their shape. In another approach, cerebral angiography, an X-ray-opaque dye is injected into the bloodstream so that pathological displacement of the blood vessels in the brain can be observed with X rays. Conventional radiography, invaluable as it is, suffers from a major drawback: on the developed film the X-ray projections of abnormalities can overlap those of the normal structures, making it difficult or even impossible to distinguish them from one another. This is particularly true when the X-ray densities of neighboring structures are similar, as is often the case with a tumor and the surrounding healthy tissue.

The development of the CAT scan (computed axial tomography) has surmounted that shortcoming. The CAT scan is a synthetic technique that combines X-ray readings taken from many different angles to yield a faithful representation of the internal structure of the living brain in cross section. The scan reveals enlarged and atrophied normal structures and any abnormal masses such as tumors and hemorrhages.

By the middle of this century electrical techniques had emerged as important tools for prospecting the brain. The messages the brain receives from the sense organs, the directives it sends to them and the messages between the billions of neurons within the brain are all carried by electrical signals. The electric fields near the surface of the brain can be picked up and amplified by the electroencephalograph. In this way disturbances in the electrical activity of the brain can be traced to specific locations.

Over the past two decades investigations of brain function have been extended to chemical processes. The utilization of energy by the brain can be studied by measurements of blood flow and of oxygen and glucose consumption. The recent work of Niels A. Lassen of the Bispebjerg Hospital in Copenhagen and David H. Ingvar of the University of Copenhagen makes it possible to see in cathode-ray-tube images how the circulation of blood in different regions of the brain changes rapidly in response to specific mental activities, such as reading aloud or reading silently. Louis Sokoloff and his co-workers at the National Institute of Mental Health have developed techniques for measuring the metabolism of glucose at any point in the brain. Because functional activity is closely related to blood flow and is intimately related to glucose utilization, such techniques provide a means for mapping the living brain in terms of the functional activity of its components.

At the level of the neuron, brain disorders can arise from anomalous chemical processes operating at the synapses between neurons. Disturbances in the synthesis, release or inactivation of a particular chemical transmitter or disturbances in the sensitivity of a transmitter's postsynaptic receptors can result in synaptic dysfunction. Such dysfunction need not be accompanied by morphological changes on either the gross or the microscopic level. The recent development of histofluorescent and immunofluorescent techniques, which in effect stain for specific transmitters or their enzymes, has made it possible to demonstrate and measure the effect of a transmitter on individual neurons. New chemical techniques employing radioactive isotopes can assay the number and the sensitivity of postsynaptic receptors, and powerful analytical instruments can examine brain fluid, cerebrospinal fluid, blood and urine for almost infinitesimal traces of transmitters and their metabolites.

Perfectly tuned and smoothly functioning synapses are essential to the successful operation of such complex mental processes as perception, cognition, affect and judgment. Since such processes are often disturbed in mental illness increased knowledge of them should help to unravel the mysteries of mental disorders. Only recently have these new techniques for studying the chemistry of the synapse been applied to mental disorders such as schizophrenia and manic-depressive psychosis. I think it is quite possible that these investigative tools may do for psychiatry what the older techniques have done for neurology.

Pathological processes in the brain can be brought about by a wide variety of proximate and remote causative factors that are often classified as being either genetic or environmental. Since every characteristic of a living organism ultimately depends on a complex interaction of genetic and environmental influences, it may seem futile to try to disentangle them. It is nonetheless possible to differentiate them by seeing how much each influence contributes to the variance in a particular characteristic. For example, language ability requires a highly developed mechanism in the brain, a mechanism that clearly depends

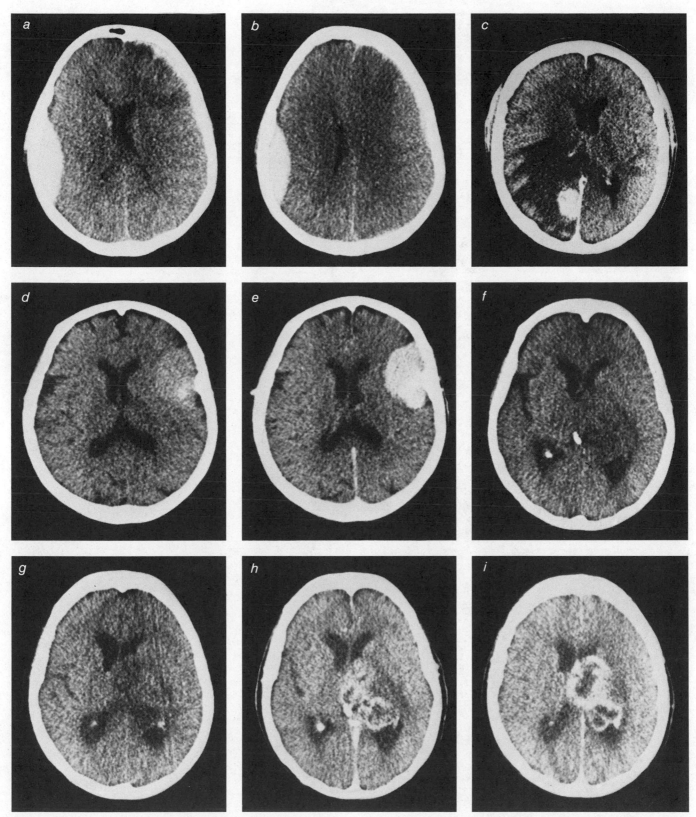

CAT SCAN (computed axial tomography) combines X-ray readings taken from many different angles to yield a representation of the living brain in cross section. The injection of an iodine solution into the venous system improves the contrast between different structures appearing in the scan. In scans *a* and *b* iodine was not needed to bring out a dense fresh blood clot between the brain and the skull. The hemorrhage was caused by a blow to that part of the skull. Diagonally opposite the clot is a shallow pool of blood on the surface of the brain or just inside it. The pool resulted from "contra coup" injury to the brain on the side opposite the blow. The ventricles (*center*) were compressed by the swelling of both halves of the brain. In scan *c* iodine brought out a tumor (*lower center*) of a patient suffering from cancer metastases. To the right of the tumor nodule is a normal vein, which stands out because it contains iodine-enriched blood. The ventricles

have been displaced by the swelling of the tissues surrounding the tumor. In scan *d* a meningioma (a benign tumor) is fairly faint without iodine. Inside the tumor is a small island of calcium. Hyperostosis, an accumulation of bone close to the tumor, is characteristic of a meningioma. In scan *e* iodine greatly enhanced the same tumor. The thin white line running through the tumor was generated by the scanning apparatus for measurement purposes. In scans *f* and *g* a malignant tumor (*center*) can scarcely be seen without the aid of iodine, but in scans *h* and *i*, made with iodine, it shows up clearly as a patchy area. The ventricles have been displaced and indented. In scan *f* a calcified pineal gland (*center*) has also been slightly displaced. The white ringlike zones of iodine enhancement are characteristic of a malignant tumor. The nine CAT scans were provided through the courtesy of Fred J. Hodges III of the Johns Hopkins University School of Medicine.

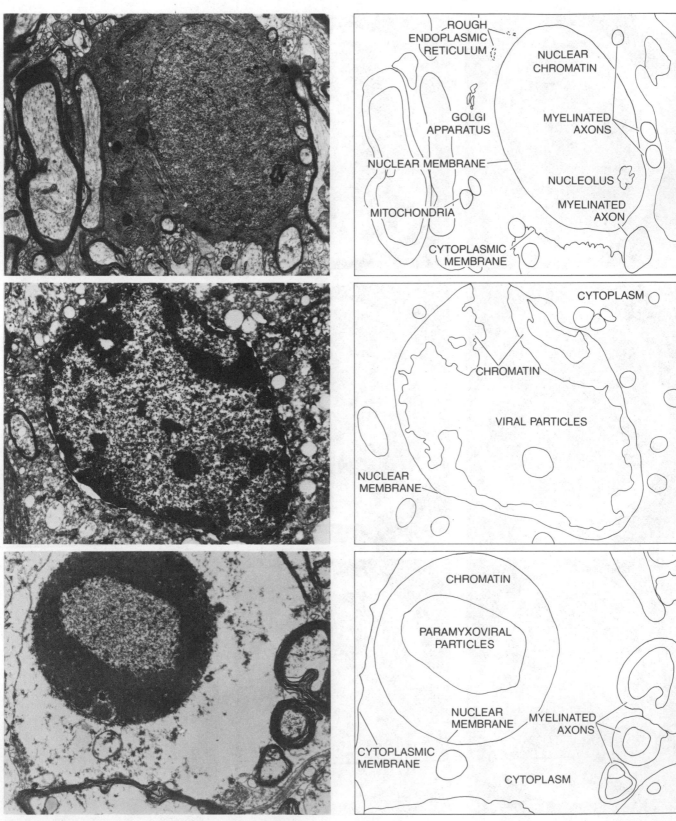

GLIAL CELL, which manufactures and maintains the fatty layer of myelin that sheathes the axons of the central nervous system, can be implicated in brain disorders. At the top left is an electron micrograph of a normal glial cell; it is a relatively dark cell with densely packed intracellular organelles, including mitochondria, "rough" endoplasmic reticulum and a well-defined Golgi apparatus. At the top right is a map of the organelles. In this normal cell chromatin, which incorporates the genetic material, is evenly dispersed throughout the nucleus. At the periphery of the cell are parts of several myelinated axons; the myelin is a direct extension of the glial cell's specialized cytoplasmic membrane. At the middle left is a glial cell from a person suffering from chronic lymphocytic leukemia. The organelles of the cell are much disrupted. The cell, which is in tissue removed at autopsy, has an enlarged and displaced nucleus, condensed chromatin and numerous viral particles that were destroying the cell. As a result the myelin of the axons was no longer being maintained. The progressive demyelination of major neural pathways gives rise to disease symptoms. About four months before the patient died he complained of decreased vision (which progressed to blindness in his left visual field), of inability to recognize faces and of inability to read. He suffered ultimately from complete blindness, mild confusion and bilateral motor dysfunction. At the bottom left is a glial cell, which is in tissue removed at autopsy, from a person suffering from subacute sclerosing panencephalitis. Here the individual organelles in the glial cell can no longer be distinguished, although the adjacent myelinated axons are still distinct. The chromatin is clumped and is displaced by particles characteristic of a paramyxovirus. The electron micrographs were made by Jerry S. Wolinsky of the Johns Hopkins School of Medicine.

on genetic processes. Yet the particular language a person speaks is not genetically determined but is accounted for almost entirely by the environmental factor of acculturation. On the other hand, there are genetic defects affecting the brain that require specific dietary conditions to bring them on. If these conditions are ubiquitous, the variance between the normal individual and the abnormal one will be entirely accounted for by the genetic factor; hence the disorder is classified as a genetic disease. Of course, most human characteristics cannot be categorized so easily. They seem to fall somewhere between the two extremes.

Genes determine the amino acid sequences that form proteins. It is these protein molecules, synthesized at specific sites and times, that serve as the structural materials and the enzyme catalysts responsible for the development and operation of the brain. Many disorders of the central nervous system, particularly those resulting in mental retardation, are known to be genetic in origin. For example, phenylketonuria and galactosemia are both caused by genetically determined enzyme deficiencies. In both diseases an enzyme deficiency makes toxic a component of the diet that is ordinarily beneficial. An infant born with phenylketonuria lacks the enzyme phenylalanine hydroxylase, which is responsible for the further metabolism of phenylalanine in the body. As a result excessive quantities of this essential amino acid accumulate in the blood and tissues, interfering with the development and operation of the brain.

In galactosemia the infant appears normal at birth, but within a few days or weeks of milk feeding it develops anorexia, vomiting and growth failure that may lead to death from wasting and inanition. Untreated survivors are often stunted and mentally retarded. Galactosemia is caused by the absence of an enzyme essential to the further metabolism of the sugar galactose, which therefore accumulates in abnormal amounts. The deleterious effects of these diseases can be eliminated by altering the environment, namely by removing the offending substance (phenylalanine or galactose) from the diet for at least the period of infancy when the brain grows and develops the most.

Some genetic disorders are sex-linked. Lesch-Nyhan syndrome, characterized by purposeless and uncontrollable movements, mental retardation and self-destructive psychotic behavior, is the result of an enzyme deficiency. An absent or defective gene on the X chromosome is responsible. The disorder affects only males because they have only one X chromosome. (In females, who have two X chromosomes, the absent or defective gene, if it is present on one X chromosome, has no effect because

15:381 (3.9%)

1:353 (.3%)

BIOLOGICAL RELATIVES
OF DEPRESSED ADOPTEES

BIOLOGICAL RELATIVES
OF CONTROL ADOPTEES

1:168 (.6%)

1:166 (.6%)

ADOPTIVE RELATIVES
OF DEPRESSED ADOPTEES

ADOPTIVE RELATIVES
OF CONTROL ADOPTEES

HIGHER INCIDENCE OF SUICIDE in biological relatives of adoptees who suffered from depression compared with the incidence in their adoptive relatives and in the relatives of control adoptees who had no mental illness suggests a genetic factor in suicide. Each ratio shows the number of relatives who committed suicide with respect to the total number of relatives. Data come from a study by the author, David Rosenthal of National Institute of Mental Health, Fini Schulsinger of University of Copenhagen and Paul H. Wender of University of Utah.

there is a normal gene on the other X chromosome.)

Brain disorders can result not only from a deficiency of genetic material but also from an excess. Extra X or Y chromosomes are associated with syndromes involving mild intellectual and personality disorders. In Down's syndrome, which afflicts about one out of every 700 newborn infants, there is an extra chromosome No. 21. Such children suffer from retarded physical and mental development.

Genetic disorders do not necessarily reveal themselves at birth. For example, the symptoms of Huntington's chorea, namely uncontrolled movements and mental deterioration, appear for the first time between the ages of 30 and 50. The disease, which depends almost entirely on a dominant genetic trait, leads to gross atrophy of the corpus striatum in the brain and to neuron degeneration in the caudate and the other deep neural nuclei and in the frontal cerebral cortex.

In 1968 Linus Pauling proposed that

there are genetically determined differences in the amount of vitamins people need. He suggested that the differences might result in disorders of the central nervous system, including the brain. This hypothesis is exemplified by several rare childhood neurological syndromes in which a genetically determined failure to absorb or process a particular vitamin creates a severe vitamin deficiency that adversely affects the central nervous system. These syndromes can be treated successfully by administering large doses of the particular vitamin involved. Pauling suggested that such a mechanism might be the cause of schizophrenia, but there is little evidence that an increased requirement of any vitamin is characteristic of the disorder.

The major psychoses, including schizophrenia and the affective disorders, are considerably commoner than the disorders mentioned above. In these psychoses genetic factors seem to play a

124   SEYMOUR S. KETY

major role, although their biological consequences have not yet been identified, as they have been for many other brain disorders. Ever since schizophrenia and manic-depressive illness were first described nearly a century ago, they have been known to run in families. Roughly 10 percent of the parents, the siblings and the offspring of an afflicted individual also suffer from the disorder. That was often taken to mean that such disorders are hereditary.

A family, however, shares environmental influences as well as genetic ones, and so the mere fact that a disease runs in families says little about its etiol-

ogy. Pellagra, a vitamin-deficiency disease that in the early decades of this century accounted for 10 percent of the mentally ill in the U.S., also afflicts families, so that it was once thought to be hereditary. In 1915 Joseph Goldberger of the U.S. Public Health Service demonstrated that the principal cause of pellagra is a severe deficiency in the diet of the B vitamin niacin. Since members of a family usually eat the same kinds of food, the disease ran in families. Pellagra has been almost entirely eradicated by dietary intervention.

Evidence of a genetic etiology for schizophrenia and for manic-depressive

disease comes from studies of the incidence of these disorders in identical twins (who share all their genes) and in fraternal twins (who share about half of the same genes). In identical twins both disorders show a high concordance rate (almost 50 percent), but in fraternal twins the rate (about 10 percent) is no different from that in all siblings. Recent studies have concentrated on adopted individuals whose genetic endowment can be investigated through their biological relatives and whose environmental influences can be examined through their adoptive relatives.

Such studies indicate that both schizo-

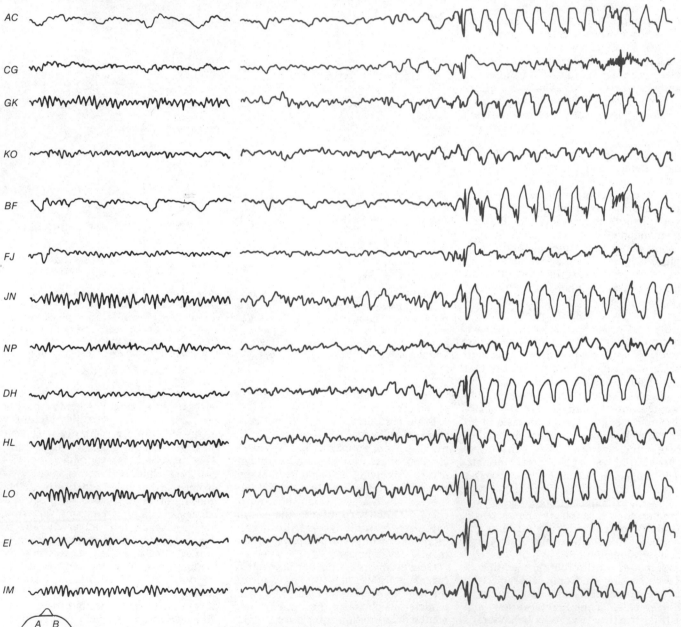

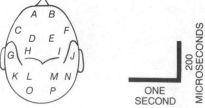

ELECTROENCEPHALOGRAM OF AN EPILEPTIC (*color*) shows normal electrical activity of the brain until the onset of a seizure at about the halfway point of the colored traces. The first half of the colored traces resembles the electroencephalogram (*black*) of a person who does not have epilepsy. Each trace records how the voltage between two areas of the head (labeled with two letters that correspond to the areas on the diagram of the head) changed in time. Below curves is a calibration mark, with horizontal line representing one second and vertical line 200 microvolts. Traces were provided by Robert R. Young of Harvard Medical School.

phrenia and manic-depressive disorder run in the biological families and not in the adoptive ones. The rate of mental illness in the adoptive relatives who lived with the affected adoptee is the same as the rate of mental illness in the general population. This finding in conjunction with the higher concordance rate in identical twins indicates the importance of genetic factors in schizophrenia and manic-depressive disorder, although it does not rule out the possibility of various environmental factors also playing a major etiological role. Since genes can express themselves only through biochemical mechanisms, the importance of genetic factors in mental disorders constitutes compelling evidence for biochemical substrates in these disorders, although such substrates have not yet been specifically identified.

Studies of biological and adoptive families suggest the presence of a significant genetic factor in chronic alcoholism, in which an environmental agent, namely alcohol, has an obvious role, and in suicide, in which many kinds of environmental influences are undoubtedly involved. The genetic factors in such disorders might explain why not everyone exposed to alcohol becomes addicted and why only a fraction of the people who find themselves in apparently hopeless situations choose to commit suicide.

Since all etiological factors that are not genetic must be environmental, the latter category spans a broad range of influences that differ in quality, intensity and the times in the life of an individual during which they exert their effects. Such factors first come into play in the uterine environment. In the complex metamorphosis from the fertilized ovum to the newborn infant, chemical and physical processes operate at every stage to allow the expression of the genetic program. All kinds of environmental deficiencies and disturbances can interfere with this expression and thwart the normal development of the central nervous system.

Many forms of cerebral palsy and mental retardation owe their origin to abnormalities in the fetal environment or in the process of birth. If rubella, or "German measles," is transmitted from the mother to the fetus in the first trimester of pregnancy, the disease can cause mental retardation and possibly infantile autism. If cytomegalovirus, which in adults is fairly common and usually innocuous, infects the brain of the fetus, it may lead to deafness and subnormal intelligence. Kernicterus, a fetal jaundice resulting from Rh incompatibility between the mother and the fetus, can cause hearing loss, cerebral palsy and mental retardation, although the incidence of such complications has been greatly reduced by diagnostic and prophylactic intervention. Hormonal disorders in the mother and her exposure to certain drugs and other foreign substances have been shown to give rise to abnormalities in the fetus. It is also likely that severe malnutrition or maternal exposure to alcohol and other toxins could disturb the normal development of the fetal brain.

Bacterial infections are a chief cause of cerebral disorders at all stages of life, although the control of infection by antibiotics has almost entirely eradicated many severe disorders, such as the general paresis, or extreme insanity, that resulted from syphilis and the often fatal meningitis, or inflammation of the membranes enclosing the brain, that resulted from tuberculosis and other bacterial infections.

Viral diseases cannot be treated as effectively as bacterial infections can, so that acute and often fatal encephalitis is occasionally associated with such viral diseases as measles, mumps, influenza and herpes. Poliomyelitis, an infection of the motor neurons, is a viral disorder of the central nervous system that has been almost completely eradicated by the development of effective vaccines. The influenza epidemic that swept the world in 1918 left in its wake countless people who gradually developed a form of Parkinson's disease, characterized by a severe dysfunction of motor control. The strain of influenza virus had a special predilection for invading the extrapyramidal system of the brain and seems to be the first recorded example of a viral infection of the nervous system that lay dormant for several years before giving rise to deleterious effects.

Recently the cause of several other disorders has been traced to latent or slow viral infections of the nervous system. For example, kuru is a slowly progressive neurological disorder that is limited to a small tribe in New Guinea. Kuru runs in families, and so it was thought to be genetic until D. Carleton Gajdusek of the National Institutes of Health established its viral etiology by showing that chimpanzees inoculated with brain tissue from infected individuals also developed the disease.

Creutzfeldt-Jakob disease, a rare dementia of middle age, is another slowly progressive disorder that is viral in origin. Alzheimer's disease, a much commoner type of senile dementia, resembles Creutzfeldt-Jakob disease in many of its clinical and neuropathological features. Several laboratories are investigating the possibility that a viral agent is responsible for Alzheimer's disease. Herpes and cytomegalovirus are examples of other viruses that can remain dormant in the nervous system for years before producing neurological or mental symptoms. There is also evidence that some forms of schizophrenia may be viral in origin.

The history of psychiatry and neurology provides numerous cases of cerebral disorders caused by toxic chemicals. The Mad Hatter was not a creature of Lewis Carroll's remarkable imagination but a fictional victim of an occupational disease of the 18th and 19th centuries. Hatmakers who were exposed daily to mercury used in the preparation of felt suffered a toxic psychosis. Other heavy metals are also known to disturb the nervous system. Manganese causes a form of Parkinson's disease and lead causes disturbances of the peripheral nerves and the brain. Lead poisoning in children (chiefly from the ingestion of lead-based paint) can give rise to behavioral abnormalities and learning disabilities.

In the Middle Ages bread made of rye infested with ergot, a parasitic fungus, was responsible for epidemics of madness. This plant parasite is now known to contain several alkaloids that have a potent effect on the nervous system. The powerful hallucinogen LSD is a synthetic derivative of one of them.

In addition to exogenous poisons and drugs, endogenous substances that are made in the body as the result of some disease can be toxic to the brain. Untreated diabetes and severe or terminal kidney or liver failure can result in the production of toxic substances that cause confusion, delirium and ultimately coma. Porphyria is a rare metabolic disorder of genetic origin in which the buildup of porphyrins interferes with mental processes. The madness of King George III has been attributed to porphyria.

Although the processes of immunity defend the body against infection, the immune response occasionally goes awry, resulting in a variety of disorders, some of which involve the brain. Allergic disorders such as asthma and hay fever are the commonest immune diseases. The root of disorders such as rheumatoid arthritis, lupus erythematosus and other collagen diseases is a faulty immune response directed against normal tissue. Such an autoimmune process has been definitively implicated in one neuropsychiatric illness: myasthenia gravis, a severe neuromuscular disorder characterized by sporadic muscular fatigability and weakness. The disease invades the neuromuscular junction, where the transmitter acetylcholine is released and acts on receptors in muscle-cell membranes in order to trigger muscular contraction. Recent work indicates that in this disorder an autoimmune process impairs receptor function and reduces the efficiency of the neuromuscular junction. It is also possible that an autoimmune process is responsible for multiple sclerosis. The evidence comes from a laboratory-animal model of an autoimmune disease, called experimental allergic encephalomyelitis, that resembles multiple sclerosis in its behavioral symptoms and neuropathology.

The most prevalent brain disorders are due to deficiencies in the supply of blood. The energy requirements of the brain are among the highest in the body. The brain needs a fifth of the heart's output of blood and a fifth of the oxygen consumed by the entire body at rest. Although rare congenital defects can disturb the vascular system of the brain, the commonest disturbance is atherosclerosis, the poorly understood disorder of the blood vessels that can affect the heart, the kidneys and the limbs as well as the brain. Atherosclerosis can lead to a narrowing of the bore and an eventual thrombosis of a blood vessel, which results in a gradual or a sudden diminution in the blood supply of an area of the brain and hence in abnormal functioning of that area. The wall of an atherosclerotic vessel can also rupture, causing a cerebral hemorrhage. The symptoms of thrombosis or cerebral hemorrhage vary greatly, depending on what areas and processes of the brain are affected. Some of the effects of a hemorrhage are the result of pressure, which acts to oppose the blood flow and to displace and distort the complex architecture of the brain. Tumors and head injuries can operate the same way.

Epilepsy, characterized by the simultaneous and rhythmic firing of large numbers of neurons, is a neuropsychiatric disorder for which the primary and proximate causes are still largely unknown. The origin of one kind of epilepsy has been traced to a scar, usually on the surface of the brain, that is the result of injury or infection. The scar tissue serves as the focus of abnormal electrical activity, which spreads over a large field of adjacent normal neurons. In most kinds of epilepsy, however, scars or other lesions have not been found. Here there is accumulating evidence that the defect is a chemical one involving one or more transmitters, particularly GABA (gamma-aminobutyric acid), the major inhibitory transmitter in the central nervous system.

As for the major psychoses (schizophrenia and manic-depressive illness), their etiology is still not known. In their severe and classical form they can resemble disorders of the brain. The individual symptoms or the entire syndrome of a psychiatric disorder can sometimes be seen in the early stages of a recognized neurological disorder such as Huntington's chorea.

A chemical dimension of mental illness is most clearly suggested by the studies I have mentioned that revealed the importance of genetic factors in the etiology of the major psychoses. The biochemical processes through which these genetic factors express themselves have not been established, although there are promising indications that they operate at certain synapses in the brain. Drugs that act on the brain can alleviate the symptoms of depression, mania and schizophrenia as well as create them. Such drugs act specifically on synaptic processes. The drugs that remove certain transmitters (dopamine, norepinephrine and serotonin) from their synapses cause depression, whereas the drugs used to treat clinical depression all tend to elevate the levels of these transmitters or to enhance their function. The hypothesis that some forms of depression are the result of a deficiency of these transmitters or of other transmitters that interact with them is a plausible one, and studies of metabolites in urine and cerebrospinal fluid tend to support it.

By the same token the drugs that are effective in relieving the psychotic symptoms of schizophrenia all damp the activity of dopamine synapses,

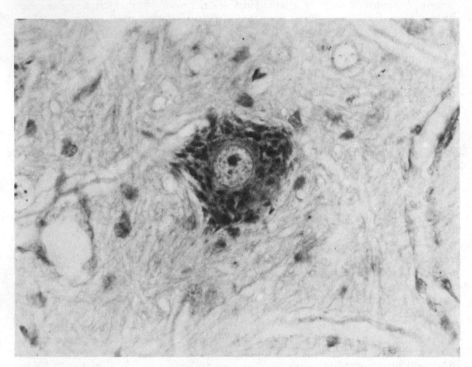

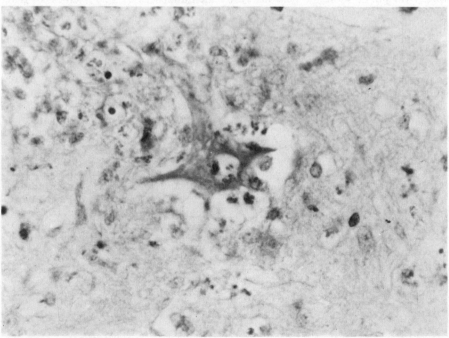

POLIOMYELITIS, a viral infection of the motor neurons, has been almost eradicated by the development of vaccines. In the electron micrograph at the top is a normal anterior-horn cell in the spinal cord of a rhesus monkey; it is characterized by massive Nissl bodies in the cytoplasm, a centrally located nucleus and dispersed chromatin. In the micrograph at the bottom is an anterior-horn cell from a monkey in a late stage of poliomyelitis. The cell is irreversibly injured. The micrographs were provided by David Bodian of Johns Hopkins School of Medicine.

whereas amphetamine, which gives rise to a toxic psychosis that closely resembles schizophrenia, increases the level of dopamine at these synapses. Although clear evidence of an excess of dopamine in the brain of schizophrenics is lacking, it is possible that other conditions might exist in the brain of schizophrenics that would have an effect similar to the one produced by an excess of dopamine, conditions such as an oversensitivity of dopamine receptors or a deficiency in the activity of another transmitter that normally opposes dopamine. All these possibilities call for much further investigation.

Psychological and social factors undoubtedly play an important role in these psychiatric disorders. There can be no doubt that such influences alter the manifestations, severity, duration and course of such disorders, and that in many instances they can precipitate them. Several plausible hypotheses have been put forward on a possible interaction between environmental factors and a biological predisposition for mental illness. The environmental influences that have been suggested or implicated as playing some etiological role in mental illness include, in addition to psychological factors, physiological difficulties during the prenatal period, birth injuries, infectious disease and certain toxins. Such influences have a differential social distribution. Most are commoner among the lower socioeconomic groups because of crowding, poor hygiene and inadequate medical care. Schizophrenia in particular is known to be twice as prevalent among the poor who live in large cities than it is in the rest of the population.

The successful treatment or prevention of a brain disorder depends largely on how much is known about it. The effects of a tumor or of a sclerotic blood vessel can sometimes be alleviated by corrective measures, but more specific treatment or prevention of a disorder calls for an understanding of the fundamental mechanisms involved. Parkinson's disease, whose symptoms cripple about 50,000 people in the U.S. per year, is a good example of how knowledge of the underlying neurobiological processes at fault in a particular disorder can give rise to a successful method of treatment. Parkinson's disease is a progressive chronic condition that once meant death or severe disability for its victims. The disease begins with an involuntary shaking of the arms. The jerky tremor spreads to the other extremities and to the neck and the jaw. The back stiffens and the muscles become so rigid that the sufferer walks with a strange shuffle. In the final stages of the disease the sufferer is bedridden, unable to walk or feed himself and unable to talk because of facial paralysis.

The work of Arvid Carlsson of the University of Göteborg and Oleh Hornykiewicz of the University of Vienna revealed that the cause of the disease is the progressive destruction of the neuron pathways that are characterized by the transmitter dopamine. As a result a deficiency of dopamine was found at the pathway synapses in the corpus striatum, a structure near the center of the brain that modulates movement.

This information enabled investigators to develop an effective treatment. It was known that although dopamine itself would not pass through the membrane that separates brain tissue from the blood, its chemical precursor, L-DOPA, would. When L-DOPA is administered orally, it enters the bloodstream from the intestine and travels to the brain, where it is taken up and converted into dopamine. In clinical trials with large doses of L-DOPA George C. Cotzias of the Brookhaven National Laboratory found that the symptoms of the disorder were dramatically relieved. The therapeutic doses of L-DOPA are quite large (as much as 8,000 milligrams a day), so that many adverse side effects result from the action of dopamine on other parts of the body. Modified forms of the treatment have been developed recently that introduce fewer adverse complications.

The treatment of Parkinson's disease constitutes one of the major medical triumphs that resulted from fundamental research in biochemistry and neuroscience. Yet even before the underlying mechanism of a brain disorder is understood an effective treatment will sometimes be discovered fortuitously. That was the case with the antidepressant and antipsychotic drugs that sparked the development of psychopharmacology, revolutionizing the treatment of mental illness. Knowledge of the actions of these drugs on chemical synapses facilitates the development of more effective drugs with fewer side effects. Epilepsy, whose underlying causes and mechanisms are still not understood, is successfully treated with Dilantin, a drug that was discovered in a systematic search with electrophysiological techniques.

As understanding of a particular disorder increases with deliberate investigation and the steady accumulation of basic knowledge, new treatments and ultimately methods of prevention are developed. That has been the case with infectious diseases of the brain, such as general paresis, poliomyelitis, meningitis and certain kinds of encephalitis, where identification of the etiological agent made possible vaccine prophylaxis and antibiotic therapy. It was the case even earlier with pellagra. One may reasonably expect it will also happen for those brain disorders that are still shrouded in mystery.

XI

Thinking About the Brain

Thinking about the Brain

BY F. H. C. CRICK

Reflecting on itself, the human brain has uncovered some marvelous facts. What appears to be needed for understanding how it works is new techniques for examining it and new ways of thinking about it

The reader of the preceding articles in this book will have seen how the brain is being studied at many levels, from the molecules at its synapses up to complex forms of behavior, and by diverse approaches—chemical, anatomical, physiological, embryological and psychological—to the nervous system in many different animals, from simple invertebrates to man himself. And yet the reader will also have noted that in spite of the steady accumulation of detailed knowledge how the human brain works is still profoundly mysterious. The editors of *Scientific American* have asked me, as a newcomer to neurobiology, to make some general comments on how the subject strikes a relative outsider. I have been interested in neurobiology for more than 30 years, but only in the past couple of years have I attempted to study it seriously.

In approaching a new discipline it is a useful exercise to attempt to separate those topics that, although far from being understood, appear at least capable of explanation by familiar approaches of one kind or another from those for which no ready explanation, even in outline, seems available at the present time. (It was such an analysis that led James Watson and me to search for the structure of DNA.) In the first category I would put topics such as the chemical and electrical nature of neurons and synapses, the habituation and sensitization of single neurons, the effects of drugs on the nervous system and so on. In fact, I would put in it almost all of neuroanatomy and neuropharmacology and much of neurophysiology. Even the development of the brain does not seem to me to be essentially mysterious, in spite of our ignorance of the exact processes at work in the growing embryo.

On the other hand, there are some human abilities that appear to me to defeat our present understanding. We sense there is something difficult to explain, but it seems almost impossible to state clearly and exactly what the difficulty is. This suggests that our entire way of thinking about such problems may be incorrect. In the forefront of the problems I would put perception, although here others might substitute conception, imagination, volition or emotion. All of these have in common that they are part of our subjective experience and that they probably involve large numbers of neurons interacting in intricate ways.

To understand these higher levels of neural activity we would obviously do well to learn as much as possible about the lower levels, particularly those accessible to direct experiment. Such knowledge by itself, however, may not be enough. It seems certain that we need to consider theories dealing directly with the processing of information in large and complex systems, whether it is information coming in from the senses, instructions going out to the muscles and glands or the flow of information in the vast amount of neural activity between these two extremes.

The reason I emphasize perception, and in particular visual perception, is that, as the article by David Hubel and Torsten Wiesel in this issue shows clearly [see "Brain Mechanisms of Vision," by David H. Hubel and Torsten N. Wiesel, page 84], it seems more accessible to direct experiment. In addition our internal picture of the external world is both accurate and vivid, which is not surprising in view of the fact that human beings are highly visual animals. The human sense of smell, in contrast, is much vaguer. Curiously, much of this visual picture is built up in ways that require little effort on our part. When we try to think of a genuinely difficult task, we usually pick something such as chess or mathematics or learning a foreign language. Few people realize what an astonishing achievement it is to be able to see at all. The main contribution of the relatively new field of artificial intelligence has been not so much to solve these problems of information handling as to show what tremendously difficult problems they are. When one reflects on the computations that must have to be carried out before one can recognize even such an everyday scene as another person crossing the street, one is left with a feeling of amazement that such an extraordinary series of detailed operations can be accomplished so effortlessly in such a short space of time.

The advent of larger, faster and cheaper computers, a development that is far from reaching its end, has given us some feeling for what can be achieved by rapid computation. Unfortunately the analogy between a computer and the

VISUAL CORTEX OF THE OWL MONKEY exemplifies the tendency of the cerebral cortex to be "mapped" into areas geometrically related to their function. The cortex of the animal has a left hemisphere consisting of nine areas that are orderly maps of the monkey's visual field (and three areas that respond to stimuli from the visual field but do not seem to represent it in an orderly way). In the highly schematic diagram at the top the visual cortex, which constitutes the posterior third of the cortex, has been unfolded so that it can be viewed from above. The geometric relations between the visual field and the various areas of the visual cortex were found in electrophysiological experiments in which microelectrodes inserted into the visual cortex recorded the response of small groups of neurons to stimuli from particular regions of the visual field. The chart at the bottom left shows the right half of the visual field. The squares mark the horizontal meridian of the visual field, the circles mark the vertical meridian and the triangles mark the extreme periphery of the field. These symbols have been superposed on those areas of the brain that respond to the parts of the field the symbols represent. The nine organized visual areas are as follows: the first visual (V1), the second visual (V2), the dorsolateral crescent (DL), the middle temporal (MT), the dorsointermediate (DI), the dorsomedial (DM), the medial (M), the ventral posterior (VP) and the ventral anterior (VA). The three apparently unorganized visual areas are the posterior parietal (PP), the temporoparietal (TP) and the inferotemporal (IT). Plus signs indicate the upper part of the visual field, minus signs the lower part. Dorsolateral view of the brain (*bottom right*) shows the position of the left hemisphere of cortex and visual areas within it. The mapping of the owl monkey was done by John M. Allman of California Institute of Technology and Jon H. Kaas of Vanderbilt University.

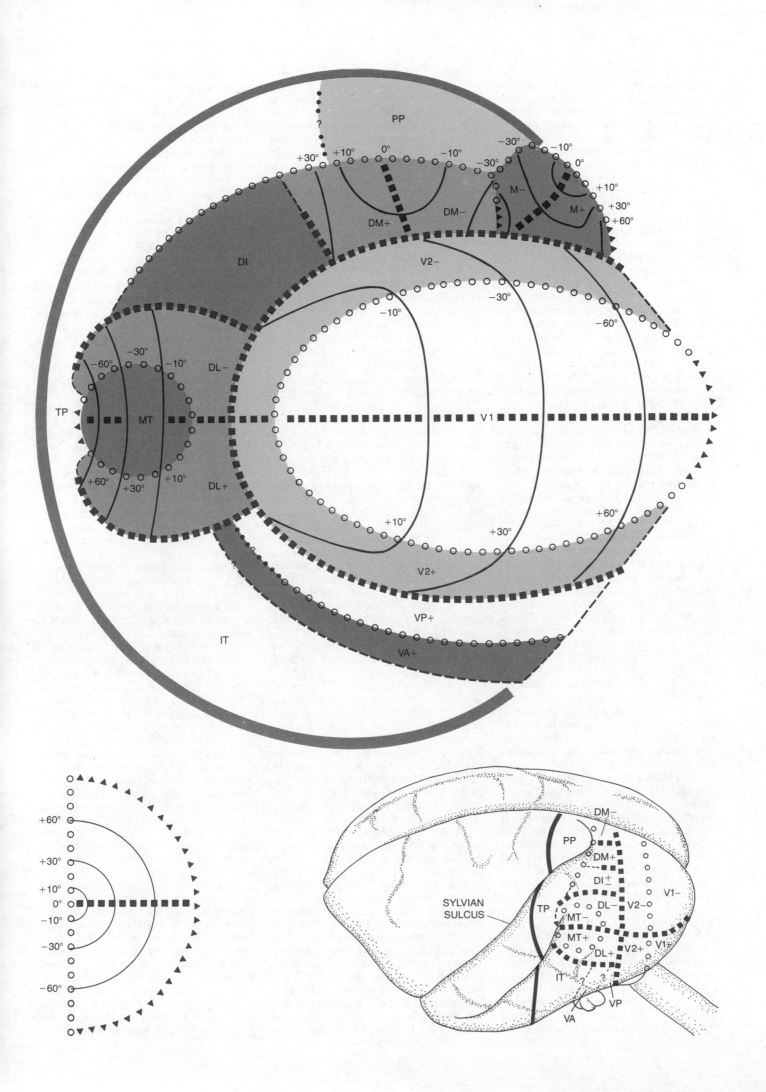

brain, although it is useful in some ways, is apt to be misleading. In a computer information is processed at a rapid pulse rate and serially. In the brain the rate is much lower, but the information can be handled on millions of channels in parallel. The components of a modern computer are very reliable, but removing one or two of them can upset an entire computation. In comparison the neurons of the brain are somewhat unreliable, but the deletion of quite a few of them is unlikely to lead to any appreciable difference in behavior. A computer works on a strict binary code. The brain seems to rely on less precise methods of signaling. Against this it probably adjusts the number and efficiency of its synapses in complex and subtle ways to adapt its operation to experience. Hence it is not surprising to find that although a computer can accurately and rapidly do long and intricate arithmetical calculations, a task at which human beings are rather poor, human beings can recognize patterns in ways no contemporary computer can begin to approach.

It would not be too surprising if the proper theoretical tool for approaching such problems turned out to be communication theory. So far the application of communication theory to visual perception has mainly been in the earlier steps along the visual pathway. For example, two theorems of information processing—the sampling theorem and Logan's zero-crossing theorem—are being invoked to explain how information sent along a limited channel, such as the optic nerve, can in principle be expressed in more detail in the visual cortex of the brain. In addition David Marr of the Massachusetts Institute of Technology has sketched some of the kinds of computation the brain must perform in order for us to see things as we do. This has made us realize the complex nature of the problem but has not so far led to any dramatic clarifications of the mechanisms involved. In particular we do not yet have any description of conscious perception that illuminates our very direct experience of it. There is more than a suspicion that such phenomena result from the computation pathways' acting in some way on themselves, but exactly how this happens is not known. Since this central problem is baffling, we can only turn to more local and detailed problems, hoping that in tackling them we may stumble on the right approach to the more difficult global ones.

What apparatus, in general terms, enables the brain to implement its remarkable performance? The number of components (neurons) in the brain is probably about 10^{11}. The number of synapses, or contacts, between them is perhaps 10^{15}. On the average every neuron receives some thousands of distinct inputs and itself connects to many other neurons. The physical layout of most of the components is not particularly neat. The dendrites, or short fibers, of neighboring neurons are intricately interlaced, even though they usually do not touch one another. Among the dendrites ramify the axons, or long fibers of the neurons, many of them often with thousands of contact points. Clearly a wiring diagram of these fibers, if one could be produced, would be extremely intricate.

How might one make some headway through this impossible jungle? One traditional method is to remove portions of the brain and see how behavior is changed. This can be done with experimental animals, although few of the dissections are as precise as one would wish. In human beings such experiments are inadvertently performed by strokes, tumors and wounds, but here it is even harder to define the damage exactly. Nevertheless, such experiments have yielded much valuable information. Two major conclusions emerge. The first is that different regions of the brain do different jobs. A deficit in performance resulting from damage in one region is often quite unlike one resulting from damage to a different region. The second conclusion is somewhat unexpected. Some experiments show that the brain handles information in ways quite different from those we might have guessed at. Processes we might have assumed to operate in one place, such as the recognition of letters and the recognition of numbers, appear to operate in different places. The converse may also be true: processes we might have guessed to be separate may be influenced by damage to a single area.

This leads us to one of the most important warnings a student of the brain must absorb. We are deceived at every level by our introspection. This applies not only to complex processes but also to apparently straightforward ones. A person who has not reflected on such matters may believe he has a detailed view of all parts of the world simultaneously before his eyes. Although he does know that something he sees "out of the corner of the eye" is not seen very clearly, he may fail to appreciate just how narrow is the high-acuity window through which he builds up much of his picture of the visible world. Since by moving his eyes he can at will summon up the details of any part of the world before him, he has the general impression that it is "there all the time."

Perhaps a more dramatic illustration is the presence of a blind spot in each eye. Not everyone realizes he has a blind spot, although it is easy to demonstrate. What is remarkable is that we do not see a hole in our visual field. The reason is partly that we have no means of detecting the edges of the hole and partly that our brain fills in the hole with visual information borrowed from the immediate neighborhood. Our capacity for deceiving ourselves about the operation of our brain is almost limitless, mainly because what we can report is only a minute fraction of what goes on in our head. This is why much of philosophy has been barren for more than 2,000 years and is likely to remain so until philosophers learn to understand the language of information processing.

This is not to say, however, that the study of our mental processes by introspection should be totally abandoned, as the behaviorists have tried to do. To do so would be to discard one of the most significant attributes of what we are trying to study. The fact remains that the evidence of introspection should never be accepted at face value. It should be explained in terms other than just its own.

The basic problem is that almost any process we can study by observing overall behavior (reading, say) involves the complex interaction of many different regions of the brain, each with its own way of handling information. We know only in the barest outline how these distinct regions should be recognized and classified. Although our knowledge of how they are interconnected is growing rapidly, it is far from complete, both qualitatively and quantitatively. Moreover, we seldom know what operation each region is performing, that is, what relates the outputs to the inputs, and in some instances we do not have even the faintest idea of what is going on.

This is the main reason pure psychology is, by the standards of hard science, rather unsuccessful. It is not that it cannot be quantitative. The branch of it called, rather curiously, psychophysics is certainly quantitative, often quantitative in a sensible and imaginative way. The basic difficulty is that psychology attempts to treat the brain as a black box. The experimenter studies the inputs and outputs and tries from the results to deduce the structure and operation of the inside of the box. Such an approach is not necessarily a bad one. For many years genetics was a black-box subject. It tried, with some success, to deduce the structure and function of the genetic material by studying breeding patterns. Indeed, much good biology is done by the black-box method. This can happen at all levels. To the previous generation of biochemists an enzyme was a black box. Nowadays many enzymologists study the structure of an enzyme to try to correlate the structure with the enzyme's behavior. One man's black box is another man's problem.

The difficulty with the black-box approach is that unless the box is inherently very simple a stage is soon reached where several rival theories all explain the observed results equally well. Attempts to decide among them often prove unsuccessful because as more experiments are done more complexities are revealed. At that point there is no choice but to poke inside the box if the matter is to be settled one way or the other.

What we know of the brain, as is indicated by the other articles in this issue, tells us two things. The brain is clearly so complex that the chances of being able to predict its behavior solely from a study of its parts is too remote to consider. The same complexity also warns us that the black-box approach of pure psychology will have to be lucky if it is not to bog down. Psychology is essential. What the organism actually does we can learn only by observing it. Psychology alone, however, is likely to be sterile. It must combine the study of behavior with parallel studies of the inside of the brain. A good example is the work of Roger W. Sperry and his colleagues at the California Institute of Technology on "split brain" patients: people in whom the connections between the cerebral hemispheres have been severed. Another is the use of deoxyglucose to mark regions of the brain that are more active than the average while an experimental animal is performing some particular task. Thus can the study of neuroanatomy and neurophysiology be combined with behavioral studies. We must study both structure and function but study them within the black box rather than only from the outside.

The novice in such matters is gratified to discover, after having recoiled in horror from the complexities of neuroanatomy, that this subject has recently become one of the most exciting in neurobiology. The reason is that even though, speaking broadly, the wiring diagram of the brain is a mess, recent studies have shown that the wiring is far more orderly than anyone realized only a few years ago. This revolution is coming about largely because of new experimental techniques introduced from biochemistry, in particular the use of amino acids labeled with radioactive atoms and of the enzyme horseradish peroxidase for tracing connections, and the use of radioactively labeled deoxyglucose for marking regions where neurons are particularly active. In addition the use of specific antibodies for staining a particular class of neurons has been fruitful. The powerful new technique of monospecific (monoclonal) antibodies just coming into use will, one hopes, be even more helpful in classifying neurons into meaningful types and revealing their three-dimensional distribution. The problems are so formidable, however, that one can say with a fair degree of confidence that without still more new methods progress may be slow. The tremendous new surge in molecular biology has been powered by the deliberate search for novel methods (for example methods of rapidly determining the sequence of bases in DNA).

Like neuroanatomy, neurophysiology has been developing steadily, particularly in the years since it became possible to record impulses from single neurons rather than from groups of cells. The classical work of Hubel and Wiesel on the visual cortex is a good example. Here again, however, one suspects that a change of pace will be needed. In particular it may be important to record from many neurons independently and simultaneously, exploiting the new opportunities made available by microelectronic technology. This would also make it possible to study more efficiently the responses to more complex patterns, for example the response to two or three parallel lines in the visual field rather than the response to just one.

In both neuroanatomy and neurophysiology the rate at which new information is being obtained is low compared with the total information contained in the system. Hence an important role for theory in neurobiology is not merely trying to create correct and detailed theories of neural processes (which may be an extremely difficult task) but pointing to which features it would be most useful to study and in particular to measure, in order to see what kind of theory is needed. It is no use asking for the impossible, such as, say, the exact wiring diagram for a cubic millimeter of brain tissue and the way all its neurons are firing. The trick is to try to spot what easily obtainable information would be the most useful and, more difficult, what might be obtained within a reasonable time by the introduction of feasible new methods. Sometimes stating a requirement clearly is halfway to seeing how to implement it. For example, a method that would make it possible to inject one neuron with a substance that would then clearly stain all the neurons connected to it, and no others, would be invaluable. So would a method by which all neurons of just one type could be inactivated, leaving the others more or less unaltered.

How far has all of this taken us to date? The articles in this issue give a good general idea of the progress that has been made. What is conspicuously lacking is a broad framework of ideas within which to interpret all these different approaches. Biochemistry and genetics were in such a state until the revolution in molecular biology. It is not that most neurobiologists do not have some general concept of what is going on. The trouble is that the concept is not precisely formulated. Touch it and it crumbles. The nature of perception, the neural correlates of long-term memory, the function of sleep, to give a few examples, all have this character.

How then should a general theory of the brain be constructed? There appear to be three broad constraints. The first is the nature of the physical world. The daily world we live in is not an amorphous mess. It consists of objects, which usually occupy space and which, although they may move with respect to other objects, usually retain their size and shape. Visually an object has surfaces, outlines, color and so on. It may emit a sound or a smell. Without laboring the point one would certainly expect that whatever processing is done on the information coming into the brain will be related to the invariants or semi-invariants in the external world accessible to the senses.

Experiment shows this to be the case, often in unexpected ways. A good example is the kind of color perception brought out in the experiments of Edwin H. Land. One might have imagined that for a large patch of color one would perceive the color of the light actually coming from it and falling on the retina. Actually the color is in most cases produced by a combination of the color of the light incident on an object and the color reflectivity of that part of the object's surface. Remarkable as it may seem, the brain manages to extract the latter information from the visual input. It can compensate to a large extent for the nature of the incident light. What we perceive corresponds more closely to the reflectivity of the surface, which is a property of the object itself.

There is a striking demonstration of this kind of phenomenon in the Exploratorium in San Francisco, although in this case the surfaces are in different shades of gray, ranging from nearly white to fairly black. The illumination, the source of which is concealed, is uneven, being much greater at the bottom of the display than at the top. One area near the bottom looks very black. Another at the top appears almost white. Small tubes allow one to view each patch separately. Looking through the tubes in this way shows that the two patches are exactly the same shade of gray! When my wife, who is an artist, saw the demonstration, she was flabbergasted and declared it was a trick. What she had not realized is that in a certain sense everything she sees is a trick played on her by her brain.

The second constraint is the one imposed by biochemistry, genetics and embryology. The nervous system is made not of metal or inorganic semiconductors but of specialized cells. The impulse moving down an axon travels at modest speeds compared with the velocity of light (even though the neuron may use tricks to speed it up), a limitation imposed by biochemistry. Although inorganic ions such as those of sodium and potassium play a large role in neuronal activity, it is not surprising to find that the molecules that transmit the nerve impulse from one neuron to the next are small organic ones, because a variety of them can be easily manufactured. The surprise is that the same transmitter serves in so many different places, a constraint probably imposed by evolution.

The far end of an axon is a long way from the nearest site of protein synthesis (apart from the mitochondria within the axon) and this fact may impose limitations on the speed with which certain biochemical changes can take place there. There are probably some types of neural circuit the organism can implement with relative ease and other types beyond its powers. For all we know it may be difficult for the genes of a higher organism to impose more than a limited degree of precision on the wiring diagram, particularly if very large numbers of cells are involved. For example, the exact wiring needed for accurate stereoscopic vision may be difficult to achieve without the benefit of some exposure to the real external world, perhaps because the systems associated with the two eyes probably cannot be built with the required precision.

There may be other limitations. It may be difficult for the neuron to arrange matters so that one transmitter is released at one branch of its axonal tree and a second transmitter is released at another branch (as Sir Henry Dale suggested many years ago). This principle may be behind the case described by Eric Kandel in this issue [see "Small Systems of Neurons," by Eric R. Kandel, page 28], where a transmitter produced by one cell excited some cells, inhibited other cells and had a mixed influence on a third kind of cell.

The third constraint is one imposed by mathematics and in particular by communication theory. Some such results may at first seem counterintuitive. Under some circumstances a distribution or pattern can be perfectly reconstructed from a small sample of it taken at regular intervals. Information can be stored in a distributed form, as in a hologram, such that removing part of the store does not remove part of the picture, although it degrades the quality of the entire picture somewhat.

There is a fourth constraint that one might be tempted to introduce if experience had not shown it to be unreliable. This is the constraint imposed by evolution. It is certainly true that all organisms and their components are the result of a long evolutionary process and that this fact should never be forgotten. It is unwise, however, to assert that evolution could not have done this or must have done that, except in the broadest possible terms. It is a good working rule for the biologist that evolution is a lot cleverer than he is. This is not to say that comparative biological studies may not suggest that a certain structure is often associated with a particular function. The taxonomic comparison of the products of evolution may be suggestive, but

such hints should always be confirmed by direct experiment.

Be this as it may, our understanding of the first three constraints is only partial. The process of analyzing the world around us into its significant features is not always straightforward. Many major questions in embryology are unanswered. Information theory is a comparatively new branch of knowledge. Therefore although it is possible to get clues and hints from all three constraints, one seldom finds oneself with so many constraints that a theory practically selects itself. There are so many possible ways in which our brains might process information that without considerable help from direct experimental facts (which are usually rather sparse) we are unlikely to hit on a correct theoretical description.

Is there any idea we should avoid? I think there is at least one: the fallacy of the homunculus. Recently I was trying to explain to an intelligent woman the problem of understanding how it is we perceive anything at all, and I was not having any success. She could not see why there was a problem. Finally in despair I asked her how she herself thought she saw the world. She replied that she probably had somewhere in her head something like a little television set. "So who," I asked, "is looking at it?" She now saw the problem immediately.

Most neuroscientists believe there is no homunculus in the brain. Unfortunately it is easier to state the fallacy than to avoid slipping into it. The reason is that we certainly have an illusion of the homunculus: the self. There is probably some good reason for the strength and persistence of this illusion. It may reflect some aspect of the overall control of the brain, but what the nature of this control is we have not yet discovered.

There is one other general fallacy one would do well to avoid. It might be called the fallacy of the overwise neuron. Consider a neuron that sends its signal for some distance down its axon. What does the signal convey to a recipient synapse? The signal is of course encoded in the frequency of nerve impulses, but what does the message mean? It is easy to slip into the habit of thinking the message conveys more than it actually does.

Take, for example, a neuron in the visual system that is said to be color-sensitive. Suppose it fires best when it is exposed to a yellow patch of light. We are inclined to believe it is telling us that the color of the light at that point is yellow. This, however, is not really true, because most color receptors have a broad response curve and will fire, at least to some extent, over a rather wide range of wavelengths. Therefore a particular rate of firing might have been caused either by a weak yellow light or by a strong red one. In addition the firing

of that particular neuron may have been influenced by the amount of movement of the spot of light and by its exact shape and size. In short, many different, although related, inputs will yield the same rate of firing.

Since the relevant sensory input to the neuron has many features and its output (roughly speaking) has only one feature, the information relayed by a single neuron is bound to be ambiguous. Notice, however, that we can extract more information by comparing the firing of one neuron with that of one or more other neurons. With one type of color receptor (rods, say) we cannot perceive color at all. We see only shades of gray. To perceive the light as being colored we need at least two types of receptor, each of which has a wavelength response curve differing from that of the other. Experiment shows this to be true: we can perceive color with rods and one type of cone.

Notice that the argument is not peculiar to color. A single "edge detector" does not really tell us that an edge is there. What it is detecting is, loosely speaking, "edginess" in the visual input, that is, a particular type of nonuniformity in the retinal image that might be produced by many different objects. One of the objectives of theoretical neurobiology is to try to turn such vague concepts as "edginess" into mathematically precise descriptions.

This general argument applies at all levels of the nervous system. It shows clearly why we need to process the neural input in so many different ways in order to extract useful information from it.

Can we nonetheless paint some broad picture of how the information is processed? Perhaps the easiest way to do so is to consider the visual system and in particular the visual cortex of the cerebrum. At first glance a map of visual responses in the striate cortex (area 17) appears to be a rather straightforward map of half of the visual field. It is true the map is systematically distorted so that a large proportion of it is devoted to the high-acuity central region of the retina (the fovea) and less to the periphery. The map is nonetheless fairly well ordered and moderately precise.

Closer inspection shows that things are not that simple. The input from the left eye is interlaced in stripes with that from the right eye. Moreover, there are three distinct types of input (from the lateral geniculate nucleus) for each eye, one input mainly for the Y cells of the retina (which respond rather transiently) and the other two inputs for the X cells. In addition there are major inputs from areas such as the pulvinar and from other areas of the visual cortex. The outputs are also multiple. There is not one output from this area but an entire series, partly outputs to neurons that form maps in other visual areas of the cortex and partly outputs to subcortical areas, including a relatively large output back to the lateral geniculate nucleus, where much of the input came from in the first place. Hence this bit of cortex is a region of multiple inputs and multiple outputs. In addition each single input or output involves large numbers of individual axons (in the millions) over the entire area.

What processing does the striate cortex (the first visual area) carry out? As the article by Hubel and Wiesel shows, the main function of the striate cortex is to respond to the orientation of forms in the visual field. In each "column" of the striate cortex the neurons respond to one orientation only, although the response can be any one of a variety of types. The input, thus transformed, is then sent out to other places.

How much does the processing spread sideways in the cortex? The remarkable thing is that the processing is fairly local. Beyond a range of a couple of millimeters there are relatively few interconnections, except for axonal connections of a diffuse nature from the brain stem. Within any one small region there are many neurons connected together (there are some 100,000 neurons per square millimeter of cortical surface), but they hardly connect at all, in a direct way, to those dealing with more distant parts of the visual field. (In the macaque monkey the total surface area of the striate cortex on one side is about 1,400 square millimeters.)

Notice that there is as yet no firm evidence that there are discrete modules within the area. The relation is rather like one between people living in an imaginary city all of whom are forbidden to travel more than half a mile from their home. They can interact with their neighbors within a mile, particularly their close neighbors, but have no direct contact with anyone farther away.

The remarkable thing is that this description, in its most general terms, seems to apply to much if not all of the cerebral cortex. There are known to be a good number of distinct visual areas, each with some kind of "map" of the visual field. The owl monkey has at least eight cortical areas that are primarily visual, and there are probably more. When we look at the auditory areas or the somatic sensory areas we find the same story. The auditory cortex in the monkey has at least four distinct areas "mapped" for frequency and probably for amplitude. The body surface of the monkey is mapped several times in the somatic sensory regions. In all cases the inputs, most of which lead into the middle layers of the cortex, consist of alternating stripes of one type or another. These inputs get mixed together in the processing that takes place in the upper and lower layers. The outputs of the

processing arc sent in a systematic way to several other places in both the cortex and the subcortical areas. It is a reasonable hypothesis that when two areas are connected in this manner, the output of one area is mapped in a regular but not necessarily uniform way into the surface of the other one. Moreover, there is often a reverse connection. In the monkey area 17 sends a mapped projection to area 18, but area 18 also sends some of its output back to area 17. The return connections are probably not diffuse but constitute a reverse mapping. Exactly how closely a mapping and its reverse correspond is not known. One might guess that the correspondence would be fairly precise.

There is an interesting exception to the rule that obvious clusters of neurons are not found within a cortical sheet. It is the barrel spindles, studied by Thomas A. Woolsey and his colleagues at the Washington University School of Medicine and mentioned in the article in this issue by Maxwell Cowan [see "The Development of the Brain," by W. Maxwell Cowan, page 56]. Each barrel spindle is some 200 millimicrons across, and although adjacent barrels are connected, the connections within a barrel are much richer. This illustrates how the cortex can handle smallish inputs that are spatially discrete rather than continuous.

Can it be that there is a fixed, countable number of discrete areas in the cortex? It certainly seems to be true for the sensory areas and probably for the motor ones. The illustration on page 131 shows a recent map of the visual cortex of the owl monkey, made by John M. Allman and his colleagues at the California Institute of Technology. It shows the eight discrete areas that have been mapped in that region. Note that the mapping shows that although each area has a fairly well-defined boundary, so that the definition of an area is in these cases fairly unambiguous, there are no obvious insulating boundaries in the cortex at these points. The cortex in each hemisphere is a continuous sheet with a single edge. There are no slits in it. It is therefore not surprising to find that at the boundaries there is, loosely speaking, a local mirror plane in the mapping. In other words, the two maps, one on each side of the boundary, are related. They are similar on each side as one moves along the boundary. As one proceeds away from the boundary at right angles to it, the direction of movement in the visual field is the same in one map as it is for a movement away from the boundary in the other map. Careful inspection of the illustration will show that this rule is violated in only one place. The local-mirror-plane rule is also obeyed in the mapping of both the auditory and the somatic sensory system, again with a few exceptions. This is exactly what one might expect if there

were a series of discrete maps that nonetheless interacted to some extent at their edges. It suggests, incidentally, that when new functional areas of the brain arise in evolution, they arise in pairs.

Is this mapping into discrete areas true for the rest of the cortex, particularly the frontal regions and what are called the association regions? At the moment nobody knows, not even for a monkey, let alone for a man. What is already clear is that for a monkey most of the cerebral cortex can be mapped in this way. Although it is easy to think of ways in which the area concept could break down (an area is a useful concept only if several distinct definitions of it lead unambiguously to the same parcellation into areas), I rather suspect it may hold almost everywhere in the cortex. If it does hold, how many areas are there in the human cortex? More than 50? Perhaps less than 100? If each area could be clearly stained postmortem, so that we could see exactly how many there are, how big each one is and exactly how it is connected to other areas, we would have made a big step forward.

So far I have spoken only of the cerebral cortex, but the cortex of the cerebellum appears to be similar. Again the input is orderly and forms more than one map. Both major inputs seem to be in stripes. There is something in embryology that likes stripes. This has been dramatically shown by Martha Constantine-Paton of Princeton University, who by embryological manipulation has constructed frogs with a third eye. Normally only one eye projects to one optic tectum, but in this case two eyes may do so. When that happens, the inputs sort themselves into stripes, a situation that does not arise in a normal frog.

In addition, if we look at subcortical regions such as the thalamus, again we find some evidence for regular mappings. Each cortical area tends to map its own special region of the thalamus, often with some kind of patchy distribution. There appear to be regular mappings in other parts of the central nervous system, such as the basal ganglia, the brain stem, the spinal cord and so on. In each case we need to know exactly how to parcel out the vast array of neurons into the smallest meaningful units, even if these units interact to some extent with their neighbors. In many cases the units are sheets or parts of sheets. In other cases they appear to have a more compact shape. Their inputs and outputs are not always as tidily arranged as they are in the cortex, and so the job will not always be a simple one.

Armed with a very rough picture of the higher parts of the brain, we can address ourselves to the general questions of the nature of the connections. To do this we need two rather simple concepts: precision wiring and associative nets. Where it sometimes seems that in the brain everything is connected to every-thing else, in precision wiring the con-nections are made in a definite, orderly manner. Only certain cells are connect-ed to certain other cells, and the pattern of connections is often the same from one individual animal to another. Preci-sion wiring is often found when rather small numbers of cells are involved, as in simple invertebrates such as *Aplysia,* discussed in this issue by Kandel. The small nematode worm *Caenorhabditis elegans* studied by Sydney Brenner and his colleagues at the Medical Research Council Laboratory of Molecular Biol-ogy at Cambridge in England is a good example. The species has exactly 279 neurons wired, to a good approxima-tion, in exactly the same way in every in-dividual. Larger numbers of neurons can also be precisely wired, particular-ly if the cellular pattern is repetitive, as it is in the fly's eye. Precision wiring does not imply that learning cannot take place, as Kandel's article shows clearly, because the strength of the connections can be changed by experience.

On the other hand, when we look at the wiring diagram (as far as it is known) of a brain area in a more com-plex animal, say an area in the visual cortex of a monkey, we see two things. There are many more cells and their wiring appears to be far less precise. One side of a monkey's head is certainly not wired exactly the same way as the other side. Nevertheless, the connections from the eye to the visual cortex are by no means completely random. As Hubel and Wiesel write in their article, the con-nections form a topographical map, al-though it is not an exact one. The neu-rons are of a number of distinct types that are not connected haphazardly, al-though the precise degree of order in the connections is hard to define. Within one small region one gets the impression that the exact connections are partly a matter of chance. Moreover, one simple signal to the eye—say a short line at one point in the visual field—will cause not just one edge detector to fire but possi-bly several thousand such detectors. In short, the wiring not only is designed to extract particular features from the in-put but also appears to have some of the properties of an associative net.

An associative net is an abstract wir-ing diagram that has been studied by theoreticians such as Marr, Christopher Longuet-Higgins, Leon Cooper and oth-ers. Such a net has a set of input chan-nels (sometimes more than one set) and a set of output channels. Every input channel is connected to every output channel, but the strengths of the connec-tions vary. The exact arrangement de-pends on the type of net being consid-ered. The strength of the connections is adjusted "by experience" on the basis of certain well-defined rules, usually so that pathways that are often activated

together are strengthened in some way. Such nets can serve to fine-tune a sys-tem that has been partly precision-wired or to assist in the recall of a complex output when an input (or better still a partial input) of something often associ-ated with it arrives. Seeing a person's face, you remember that person's name (although, alas, not in all cases). You may still be able to do it even though you have seen only part of the per-son's face.

The higher nervous system appears to be an exceedingly cunning combination of precision wiring and associative nets. It is not wired so that every input chan-nel is directly connected to all other in-put channels. Nor, in higher animals, does it seem to be wired in a precise way. The system relies on two stratagems to achieve its ends. There is the stratagem of multiple and successive mapping (in-cluding reciprocal mapping), that being the component approximating the pre-cision wiring. The system also, how-ever, appears to organize the wiring so that locally—within one small region—it does, roughly speaking, connect ev-erything with everything. In each region there is an entire family of local, over-lapping associative nets. Hence in the early stage of signal processing some signals (one set from the eye, say, and one from the ear) do not relate to one another. But as the signals proceed from one map to another the original map-ping becomes both more diffuse and more abstract (the response is better to orientations than to spots, for example), so that the signal is analyzed in succes-sively more complex ways in associa-tion with signals from other inputs.

When the system is described this way, we can see immediately that it is not just one immense associative net. A net in which each neuron reacted direct-ly with every other neuron would be far too difficult to wire up and would take up far too much space. Therefore the net is broken down into many small sub-nets, some in parallel, others arranged more serially. Moreover, the parcella-tion into subnets reflects both the struc-ture of the world, external and internal, and our relation to it. Each local net is made to perform those particular opera-tions on its input that are most needed at that point to extract meaningful new in-formation. Seen this way many broad features of the brain—the numerous functional areas, the many connections to each neuron—begin to make some kind of sense.

There is of course much more to the performance of the brain than the processes I have sketched so far. There must be mechanisms for attention, par-ticularly localized attention, so that the activity of small parts of the brain can be increased. There must be some kind of overall control system. In case my oversimplified account should mislead

the reader I advise him to refer to the article in this issue by Walle Nauta and Michael Feirtag, which shows clearly how complex the entire arrangement really is [see "The Organization of the Brain," by Walle J. H. Nauta and Mi-chael Feirtag, page 40]. Nevertheless, the scheme I have outlined should show at least some of the things we may ex-pect to find as we explore neural proc-essing in more detail.

What system or what level is most likely to yield most easily to experimen-tal attack? This is always a difficult ques-tion to answer. As Kandel points out, invertebrates with large cells connected in a rather precise way have many ad-vantages, and it is virtually certain that some of the results, insights and tech-niques that come from studying them will be useful in understanding the ner-vous systems of higher and more com-plex organisms. It is doubtful, however, that all the answers can be obtained from lower animals. What animal is the best model for man and what part of the brain is easiest to study are also difficult questions to answer. The visual system of the macaque monkey appears to be very similar to ours. The visual system of the cat is less so, but cats have other experimental advantages. The argument over whether the cerebellum or the visu-al cortex is the better system for study has been rumbling for years. (The input to the visual system is easier to control, but its neural structure is nothing like as regular as that of the cerebellum.)

How should one decide, for example, whether it is more opportune to study one or more cortical areas in detail in order to explain accurately the observed processing going on in them in terms of both their neuroanatomy and neu-rophysiology, or alternatively to treat each area as a small black box and con-centrate on the relations between corti-cal areas? It could well be maintained that regions that control more diffuse "enabling" systems, such as the system projecting from the locus coeruleus, may yield more easily than systems concerned with the detailed processing of information. Whatever choices are made about what to tackle first, it seems that we have a long way to go to reach even an outline understanding of brain function that is solidly based on both experiment and theory.

What prospects, then, are there for early progress in our understanding of the brain? As knowledge accumulates can we expect some kind of break-through? That is always possible, but the prospects are not very encouraging. It is sometimes forgotten that neurobiology has already had several breakthroughs. The discovery that the nerve impulse was propagated down the axon as a "spike" of roughly uniform amplitude and velocity was one such break-through. The realization that most syn-apses involve chemical transmission, and particularly that synapses can be inhibitory as well as excitatory, was another. Both of these discoveries bear on phenomena that originated at an early stage in animal evolution. It is sobering to note that the major breakthroughs in molecular biology also have to do with mechanisms that originated very long ago. There are often simple processes underlying the complexities of nature, but evolution has usually overlaid them with baroque modifications and additions. To see through to the underlying simplicity, which in most instances evolved rather early, is often extremely difficult.

There is an additional problem. An analysis of which parts of molecular biology have proceeded most rapidly shows that they are those parts of the subject that deal with one-dimensional arrangements (such as determining the sequence of bases in a nucleic acid or of amino acids in a protein) or that depend on being able to separate a small part of a system (such as an enzyme) and study it in comparative isolation from the rest of the system. Problems that involve a large number of almost simultaneous parallel interactions, such as the problem of predicting how a chain of amino acids will fold up, have made little progress. Such an analysis does not augur well for problems of understanding the higher nervous system, which are mainly of the latter type.

There was, however, one breakthrough in genetics, the one that began with Mendel, that resulted from the black-box approach (the breeding pattern of a plant) and yielded information at a high level of organization (the chromosome). Therefore if a breakthrough in the study of the brain does come, it is perhaps likely to be at the level of the overall control of the system. If the system were as chaotic as it sometimes appears to be, it would not enable us to perform even the simplest tasks satisfactorily. To invent a possible, although unlikely, example, the discovery that brain processing was run phasically, by some kind of periodic clock, as a computer is, would probably constitute a major breakthrough.

What this *Scientific American* book shows is that the brain is being studied successfully from many different angles and that much interesting and exciting new work has resulted. It is only when we reflect on how intricate the entire system is and how complicated the many different operations it has to perform are (only some of them have been touched on in this article) that we realize we have a long way to go. But new methods bring new results and new results foster new ideas, and so we should not be too easily discouraged. There is no scientific study more vital to man than the study of his own brain. Our entire view of the universe depends on it.

The Authors
Bibliographies
Index

The Authors

DAVID H. HUBEL ("The Brain") is George Packer Berry Professor of Neurobiology at the Harvard Medical School. Born in Windsor, Ont., he received his B.Sc. and M.D. degrees at McGill University. He then studied clinical neurology for three years at the Montreal Neurological Institute, coming to the U.S. in 1954 for a year's residency in neurology at the Johns Hopkins Hospital. The following year he began neurophysiological research at the Walter Reed Army Institute of Research in Washington, and in 1958 he joined the physiology faculty of the Johns Hopkins School of Medicine. He moved to the Harvard Medical School in 1960.

CHARLES F. STEVENS ("The Neuron") is professor of physiology at the Yale University School of Medicine. He did his undergraduate work in experimental psychology at Harvard University and obtained his M.D. at the Yale School of Medicine and his Ph.D. in biophysics from Rockefeller University in 1964. From 1963 through 1975 he was on the physiology and biophysics faculty of the University of Washington School of Medicine, taking a sabbatical leave during the 1969–70 academic year at the Lorentz Institute for Theoretical Physics at the University of Leiden.

ERIC R. KANDEL ("Small Systems of Neurons") is professor of physiology and psychiatry and director of the Division of Neurobiology and Behavior at the Columbia University College of Physicians and Surgeons. He was born in Vienna and came to the U.S. in 1939. He was graduated from Harvard College in 1952 and received his M.D. at the New York University School of Medicine in 1956. After a year of internship at Montefiore Hospital in New York he spent three years as a postdoctoral fellow at the National Institute of Mental Health, working on a cellular study of the hippocampus, a part of the mammalian brain thought to play a role in memory. He was a resident in psychiatry at

the Massachusetts Mental Health Center and the Harvard Medical School from 1960 to 1962 and again from 1963 to 1964. In the intervening year he was a National Institutes of Health special fellow at the Institute Marey in Paris. There, seeking to work on a simple organism in which it might be possible to study the neural mechanisms of behavior and learning more directly than is possible with complex organisms, he began to do research with Ladislav Tauc on the nervous system of the marine snail *Aplysia*. Kandel has continued to work with *Aplysia* since then. In 1965 he returned to the New York University School of Medicine to develop a neurobiology group, and in 1974 he moved to Columbia.

WALLE J. H. NAUTA and MICHAEL FEIRTAG ("The Organization of the Brain") have collaborated for more than four years on a textbook of neuroanatomy. Nauta is Institute Professor in the department of psychology at the Massachusetts Institute of Technology and staff neuroanatomist at McLean Hospital in Belmont, Mass. Born in Indonesia, he was educated at the University of Leiden and the University of Utrecht, where he obtained his M.D. in 1942 and his Ph.D. in anatomy and neurophysiology in 1945. After teaching at the universities of Utrecht, Leiden and Zurich he worked from 1951 to 1964 as a neurophysiologist at the Walter Reed Army Institute of Research in Washington and taught for part of that time in the department of anatomy at the University of Maryland. In 1964 he joined the M.I.T. faculty. Nauta has received the Research Career Award of the National Institute of Mental Health and the Karl Spencer Lashley Award for research in neurobiology of the American Philosophical Society. Feirtag is an editor of *Technology Review*, a magazine published by M.I.T.

W. MAXWELL COWAN ("The Development of the Brain") is Edison Professor of Neurobiology and head of the

department of anatomy at the Washington University School of Medicine. A native of South Africa, he received his undergraduate education at the University of the Witwatersrand. In 1953 he went to the University of Oxford to obtain his Ph.D. and complete his medical training, and from 1958 until 1966 he was a fellow of Pembroke College. In 1966 he emigrated to the U.S. and taught at the University of Wisconsin; after two years he moved to Washington University. Much of Cowan's scientific work has been on the organization of the limbic system and the development of the visual system.

LESLIE L. IVERSEN ("The Chemistry of the Brain") is director of the Medical Research Council Pharmacology Unit at Cambridge in England. He did his undergraduate work at Trinity College of the University of Cambridge and went on to receive his Ph.D. in biochemistry and pharmacology in 1964. The following year he came to the U.S. on a postdoctoral fellowship in the laboratories of Julius Axelrod at the National Institute of Mental Health and of Steven Kuffler at the Harvard Medical School. He then returned to England to become a research fellow in the department of pharmacology at Cambridge. In 1967 he was elected a Locke Research Fellow of the Royal Society, and in 1971 he became director of the Neurochemical Pharmacology Unit. Iversen is chief editor of the *Journal of Neurochemistry* and president of the European Neuroscience Association.

DAVID H. HUBEL (see first column) and TORSTEN N. WIESEL ("Brain Mechanisms of Vision") have collaborated on studies of the mammalian visual system for nearly 20 years. Wiesel is Robert Winthrop Professor and chairman of the department of neurobiology at the Harvard Medical School. Born in Sweden, he obtained his M.D. in 1954 at the Karolinska Institute in Stockholm. After a year as an instructor of physiology there he came to the U.S. to join the faculty of the Johns Hopkins University School of Medicine. He moved to the Harvard Medical School in 1959.

EDWARD V. EVARTS ("Brain Mechanisms of Movement") is chief of the Laboratory of Neurophysiology of the National Institute of Mental Health. He obtained his M.D. at the Harvard Medical School in 1948 and received clinical training in psychiatry and neurology at Peter Bent Brigham Hospital in Boston, the National Hospital in London and the Payne Whitney Clinic in New York. During a year of research with Karl Spencer Lashley at the Yerkes Laboratories of Primate Biology in Florida he became interested in brain science. In 1953 Evarts began his research at the National Institutes of Health, where he combined the behavioral techniques he had learned at Yerkes with techniques for recording the activity of single neurons in the brain of freely moving monkeys. Since then he has expanded the technique of studying brain activity during volitional movement to explore higher brain functions such as attention, memory and motivation.

NORMAN GESCHWIND ("Specializations of the Human Brain") is James Jackson Putnam Professor of Neurology at the Harvard Medical School and director of the Neurological Unit at Beth Israel Hospital in Boston. He is also professor in the department of psychology and in the School of Health Sciences and Technology at the Massachusetts Institute of Technology. He obtained his bachelor's degree from Harvard College and his M.D. at the Harvard Medical School and then received postgraduate training in Boston and London. Geschwind's research has focused on the relation between the anatomy of the brain and behavior, including the cerebral organization of language, aphasias, emotional changes resulting from brain lesions, the evolution of language and the functional asymmetry of the brain.

SEYMOUR S. KETY ("Disorders of the Human Brain") is professor of psychiatry at the Harvard Medical School and director of the Laboratories for Psychiatric Research at the Mailman Research Center and McLean Hospital in Belmont, Mass. He was educated at the University of Pennsylvania, where he obtained his bachelor's degree in 1936 and his M.D. in 1940. After a National Research Council fellowship at the Massachusetts General Hospital he returned to the University of Pennsylvania School of Medicine, where he spent eight years in the department of pharmacology and physiology. In 1942 he developed the citrate treatment for lead poisoning (a forerunner of current therapies) and in 1945 he developed a technique for measuring cerebral blood flow in man, which he subsequently applied to studies of the circulation and metabolism of the brain in health and disease. In 1951 he became the first scientific director of the National Institute of Mental Health and of the National Institute of Neurological Diseases and Stroke, and in 1956 he became chief of the Laboratory of Clinical Science at the National Institute of Mental Health. He joined the Harvard Medical School faculty in 1967. Much of Kety's research has dealt with the role of biological mechanisms in mental illness and the importance of genetic factors in the etiology of schizophrenia.

F. H. C. CRICK ("Thinking about the Brain") is Kieckhefer Distinguished Research Professor at the Salk Institute for Biological Studies in La Jolla, Calif. He did his undergraduate work in physics at University College London, but his doctoral work was interrupted in 1939 by the outbreak of World War II. Throughout the war he worked in the British Admiralty on the development of magnetic and acoustic mines. In 1947 he left the admiralty to study biology at the University of Cambridge, joining the Medical Research Council Unit that was then housed in the Cavendish Laboratory. He met James D. Watson in 1951, and their scientific collaboration led two years later to the proposal of the double-helix structure for the DNA molecule and a scheme for its replication. Crick received his Ph.D. in 1954 for his research on the X-ray diffraction of polypeptides and proteins. Over the next several years he collaborated with Sydney Brenner on genetic and biochemical studies that gave new insights into the mechanisms of protein synthesis and the genetic code. In 1962 he, Watson and M. H. F. Wilkins shared the Nobel prize in physiology and medicine.

Bibliographies

Readers interested in further explanation of the subjects covered by the articles in this issue may find the following lists of publications helpful.

THE BRAIN

HISTOLOGIE DU SYSTÈME NERVEUX DE L'HOMME ET DES VERTÉBRÉS. Santiago Ramón y Cajal. Consejo Superior de Investigaciones Científicas, Instituto Ramón y Cajal, 1952.

NERVE, MUSCLE, AND SYNAPSE. Bernhard Katz. McGraw-Hill Book Company, 1966.

THE HUMAN BRAIN AND SPINAL CORD. Edwin Sisterson Clarke and C. B. O'Malley. University of California Press, 1968.

THE NEURON

FROM NEURON TO BRAIN: A CELLULAR APPROACH TO THE FUNCTION OF THE NERVOUS SYSTEM. Stephen W. Kuffler and John G. Nicholls. Sinauer Associates, Inc., Publishers, 1976.

NEUROMUSCULAR TRANSMISSION. J. H. Steinbach and C. F. Stevens in *Frog Neurobiology: A Handbook,* edited by R. Llinás and W. Precht. Springer-Verlag, 1976.

GATING IN SODIUM CHANNELS OF NERVE. Bertil Hille in *Annual Review of Physiology,* Vol. 38, pages 139–152; 1978.

INTERACTIONS BETWEEN INTRINSIC MEMBRANE PROTEIN AND ELECTRIC FIELD: AN APPROACH TO STUDYING NERVE EXCITABILITY. Charles F. Stevens in *Biophysical Journal,* Vol. 22, No. 2, pages 295–306; May, 1978.

CONTROL OF ACETYLCHOLINE RECEPTORS IN SKELETAL MUSCLE. Douglas M. Fambrough in *Physiological Reviews,* Vol. 59, No. 1, pages 165–227; January, 1979.

SMALL SYSTEMS OF NEURONS

GENETIC DISSECTION OF BEHAVIOR. Seymour Benzer in *Scientific American,* Vol. 229, No. 6, pages 24–37; December, 1973.

THE NERVOUS SYSTEM OF THE LEECH. John G. Nicholls and David Van Essen in *Scientific American,* Vol. 230, No. 1, pages 38–48; January, 1974.

THE NEUROBIOLOGY OF CRICKET SONG. David Bentley and Ronald R. Hoy in *Scientific American,* Vol. 231, No. 2, pages 34–44; August, 1974.

CELLULAR BASIS OF BEHAVIOR: AN INTRODUCTION TO BEHAVIORAL NEUROBIOLOGY. Eric R. Kandel. W. H. Freeman and Company, 1976.

CELLULAR INSIGHTS INTO BEHAVIOR AND LEARNING. Eric R. Kandel in *The Harvey Lectures,* Series 73, pages 29–92; 1979.

THE ORGANIZATION OF THE BRAIN

NEUROLOGICAL FOUNDATIONS OF ANIMAL BEHAVIOR. C. Judson Herrick. Henry Holt and Company, 1924.

A GENERAL PROFILE OF THE VERTEBRATE BRAIN WITH SIDELIGHTS ON THE ANCESTRY OF CEREBRAL CORTEX. Walle J. H. Nauta and Harvey J. Karten in *The Neurosciences: Second Study Program.* Edited by Francis O. Schmitt. Rockefeller University Press, 1970.

NEUROLOGY. In *Gray's Anatomy,* 35th British edition, edited by Roger Warwick and Peter L. Williams. W. B. Saunders Company, 1973.

THE DEVELOPMENT OF THE BRAIN

DEVELOPMENTAL PROGRAMMING FOR RETINOTECTAL PATTERNS. R. Kevin Hunt in *Cell Patterning: Ciba Foundation Symposium 29.* Associated Scientific Publishers, 1975.

CELL MIGRATION AND NEURONAL ECTOPIAS IN THE BRAIN. P. Rakic in *Birth Defects: Original Articles Series,* Vol. 11, pages 95–129; 1975.

PLASTICITY OF OCULAR DOMINANCE COLUMNS IN MONKEY STRIATE CORTEX. D. H. Hubel, T. N. Wiesel and S. LeVay in *Philosophical Transactions of the Royal Society of London, Series B,* Vol. 278, No. 961, pages 377–409; April 26, 1977.

ASPECTS OF NEURAL DEVELOPMENT. W. Maxwell Cowan in *International Review of Physiology, Vol. 17: Neurophysiology III,* edited by R. Porter. University Park Press, 1978.

DEVELOPMENTAL NEUROBIOLOGY. Marcus Jacobson. Plenum Press, 1978.

THE CHEMISTRY OF THE BRAIN

CHEMISTRY OF SYNAPTIC TRANSMISSION: ESSAYS AND SOURCES. Edited by Zach W. Hall, John G. Hildebrand and Edward A. Kravitz. Chiron Press, 1974.

HANDBOOK OF PSYCHOPHARMACOLOGY. Edited by Leslie L. Iversen, Susan D. Iversen and Solomon H. Snyder. Plenum Press, 1975–78.

THE BIOCHEMICAL BASIS OF NEUROPHARMACOLOGY. Jack R. Cooper, Floyd E. Bloom and Robert H. Roth. Oxford University Press, 1978.

CENTRALLY ACTING PEPTIDES. Edited by J. Hughes. University Park Press, 1978.

BEHAVIORAL PHARMACOLOGY. Susan D. Iversen and Leslie L. Iversen. Oxford University Press, second edition in press.

BRAIN MECHANISMS OF VISION

MODALITY AND TOPOGRAPHIC PROPERTIES OF SINGLE NEURONS OF CAT'S SOMATIC SENSORY CORTEX. V. B. Mountcastle in *The Journal of Neurophysiology,* Vol. 20, No. 4, pages 408–434; July, 1957.

RECEPTIVE FIELDS AND FUNCTIONAL ARCHITECTURE OF MONKEY STRIATE CORTEX. D. H. Hubel and T. N. Wiesel in *The Journal of Physiology,* Vol. 195, No. 2, pages 215–244; November, 1968.

FERRIER LECTURE: FUNCTIONAL ARCHITECTURE OF MACAQUE MONKEY VISUAL CORTEX. D. H. Hubel and T. N. Wiesel in *Proceedings of the Royal Society of London, Series B,* Vol. 198, pages 1–59; 1977.

ANATOMICAL DEMONSTRATION OF ORIENTATION COLUMNS IN MACAQUE MONKEY. David H. Hubel, Torsten N.

Wiesel and Michael P. Stryker in *The Journal of Comparative Neurology,* Vol. 177, No. 3, pages 361–379; February 1, 1978.

BRAIN MECHANISMS OF MOVEMENT

MOTOR CONTROL: ISSUES AND TRENDS. Edited by George E. Stelmach. Academic Press, 1976.

CORTICOSPINAL NEURONES: THEIR ROLE IN MOVEMENT. C. G. Phillips and R. Porter. Academic Press, 1977.

THE ORGANIZATION OF VOLUNTARY MOVEMENT: NEUROPHYSIOLOGICAL MECHANISMS. Ya. M. Kots. Plenum Press, 1977.

THE PURPOSIVE BRAIN. Ragnar Granit. The MIT Press, 1977.

CONCEPTS OF MOTOR ORGANIZATION. F. A. Miles and E. V. Evarts in *Annual Review of Psychology,* Vol. 30, pages 327–362; 1979.

SPECIALIZATIONS OF THE HUMAN BRAIN

EMOTIONAL BEHAVIOR AND HEMISPHERIC SIDE OF THE LESION. G. Gainotti in *Cortex,* Vol. 8, No. 1, pages 41–55; March, 1972.

SELECTED PAPERS ON LANGUAGE AND THE BRAIN. Norman Geschwind. D. Reidel Publishing Co., 1974.

THE INTEGRATED MIND. Michael S. Gazzaniga and Joseph E. Ledoux. Plenum Press, 1978.

RIGHT-LEFT ASYMMETRIES IN THE BRAIN. Albert M. Galaburda, Marjorie LeMay, Thomas L. Kemper and Norman Geschwind in *Science,* Vol. 199, No. 4311, pages 852–856; February 24, 1978.

DISORDERS OF THE HUMAN BRAIN

THE BIOLOGY OF MENTAL DEFECT. L. S. Penrose, with a preface by J. B. S. Haldane. Grune & Stratton, 1962.

MADNESS AND THE BRAIN. Solomon H. Snyder. McGraw-Hill Book Company, 1974.

BRAIN WORK: THE COUPLING OF FUNCTION, METABOLISM AND BLOOD FLOW IN THE BRAIN. Edited by David H. Ingvar and Niels A. Lassen. Munksgaard, 1975.

THE BIOLOGICAL ROOTS OF MENTAL ILLNESS: THEIR RAMIFICATIONS THROUGH CEREBRAL METABOLISM, SYNAPTIC ACTIVITY, GENETICS, AND THE ENVIRONMENT. Seymour S. Kety in *The Harvey Lectures,* Series 71, pages 1–22; 1978.

GENETIC TRANSMISSION OF SCHIZOPHRENIA. Dennis K. Kinney and Steven Matthysse in *Annual Review of Medicine,* Vol. 29, pages 459–473; 1978.

THINKING ABOUT THE BRAIN

A REPRESENTATION OF THE VISUAL FIELD IN THE INFERIOR NUCLEUS OF THE PULVINAR IN THE OWL MONKEY (*AOTUS TRIVIRGATUS*). J. M. Allman, J. H. Kaas, R. H. Lane and F. M. Miezen in *Brain Research,* Vol. 40, No. 2, pages 291–302; May 26, 1972.

THE GENETICS OF *CAENORHABDITIS ELEGANS.* S. Brenner in *Genetics,* Vol. 77, No. 1, pages 71–94; January, 1974.

CENTRAL PROJECTION OF OPTIC TRACT FROM TRANSLOCATED EYES IN THE LEOPARD FROG (*RANA PIPIENS*). Martha Constantine-Paton and Robert R. Capranica in *Science,* Vol. 189, No. 4201, pages 480–482; August 8, 1975.

Index